Recent Advances in

Obstetrics and Gynaecology

Recent Advances in Obstetrics and Gynaecology 19
Edited by John Bonnar

Section one: **Obstetrics**

Advances in the treatment of ectopic pregnancy
A. N. Bhatt, D. J. Taylor

Low-dose aspirin: the rationale for preventing pre-eclampsia and intrauterine growth retardation: a role after CLASP?
K. A. Loudon, M. D. Kilby

The management of IUGR
R. B. Beattie, M. J. Whittle

Fetal surveillance during labour
P. R. Stone, H. G. Murray

Thromboembolic disease during pregnancy: a practical guide for obstetricians
J. R. Gray, J. S. Ginsberg

Malignant disease and pregnancy
D. N. Carney

Audit in obstetrics
J. Chapple

Section two: **Gynaecology**

Avoiding complications in minimally invasive pelvic surgery
S. Duffy

Recent advances in the diagnosis and treatment of polycystic ovary syndrome
T. J. McKenna, F. J. Hayes

Cost-effective medical treatment of endometriosis
R. W. Stones, E. J. Thomas

Investigation and management of the unstable bladder
G. J. Jarvis

The management of postoperative voiding dysfunction
T. R. Sayer

Investigation and management of faecal incontinence
J. Hill, E. S. Kiff

The management of vulval dystrophy
N. C. Gleeson

ISBN 0443 05253 0
ISSN 0143 6848

NUMBER

20

Recent Advances in

Obstetrics and Gynaecology

Edited by

John Bonnar MA MD (Hons) FRCOG FRCP(I)

Professor and Head, Department of Obstetrics and Gynaecology,
University of Dublin: Fellow of Trinity College, Dublin;
Consultant Obstetrician and Gynaecologist, St James' Hospital and Coombe
Women's Hospital, Dublin, Ireland

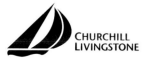
CHURCHILL
LIVINGSTONE

EDINBURGH LONDON NEW YORK PHILADELPHIA SYDNEY TORONTO 1998

CHURCHILL LIVINGSTONE
An imprint of Harcourt Brace & Company Limited

Robert Stevenson House, 1–3 Baxter's Place, Leith Walk, Edinburgh, EH1 3AF

First published 1998

ISBN 0-443-06022 3
ISSN 0143 6848

British Library Cataloguing in Publication Data
A catalogue record for this book is available from the British Library

Library of Congress Cataloging in Publication Data
A catalog record for this book is available from the Library of Congress

Medical knowledge is constantly changing. As new information becomes available, changes in treatment, procedures, equipment and the use of drugs become necessary. The editors and the publishers have, as far as possible, taken care to ensure that the information given in this text is accurate and up to date. However, readers are strongly advised to confirm that the information, especially with regard to drug usage, complies with current legislation and standards of practice.

The
publisher's
policy is to use
**paper manufactured
from sustainable forests**

Typeset by B A & G M Haddock
Printed in Singapore through Addison Wesley Longman China Limited

Contents

Section one: **Obstetrics**

1. The role of folic acid/folate in pregnancy: prevention is better than cure   1
   John M. Scott, Donald G. Weir

2. Effects of major haemoglobinopathies on pregnancy   21
   Susan M. Tuck, Carl E. Jensen

3. Inherited coagulation disorders and thrombophilia in pregnancy   35
   Isobel D. Walker

4. Fetal assessment and management of labour in twin pregnancy   65
   John C.P. Kingdom, Rekha Bajoria

5. Antenatal corticosteroids prior to preterm delivery   81
   Patricia Crowley

6. Recent advances in preterm labour   97
   Zoe J. Penn, Philip J. Steer

7. Advances in the management of severe pre-eclampsia and antihypertensive therapy   111
   James J. Walker

8. Advances in assisted vaginal delivery with vacuum extractor   125
   Richard Johanson

9. Reducing the complications of caesarean section   141
   Karl W. Murphy

10. Cerebral palsy and its relationship with pregnancy and delivery   153
    Ann Johnson

Section two: **Gynaecology**

11. The diagnosis and management of vulval intraepithelial neoplasia   167
    Ronald W. Jones

12. Advances in the treatment of ovarian cancer with paclitaxel   179
    Paul Donnellan, David Fennelly

13. Complications of laparoscopy and how to avoid them   189
    Ray Garry

14. How to avoid complications at hysteroscopic surgery   201
    Hugh O'Connor, Adam Magos

Index   215

Preface

Recent Advances in Obstetrics and Gynaecology has been published for over seventy years and is widely read in both the developed and developing countries. This 20th issue of Recent Advances contains a wealth of new information which will be of major interest to both practising specialists as well as those in training. The purpose of the book is to present new knowledge and review key areas of clinical practice, both aimed at providing the best possible patient care.

The obstetric section begins with an excellent review of folic acid metabolism in pregnancy by John Scott and Donald Weir of Trinity College, Dublin who have carried out major research in human nutrition to elucidate the biochemical role of folate and the effects of deficiency in pregnancy. Susan Tuck and Carl Jensen of The Royal Free Hospital, London, give detailed guidance on the management of haemoglobinopathy in pregnancy. Isobel Walker of the Department of Haematology at Glasgow Royal Infirmary contributes an excellent update on the management of women with inherited coagulation disorders and women with thrombophilia who are at special risk to the complications of haemorrhage and venous thrombosis.

The three chapters on haematological aspects of pregnancy are followed by six chapters dealing with specific areas of clinical obstetrics where major advances have occurred. John Kingdom now in Toronto and Rekha Bajoria of St Mary's Hospital, Manchester, present a detailed review of fetal assessment and management of labour in twin pregnancy. Pre-term labour remains the major factor in perinatal morbidity. Patricia Crowley of the Coombe Women's Hospital, Dublin, analyses the evidence for the use of antenatal corticosteroids prior to pre-term delivery and the many benefits for the infant. Zoe Penn and Philip Steer of Chelsea and Westminster Hospital, London, examine the factors responsible for pre-term labour and the possibilities for prevention. James Walker of St James's University Hospital, Leeds, has carried out sterling work in pre-eclampsia and he provides a clear account of the modern management of the patient with severe pre-eclampsia.

In the British Isles, a major part of obstetric litigation relates to complications arising from operative delivery. Richard Johanson of the City

General Hospital, Stoke-on-Trent, has a wealth of experience in assisted vaginal delivery with the vacuum extractor. He examines in detail the role of vacuum extraction and the new developments with the equipment. Current evidence based on audit indicates that the ventouse is the instrument of first choice for operative vaginal delivery. Caesarean section is now one of the most commonly performed operations but inevitably maternal morbidity and mortality are higher than vaginal delivery. Karl Murphy of St Mary's Hospital, London, reviews the various innovations and prophylactic methods which can reduce the level of morbidity. The obstetric section concludes with a chapter by Ann Johnson of the National Perinatal Epidemiology Unit in Oxford, on cerebral palsy and its relationship with pregnancy and delivery. Ann Johnson has been at the forefront of recent research on cerebral palsy and her chapter should be compulsory reading for all obstetricians and neonatologists.

In the gynaecology section, Ronald Jones of the National Women's Hospital, Auckland, discusses the increase in the incidence of vulval intra-epithelial neoplasia in younger women and the need for treatment to prevent progression to invasive cancer. Chemotherapy for ovarian cancer is constantly evolving and paclitaxel has been shown to provide significant improvement in patient management. Paul Donellan and David Fennelly, Medical Oncologists at St Vincent's Hospital, Dublin, review the recent clinical trials on paclitaxel which are aimed at providing maximum patient benefit. The last two chapters deal with gynaecological endoscopy and how to avoid complications with these surgical procedures. Ray Garry of South Cleveland, Hospital, Middlesborough, has pioneered the necessary training in laparoscopic surgery and he presents important new modifications to prevent the serious complications which continue to arise during entry to the abdominal cavity. Hugh O'Connor, now in Dublin and Adam Magos of the Royal Free Hospital, London, have worked together to investigate the role of endometrial resection in the treatment of menorrhagia. Based on their extensive experience they advise on the appropriate training, the surgical techniques, and careful patient selection which are all required for safe hysteroscopic surgery.

The contributors to the 20th issue are specialists of international standing and I thank them for providing the most up-to-date knowledge relative to patient care. I know that practising specialists will find the 20th issue of *Recent Advances in Obstetrics and Gynaecology* of major help in updating their clinical practice.

I would like to express my gratitude to Dr Gill Haddock and Churchill Livingstone for ensuring the publication of *Recent Advances in Obstetrics and Gynaecology* at a time of major change within the Company.

Dublin, 1998   **J. B.**

Contributors

Rekha Bajoria PhD MRCOG
Senior Lecturer, Department of Obstetrics and Gynaecology, St Mary's Hospital, University of Manchester Medical School, Manchester, UK

John Bonnar MD FRCOG FRCP(I)
Professor of Obstetrics and Gynaecology, Trinity Centre for Health Sciences, St James's Hopspital, Dublin, Ireland

Patricia Crowley MRCOG FRCP(I)
Senior Lecturer and Consultant, Department of Obstetrics and Gynaecology, Trinity College Dublin, Coombe Women's Hospital, Dublin, Ireland

Paul Donnellan MSc MB MRCP(I)
Research Fellow in Medical Oncology, St Vincent's Hospital, Dublin, Ireland

David Fennelly MSc MB MRCP(I)
Consultant Medical Oncologist , St Vincent's Hospital, Dublin, Ireland

Ray Garry MD FRCOG
Consultant Gynaecologist and Medical Director, The Women's Endoscopic Laser Foundation, South Cleveland Hospital, South Tees Acute Hospitals NHS Trust, Middlesbrough, Cleveland, UK

Carl E. Jensen MMed FCOG(SA) MRCOG
Senior Registrar, Department of Obstetrics and Gynaecology, University College Hospital, London, UK

Richard Johanson BSc MA MD MRCOG
Senior Lecturer in Perinatology, Academic Department of Obstetrics and Gynaecology, Maternity Department, North Staffordshire Hospital Trust, City General, Stoke-on-Trent, UK

Ann Johnson MD ERCP
Developmental Paediatrician, National Perinatal Epidemiology Unit, Radcliffe Infirmary, Oxford, UK

Ronald W. Jones FRCSE, FRCOG, FRNZCOG
Visiting Gynaecologist/Oncologist and Clinical Reader in Gynaecological Oncology, National Womens Hospital, Aukland, New Zealand

John C.P. Kingdom MD MRCP MRCOG DCH
Associate Professor, University of Toronto, Department of Obstetrics and Gynaecology, Mount Sinai Hospital, Toronto, Canada

Adam Magos BSc MD MRCOG
Consultant Obstetrician and Gynaecologist, Minimally Invasive Therapy Unit and Endoscopy Training Center, University Department of Obstetrics and Gynaecology, The Royal Free Hospital, London, UK

Karl W. Murphy MD MRCOG MRCP(I) DCH
Consultant Obstetrician and Gynaecologist, Subspecialist in Fetomaternal Medicine, St Mary's Hospital, London, UK

Hugh O'Connor BA DCH MRCP(I) MRCOG
Consultant Obstetrician and Gynaecologist, The Coombe Women's Hospital and St James's Hospital, Dublin, Ireland

Zoe J. Penn MD MRCOG
Consultant Obstetrician, Academic Department of Obstetrics and Gynaecology, Charing Cross and Westminster Medical School, Chelsea and Westminster Hospital, London, UK

John M. Scott PhD ScD MRIA
Professor of Human Nutrition, Biochemistry Department, Trinity College Dublin, Dublin, Ireland

Philip J. Steer BSc MD FRCOG
Professor and Head, Academic Department of Obstetrics and Gynaecology, Charing Cross and Westminster Medical School, Chelsea and Westminster Hospital, London, UK

Susan M. Tuck MD MRCGP FRCOG
Consultant Senior Lecturer, University Department of Obstetrics and Gynaecology, The Royal Free Hospital, London, UK

Isobel D. Walker MD FRCP FRCPath
Consultant Haematologist, Department of Haematology, Glasgow Royal Infirmary, Glasgow, UK

James J. Walker MD FRCP(E) FRCP(G) FRCOG
Head, Department of Obstetrics and Gynaecology, St James University Hospital, Leeds, UK

Donald G. Weir MD FRCP FRCP(I) FACP
Professor of Clinical Medicine, Department of Clinical Medicine, Trinity College Dublin, St James's Hospital, Dublin, Ireland

John M. Scott Donald G. Weir

CHAPTER 1

Role of folic acid/folate in pregnancy: prevention is better than cure

In the 1930s the English physician Dr Lucy Wills, while working in the slums in Bombay, made a very astute and far reaching clinical observation (Wills 1931). She described an anaemia in young pregnant mill workers. This macrocytic anaemia was identical in the presentation to that already described in pernicious anaemia (PA) some years earlier (Chanarin 1979). She consequently termed it 'pernicious anaemia of pregnancy'. However, unlike PA which was associated with the elderly and was quickly and universally fatal after diagnosis, this 'pernicious anaemia of pregnancy' regressed to a great extent when the pregnancy was over. Subsequently, PA was shown to be an autoimmune disease causing malabsorption of vitamin B_{12} (Chanarin 1979). What Dr Wills had identified was the deficiency of a hitherto unknown vitamin. Folic acid/folate was later chemically synthesised and characterised and found to be a small water soluble vitamin that acted as a cofactor to a variety of enzymes (Scott & Weir 1994). Dr Wills set the ground work not only by her clinical observations but also by producing the same anaemia in monkeys and showing that it could be treated with a yeast extract called marmite, which is a good source of folate. She is credited with the discovery of folic acid/folate and with describing its role in the anaemia that occurs in late pregnancy.

A quarter of a century later another obstetrician Bryan Hibbard felt that folate had a role in early embryonic development (Hibbard 1964). Some years later, Richard Smithells was the first to show a role for this vitamin in the prevention of early birth defects, specifically neural tube defects (NTDs) (Smithells et al 1980). Many important observations have been made subsequently, such as the UK Medical Research Council Trial (1991) and our own findings that NTDs are responsive to folate throughout the physiological range (Daly et al 1995).

John M. Scott PhD ScD MRIA, Professor of Human Nutrition, Biochemistry Department, Trinity College Dublin, Dublin 2, Ireland

Donald G. Weir, Professor of Clinical Medicine, Department of Clinical Medicine, Trinity College Dublin, St James's Hospital, Dublin 8, Ireland

Recent Advances in Obstetrics and Gynaecology 20

Folates

Folates, as discussed later, participate in two different metabolic cycles in all cells (Scott & Weir 1994). The various interconversions in these cycles mean that, in cells, folate exists not in one, but seven different forms. These all have in common two ring structures attached to the amino acid glutamate (Fig. 1.1). The circulation form in plasma has a single glutamate but all intracellular folates are attached to a chain of multiple glutamates, 5 to 11 depending upon the cell type. This conjugation is necessary for their retention within cells and also enhances their activity. The biologically active forms of the vitamin all have one of the rings (pteridine) reduced and this reduced structure may or may not have a carbon group attached, since their function is to pass a variety of carbon groups from one enzyme to another. Thus cells and, as a consequence, food is a mixture of reduced often carbon substituted folate polyglutamate, e.g. 10-formyltetra-hydrofolate, pentaglutamate, 5-methyltetrahydrofolate hexaglutamate or tetra-hydrofolatepentoglutamate. These polyglutamyl chains are broken down to a single glutamate during intestinal absorption. Also, during transit through the intestinal mucosa, the different derivatives present in food are converted to a single form. The net result of these two conversions is that the plasma folate is almost entirely in the single form of 5-methyltetrahydrofolate monoglutamate. This is taken up from the plasma by all cells and after the removal of the methyl group by the vitamin B_{12} dependent enzyme methionine synthase is converted into intracellular polyglutamates.

Folic acid

Folic acid is the synthetic form of the vitamin, chemically synthesised by the pharmaceutical industry. It does not occur in nature. Unlike all of the naturally occurring folates its pteridine ring is oxidised. Fortuitously it is reduced by an enzyme (dihydrofolate reductase) present in all cells, first to dihydrofolate and then to tetrahydrofolate. This form can then be conjugated with a poly-glutamyl chain and integrated into the cells functional folate pool. The synthetic form of the vitamin is more biologically effective than the naturally occurring forms found in food. The natural reduced forms are very susceptible to oxidative destruction during the harvesting, storage and cooking of food (Chanarin 1979). Folic acid not having a reduced ring is not susceptible to such destruction. Secondly, as mentioned above, food folates are all polyglutamate conjugates. The removal of the polyglutamate chain is not absolute during intestinal absorption. This results in these natural forms being probably only one-quarter or one-half as bioavailable as synthetic folic acid (Cuskelly et al 1996). Finally, while at physiological concentrations folic acid is converted during its transit through the gut to the circulatory plasma form 5 methyltetra-hydrofolate, this system is easily saturated and a dietary intake of folic acid greater than 300 μg per dose results in unaltered folic acid appearing in the plasma (Kelly et al 1997). Such folic acid when it is taken up by cells can be polyglutamated and retained without having to be acted upon by the vitamin

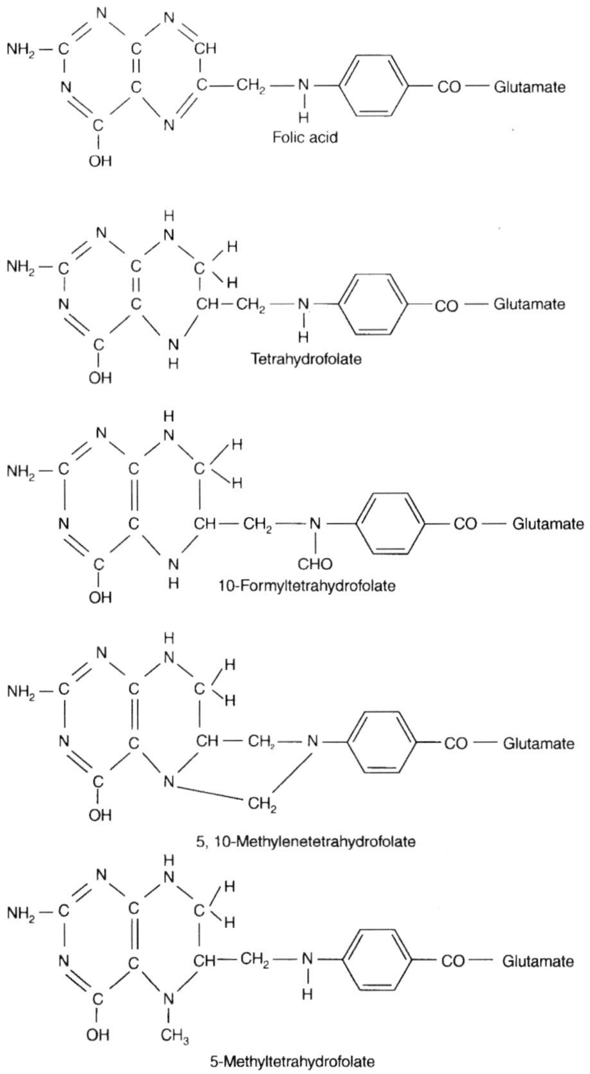

Fig. 1.1 Formulae of the synthetic (folic acid) and naturally occurring (folates) forms of the vitamin.

B_{12} dependent enzyme methionine synthase, a consideration that may be potentially important in masking the anaemia of PA and thus preventing its timely diagnosis (see later).

FUNCTIONS OF FOLATE

The seven intracellular forms of the vitamin arise because the function of the folates is to transfer so-called 'carbon one' units (Scott & Weir 1994). Three of these carbon one units are formyl (–CHO), or methylene (–CH_2–) or methyl (–CH_3). The former two are involved in purine and the latter in pyrimidine

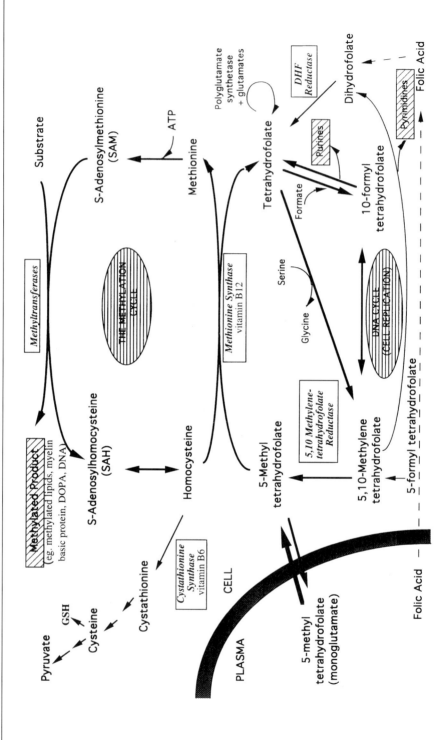

Fig. 1.2 The role of the folate cofactors in the DNA cycle and the methylation cycle.

biosynthesis (Fig. 1.1). The enzyme pathway that builds up the purine ring for two of its steps (the insertion of the carbon 2 and carbon 8 into the purine ring), must have the formyl group presented to the enzyme attached to a folate. Likewise, the enzyme thymidylate synthase, which is essential for pyrimidine biosynthesis, needs the carbon group required to make the thymidine base to be presented to it attached to folate (i.e. 5,10-methylenetetrahydrofolate). In the former two instances tetrahydrofolate is produced which can now attach another carbon group usually from the amino acid serine and repeat the cycle. During pyrimidine biosynthesis, dihydrofolate is made which is quickly reduced to tetrahydrofolate by the enzyme dihydrofolate reductase, thus completing the cycle (Fig. 1.2). The purines and pyrimidines so synthesised, with the involvement of the folate cofactor, go on to form the building blocks of RNA and, more importantly, DNA.

It is apparent from Figure 1.2 that 5,10-methylenetetrahydrofolate, once formed from serine and tetrahydrofolate, has direct involvement in pyrimidine biosynthesis and indirect involvement after, its conversion to 10-formyltetra-hydrofolate, in purine biosynthesis. It can also be converted to 5-methyltetra-hydrofolate. This represents a channel by which carbon groups can be directed from the amino acid serine up into the methylation cycle. The methylation cycle is found in all cells and involves methionine in its activated form S-adenosylmethionine which donates methyl ($-CH_3$) groups to a wide range of methyltransferase enzymes. About 30 such methyltransferases are found in most cells and they methylate a wide range of substrates ranging from the methylation of proteins, lipids and nucleic acids to the methylation of hormones, such as DOPA. The remaining intracellular folate is 5-formyltetra-hydrofolate a storage form in cells. This form, also called leucovorin, is used clinically to rescue normal cells during cancer chemotherapy with antifolate drugs, such as methotrexate.

DEFICIENCY OF FOLATE

DNA cycle

One would anticipate that the DNA cycle would be compromised during folate deficiency with a reduction in the rate of *de novo* synthesis of purines and pyrimidines in all cells and, thus, in the capacity to make DNA. This will, in turn, lead to a reduction in the rate of cell division. Clinically, this will be most relevant in cells undergoing rapid division, such as the cells produced by the bone marrow, in the red cell line leading to anaemia, in granulocytes causing neutropenia, and megakaryocytopenia producing a reduction in platelets or thrombocytopenia. The enterocytes in the gut, while less obvious, are also affected with severe folate deficiency leading to gut atrophy (Chanarin 1979).

Methylation cycle

The methylation cycle would also be expected to function to a decreasing extent during folate deficiency. The functions of the methylations carried out by this cycle are wide and varied. Methylation of proteins is involved in their structural stability. Methylation of nucleic acid in the gene switches them off with respect to cell replication. Methylation of lipids is involved in cell signalling. Thus reduction in the methylation cycle would be likely to have wide and varied results, none of which might be obvious or easily recognisable. The methylation cycle may be interrupted for a different reason, particularly in conditions of vitamin B_{12} deficiency, such as PA. Sub acute combined degeneration (SCD) is caused by a reduction in myelin leading to a neuropathy of the peripheral nerves, brain and spinal cord. This arises from inability of the nerve cells to methylate myelin basic protein (Scott & Weir 1981, Weir & Scott 1995). This protein makes up about one-third of the structure of myelin and, when not methylated, becomes unstable and degrades. SCD is not a usual presenting feature of folate deficiency as nerve cells concentrate folate at the expense of other tissues. Consequently, the effects on other tissues, such as the bone marrow, will usually be recognised and treated before involvement of the neural tissue is clinically apparent. It has been shown that patients with severe prolonged folate deficiency do get SCD (Mazoor & Runzie 1976).

CELLULAR TURNOVER (OR CATABOLISM) OF FOLATES

Folate taken into cells after conjugation would not appear to be available for re-utilization and folates are recycled after cell turnover only, i.e. there is no mobilisable folate store *per se*. In addition, a certain amount of folate is broken down or catabolised each day (McNulty et al 1994) and involves the cleavage of the folates to produce pterdines and *p*-aminobenzoate which, after acetylation, is excreted in the urine. Quantitative analysis has shown those catabolites to be increased during periods of rapid growth (McNulty et al 1994) and such increased catabolism is associated with the latter stages of pregnancy, both in experimental animals (McNulty et al 1993) and in humans (McPartlin et al 1993) leading to megaloblastic anaemia of pregnancy before term in women with inadequate folate stores.

As discussed above, severe folate deficiency will have associated with it the obvious signs of anaemia and, if prolonged, perhaps also neuropathy. However, as discussed later, certain other clinical conditions, such as neural tube defects and elevated levels of plasma homocysteine occur at folate levels which have conventionally been considered to be well within the normal range.

FOLATE AND PREGNANCY

Folate has two distinct roles in pregnancy – the long established role in the prevention of anaemia in late pregnancy and the more recently demonstrated role in early embryogenesis, particularly in relation to neural tube defects. There are also less established roles (Table 1.1).

Megaloblastic anaemia in pregnancy

During the latter stages of pregnancy, the plasma volume expands by as much as a litre. The increase of red cell volume is less, so the concentration of red cells

Table 1.1 Indications for the use of folic acid supplements or folic acid fortified foods associated with pregnancy

Indication	Benefit	Amount (daily) and duration	Comments
Anaemia	Absolute	+ 300 μg, 2nd and 3rd trimester	Current reference nutrient intake (RNI) COMA (1991) may be revised upward
Neural tube defects: occurrence	Absolute	+ 400 μg, 2–3 months preconception and 1st trimester	Department of Health, UK (1992) CDC Atlanta, GA, USA (1992)
Neural tube defects: recurrence	Absolute	+ 4.0 mg, 2–3 months periconception and 1st trimester	Department of Health, UK (1992) CDC Atlanta, GA, USA (1992)
Other birth defects	Possible	Same as prevention of NTDs (occurrence)	Covered by NTD advice
Spontaneous abortion	Probable	Same as prevention of NTDs (occurrence)	Covered by NTD advice
Intrauterine development	Probable	Same as prevention of anaemia	Covered by anaemia advice
Post natal development	Possible	Possibly for premature babies – also vitamin B_{12}	
Anti convulsant therapy	Probable	Benefit but suggestions that it will reduce control of epilepsy	Evidence not strong but a judgement is required particularly for recurrence
Alcohol abuse	Possible	Same as prevention of NTDs occurrence and of anaemia	Ideally stop alcohol but NTD and anaemia advice would help replenish stores anyway
Oral contraceptives	Possible	Same as prevention of NTD occurrence but ensure 2–3 months prior to conception	Reduction in folate status is not usually dramatic but is of unknown cause
Lactation	Absolute	+ 60 μg duration of lactation	Current reference nutrient intake (RNI) COMA (1991) may be revised upwards
Multiple pregnancies	Absolute	Same as prevention of NTDs occurrence and anaemia	The higher demand should be adequately catered for by usual pregnancy advice
Reduced status general	Absolute	Same as prevention of NTDs occurrence and anaemia	Deficiency should first be treated with 1 month of 4.0 or 5.0 mg/day
Summary to cover all indications	Absolute	400 μg preconception and 1st trimester, 300 μg 2nd and 3rd trimesters	Most circumstances are covered by + 300 μg 2–3 months prior to conception and into the first trimester. A similar amount of 400 μg or the lesser amount of 300 μg as suggested by the RNI for the duration of the pregnancy and some lesser amount during lactation

per unit volume of plasma decreases. Thus, a progressive drop occurs during pregnancy of plasma folate and red cell folate. However, as discussed below, there will also be an additional reduction in folate status as the fetus develops and, frequently in the latter stages of pregnancy, a woman's folate status may have been reduced to the point where signs of folate deficiency will appear. Initially, macrocytic red cells are seen which may progress to overt megaloblastic anaemia. In the latter MCV is raised, haemoglobin reduced beyond that due to haemodilution and the bone marrow aspirate is megaloblastic.

Several explanations for this reduced folate status have been advanced over the years. There is a small increase in initial folate lost in the urine but this would not be sufficient to reduce status to the level frequently encountered (Chanarin 1979). Earlier suggestions that pregnancy leads to malabsorption of food folate have largely been discounted (Bailey 1995), but some reduction in intake of dietary folate may be due to loss of appetite. Most frequently, a transfer of folate from the mother to the fetus has been suggested (Ek 1982). However, the total folate content of the fetus plus the placenta at term is no more than 800 μg (Iyengar & Apte 1972) and this small amount of folate would be insufficient to diminish maternal stores. In experimental animals (McNulty et al 1993) and in humans (McPartlin et al 1993), as pregnancy progresses, there is an increase in the catabolites excreted in the maternal urine. This is equivalent to some 200 μg of folate per day, increasing in the second and third trimester of pregnancy to over 600 μg per day. This doubling in the rate of destruction of folate in the later stages of pregnancy leads to a pronounced negative folate balance in relation to the available dietary folate. Thus, unless a women entering pregnancy has adequate folate stores to cover this loss, or has been given prophylactic folic acid either as supplements, or in fortified food during the latter stages of pregnancy, folate deficiency results leading to overt megaloblastic anaemia.

Prevention of megaloblastic anaemia of pregnancy

There are two schools of thought in this context. The first is that prophylaxis is necessary only for women with poor nutrition, as occurs in developing countries or with low socio-economic background in developed countries. This view would suggest that for most, if not all, women in developed communities, folate stores will be adequate to cover the period of pregnancy, that some reduction in the indices of folate status in serum and red cell folate is normal, through haemodilution, and even some real reduction through negative folate balance. The Scandinavian countries would take this view. The more widespread view, particularly in Great Britain and Ireland, is that for many women existing folate stores will not be adequate without the mother and perhaps also the fetus being at some risk (Department of Health 1991a). Previously, the presence of anaemia was used as the criterion of the prevalence of the problem. Pregnant women with anaemia varied from a few per cent in studies in the UK up to 18% in one study in Western Australia and 24% in Malaysia. Before prophylaxis with folic acid was introduced on a widespread basis in pregnancy, overt anaemia occurred in one in every 200 pregnancies and could be as high as a quarter of all pregnancies in some centres (Chanarin 1979). More recently, studies have looked for earlier indices of folate deficiency, namely plasma and red cell folate. In earlier studies, large numbers (15–54%)

had plasma levels that would be considered low even allowing for haemodilution (Chanarin 1979). Studies using the much better index of folate status, the red cell folate level, also showed cause for concern (Chanarin 1990, Sauberlich 1995). Red cell folate measures not recent folate intake but reflects the average folate status of the 120 day life of the red cell and, as such, gives a true historic picture of folate intake balanced against requirement. A recent, well conducted survey done in the US under the programme called NHANES II (Senti & Pilch 1995) showed that, in a randomly selected population of females of all social classes, some 12% had evidence of low red cell folate status and this increased to 21% among pregnant subjects. Most expert opinion would hold the view that, in any community, some women through lack of folate will be at risk of compromising their own health and that of their developing embryo. This has led to the conclusion in most centres that routine supplementation with folic acid is advisable in pregnancy (Bailey et al 1980, Smith et al 1983).

Barker and colleagues (1990) have suggested that reduction in intrauterine nutrition may be responsible for problems of the cardiovascular system or the pancreas in later life as a result of impaired intrauterine development. This had lead to concern about folate status. The most prudent course would seem to be initiation of prophylaxis with folic acid supplements of 300 or 400 µg per day from the first booking clinic to cover the second and third trimester. This represents a reasonable precaution with no risk to the mother or her developing embryo. Taken with the recommendations for prevention of neural tube defects, 400 µg per day should be recommended before and during pregnancy.

NEURAL TUBE DEFECTS (NTDS)

Between days 24 and 28 post conception, the neural plate closes to form the neural tube and the cranium. Incomplete closure of the former results in spina bifida and of the latter in anencephaly.

While anencephaly is incompatible with life, the embryo dying either *in utero* or shortly after birth, spina bifida can result in very mild to extremely severe clinical outcomes. In the latter instance, significant lack of closure can result in a marked restriction in the quality of life, with paralysis of the bladder and lower limbs and hydrocephalus due to improper drainage of CSF.

NTDs have long been known to have a strong genetic predisposition (Scott et al 1990, Scott et al 1994). The strongest evidence for this is in the marked increase in the risk of **recurrence**. A women with a previously affected pregnancy has up to a 10-fold increased risk of having a recurrence. A marked difference in prevalence is found between different ethnic groups with high levels in those of Celtic origin and very low levels in Afro-Americans (Elwood et al 1992). A non genetic factor, probably nutritional, was known to have a marked influence on prevalence. Epidemics often occurred in cycles within the same genetic pool and in some instances increases were associated with periods of malnutrition, such as during the Depression of the 1930s or after the Dutch Famine in 1945.

In recent years, it has been shown beyond any scientific doubt that this variable nutrient is the vitamin folate. The evidence has taken two forms. Trials have been done where folic acid has been given to women before they became pregnant. Alternatively, the prevalence of NTDs in women who just happened to be taking folic acid containing supplements during conception was compared to matched controls from the same community who also delivered a child at the same time period but who were not taking supplements. The earlier intervention trials were carried out by Smithells et al (1980) on the effect of folic acid in preventing the **recurrence** of an NTD birth in women who had a previously affected birth. The original intention was to do a double blind placebo controlled trial using a multivitamin multimineral supplement of nutrients called Pregnavite Forte F. Unfortunately, one of the hospital Ethics Committees to which the protocol was submitted turned it down insisting that all women in the trial should receive treatment. The possibility that specific intervention with any nutrient or nutrients would prevent NTDs was, at that point, sufficiently unproven that the rejection of the placebo design was unfortunate. This created a huge problem subsequently, when Smithells et al (1980) did an intervention study with this supplement and found a significant reduction in the prevalence of NTD in women who already had at least one affected pregnancy. Their control population was the prevalence of NTD births in women who, for one reason or another, had not taken part in the trial. Many felt that the observed difference in recurrence could be due to the difference in rates of prevalence between those women who agreed to join such a trial and those that did not. Smithells et al (1983) argued persuasively that there was no significant difference between the two groups with respect to factors that might cause the trial group to have a natural lower prevalence, e.g. social class. He also continued to add new cases and continued to show reduction of NTDs of well over half that found in his non treated control (Smithells et al 1983). Nevertheless, the benefits of such nutrient supplementation on preventing NTDs was not accepted for standard treatment.

The study of Smithells et al (1980) suggested to Laurence and colleagues (1981) to re-examine their small placebo controlled trial using folic acid (4.0 mg per day). The authors felt justified in transferring two treated pregnancies to the control group and the overall results became statistically significant. Many questioned a retrospective assignment of the two affected pregnancies. This and the small size of the trial again lead to the view that folic acid had not been shown to prevent NTDs. The UK Medical Research Council (1991) set up a multicentre trial to answer the various outstanding issues (MRC Vitamin Study Research Group 1991). The trial had a placebo arm and three treatment arms, folic acid, folic acid plus multinutrient and multinutrient alone. The latter two arms used the same mixture of vitamins and minerals at the same concentrations as in the Pregnavite Forte F used by Smithells. The level of folic acid used was much higher at 4.0 mg instead of 360 μg used by Smithells. This large amount was justified at the time to test simultaneously both the Smithells et al (1980) and the Laurence et al (1981) results. The trial was an outstanding success. Both arms containing folic acid showed a marked reduction in NTD prevalence (72%). There was no apparent benefit to taking the other vitamins or nutrients. The MRC trial on preventing **recurrence** was followed by an intervention trial by Czeizel and Dudas (1992) to prevent **occurrence**, i.e. in women who had not had a previous NTD affected pregnancy. This trial had two treatment arms and compared a multivitamin (which contained 800 μg of

Table 1.2 Recommendations

A. Recommendations from the UK Department of Health (synopsis)

To prevent first occurrence of neural tube defect

(i) Extra folate/folic acid is recommended for all women prior to conception and during the first 12 weeks of pregnancy

(ii) The three possible ways of achieving an extra intake of folate/folic acid (eating more folate rich foods, eating foods fortified with folic acid, taking folic acid as a medicinal/food supplement) are not mutually exclusive

(iii) Women who are planning a pregnancy should eat more folate rich foods and avoid over-cooking them

(iv) The range of breads and breakfast cereals fortified with folic acid should be increased (including wholemeal breads)

(v) Fortification of foods with folic acid should be restricted to breads and breakfast cereals

(vi) The present levels of folic acid fortification in breads and breakfast cereals should not be greatly exceeded

(vii) Foods which have folic acid added should where practicable indicate the level of fortification

(viii) There should continue to be a choice of unfortified breads and breakfast cereals

(ix) All women who are planning a pregnancy should be advised to take 0.4 mg (400 µg) folic acid as a daily medicinal or food supplement from when they begin trying to conceive until the twelfth week of pregnancy

(x) Women who have not been supplementing their folate/folic acid intakes and who suspect that they may be pregnant should start supplementation at once and continue until the twelfth week of pregnancy

To prevent recurrence of neural tube defect *in the offspring of women or men with spina bifida themselves, or with a history of a previous child with neural tube defect*

(i) All such women and men should be counselled about the increased risk of a future offspring being affected

(ii) Folic acid supplements at a daily dose of 5 mg (5000 µg) should be advised for all those women who wish to become pregnant or who are at risk of becoming pregnant; the daily dose should be reduced to 4 mg (4000 µg) if this preparation becomes available as a licensed product

(iii) Prescriptions of folic acid, when given for the prevention of NTD, should be free of charge

(iv) Folic acid supplementation should continue until the twelfth week of pregnancy

(v) Folic acid-only preparations are preferable to multivitamin preparations

(vi) Women in this group who are also receiving anticonvulsant therapy need individual counselling by their doctor before starting folic acid supplementation

B. Recommendations of the Centres for Disease Control, USA (synopsis)

(i) All women of childbearing age in the US who are capable of becoming pregnant should consume 0.4 mg of folic acid per day for the purpose of reducing their risk of have a pregnancy affected with spina bifida or other NTDs

(ii) Because the effects of high intakes are not well known but include complicating the diagnosis of vitamin B_{12} deficiency, care should be taken to keep total folate consumption at < 1 mg per day, except under the supervision of a physician

(iii) Women who have had a prior NTD-affected pregnancy are at high risk of having a subsequent affected pregnancy. When these women are planning to become pregnant, they should consult their physicians for advice

folic acid) with a multimineral supplement. There were six NTD affected pregnancies in the latter group with none in the former group. In parallel with these intervention trials, a series of case/control studies were reported. With one exception these showed that women taking vitamin supplements before conception have a significantly lower prevalence of NTDs than matched controls from the same community (Wald 1994). The level of folic acid in these supplements was invariably 400 μg per day.

The cumulative evidence induced the UK Department of Health (1991b) and the CDC (1991), the equivalent regulatory body in the US, to make a series of recommendations (Table 1.2). They concluded that folic acid taken periconceptionally could prevent the majority of NTDs. Since the Ceizal and Dudas (1992) trial and the case control studies looked at occurrence and because there was an obvious difference in aetiology between recurrence and occurrence NTDs, they concluded that folic acid also prevents occurrence. The question of what level to use was a problem because the MRC trial had used 4.0 mg per day, (MRC Vitamin Study Group 1991) which is some 20 times higher than the population reference intake (PRI). Because women with a previously affected pregnancy were at such high risk of a **recurrence**, the very high level was recommended. However, the bigger problem was to prevent **occurrence** of NTDs which represents 95% of all cases. Unlike women with a previously affected pregnancy, they cannot be identified in advance and, therefore, prophylactic folic acid would have to be given to all women of child bearing age. The level of 360 μg per day had apparently been effective in the earlier studies of Smithells et al (1980, 1983). The usual level in the supplements that had apparently been effective in the case/control studies was 400 μg per day and this amount was recommended to prevent **occurrence**. Both bodies suggested three ways in which this extra intake of folic acid/folate could be achieved: increase in folate rich foods; supplements (tablets); or food fortified with folic acid, such as breakfast cereals. However, realising the known benefit of folic acid in the prevention of NTD births has turned out to be more difficult than anticipated. The principal problem is that the folic acid/folate must be taken before conception.

The food option

None of the intervention trials used food folate and the synthetic form of the vitamin folic acid was used. While one or two of the retrospective case control studies did appear to show some protective effect of diet with respect to folate on the prevalence of NTDs, the effect was very weak (Bower & Stanley 1989). Recently Cuskelly et al (1996) compared the options – food folate, a food fortified with folic acid, and folic acid supplements – in a study using young female volunteers. The volunteers were randomised into five groups: group I, folic acid (400 μg) supplements; group II, 400 μg added to breakfast cereals; group III, administration of an extra 400 μg of folate by way of unfortified dietary folate; group IV, dietary advice similar to that given by the Department of Health; and group V, a control group. A statistically significant increase in folate intake was found in the first three groups but not in group IV. However, folate status, as measured by red cell folates, was significantly increased in only two groups, those on supplements (I) and fortified food (II). There was only a moderate increase in those who had been given increased dietary folate (III). The conclusion was that dietary folate even when the difficult change in dietary intake necessary to eat an extra 400 µg per day was achieved, would be unlikely to significantly improve folate status. This is presumably due to the poor chemical stability and absorption bioavailability of the reduced conjugated forms of folate found in food. Synthetic folic acid by contrast is very stable and probably totally available for intestinal absorption.

Supplement option

While this option clearly will be effective in any individual as shown by the intervention trials, the problem is that very few women actually take folic acid tablets preconceptionally. Many surveys have shown this even after fairly intensive publicity (Clark & Fisk 1994) and, in most countries, over half of all pregnancies are unplanned. Women not planning to become pregnant would be unlikely to take folic acid. In addition, it has proved very difficult to ensure that women are aware of the relationship between folic acid and NTDs. Perhaps most disappointing is that even amongst women who know that periconceptional folic acid can prevent the majority of NTDs, compliance is poor. Many women, even if they plan to become pregnant, do not comply since the concept of taking a daily tablet when they are feeling completely healthy is not accepted.

Fortification option

The addition of folic acid to some foods has been happening for many years in most countries, although forbidden in some. The most frequently fortified foods have been breakfast cereals with some containing up to the whole PRI available per serving. Some breads are also fortified, as are some fruit juices. It was originally hoped that women who did not feel inclined to take a tablet would elect to increase their intake via this means. However, the three problems remain of unplanned pregnancies, knowledge and compliance that were encountered with women not taking supplements. Compliance may be improved if women were advised that the taking of such cereals would be a protection against NTDs by general advertising or by labelling of the products. This would amount to allowing what is called a 'health claim' for a food. While such claims are permitted in a restricted manner in the US, including the claim that folic acid prevents NTDs, such health claims are totally prohibited in the UK. The concern is that, if manufacturers are allowed to make such claims about food, the practice would become widespread and be abused even if restricted by legislation, resulting in confusion amongst the general public.

An alternative within the fortification option is mandatory fortification. Here, folic acid is by legislation, or by general agreement with the industry involved without legislation, added to a staple in the diet at an agreed concentration, e.g. flour. Flour is not only present in bread but in a wide range of other foods such as pastas, confectionery, etc. In the UK, four nutrients – thiamin, niacin, calcium and iron – are all added to flour by the manufacturers. The problem is that flour (or any other staple) will have a varying level of intake depending upon an individual's dietary pattern. To enable almost all women in the UK (> 95%) to have the current target amount of folic acid (i.e. an extra 400 µg/day in their diet), a large amount would have to be added to ensure that those on very low flour intake reached this target. However, to achieve this would mean that not only women of child bearing age but many others in the community will receive much larger amounts of folic acid in order to ensure that this bottom target figure is possible. Unfortunately, high daily intakes do pose a threat in at least one specific circumstance. In the autoimmune condition pernicious anaemia (PA) there is malabsorption of not just dietary vitamin B_{12} but also the enterohepatic circulation of vitamin B_{12} is interrupted, i.e. biliary vitamin B_{12} is also unabsorbed thus producing a drain on the body's existing stores. The consequent negative balance results quickly in a very low vitamin B_{12} status after the considerable body stores have been exhausted. This results in two well established clinical sequelae, anaemia and neuropathy, the latter called SCD (Scott & Weir 1981, Weir & Scott 1995).

It is now generally agreed that the **anaemia** is due to vitamin B_{12} deficiency causing reduced activity of the enzyme methionine synthase (Fig. 1.2). This enzyme is part of the methylation cycle and continuously passes methyl groups from 5-methyltetrahydrofolate to homocysteine in order to replenish cellular methionine and SAM which is then used to maintain the methyltransferase reactions. In vitamin B_{12} deficiency, it is suggested that cellular folate gets trapped in the 5-methyl form, the so called 'methyl folate trap hypothesis'. The reductase enzyme that generates this form is irreversible in vivo and, thus, the only way that the 5-methyl form once made can be recycled back to the other folate forms is via the vitamin B_{12} dependent enzyme methionine synthase whose activity in B_{12} deficiency is absent. This trapping of 5-methyltetrahydrofolate thus produces a pseudo folate deficient state which deprives the cell of the other forms of folate needed for purine and pyrimidine biosynthesis. This, in turn, reduces the cell's capacity to make DNA and thus to replicate, hence the anaemia.

The vitamin B_{12}-associated neuropathy results from interruption of the methylation cycle (Fig. 1.2). While the methylation cycle is being provided with carbon groups to the detriment of the DNA cycle, it in fact cannot utilise these since the cycle is blocked. Interruption of this cycle results in lack of methylation of a whole range of cellular components, one of them being myelin basic protein, the major protein present in the myelin sheath. In the absence of the methylation it apparently gets destabilised and degenerates resulting in a myelopathy that is seen clinically as the neuropathy called subacute combined degeneration, or vitamin B_{12}-associated neuropathy. If somebody with vitamin B_{12} deficiency is given folic acid, it will be taken into cells and converted first to dihydro and then to tetrahydrofolate (Fig. 1.2). This latter form can then accept a carbon one unit from serine and the cells can use 5,10-methylenetetrahydrofolate either directly for pyrimidine biosynthesis or, after conversion, for purine biosynthesis. If such cells are in the bone marrow, this will enable DNA biosynthesis to occur and will be reflected in a haematological response. Progressively, however, as these folates are recycled through the DNA cycle some, and eventually all, will become trapped in the methyl folate trap. Thus the haematological response would not be sustained. However, if folic acid continues to be given either during inappropriate therapy or as a result of folic acid being added to food, then the marrow response could be sustained. At first sight, the treatment of the anaemia would not appear to be a problem. However, the consequence in practice would be a 'masking of the anaemia' making the diagnosis more difficult as the presenting signs and symptoms are not expressed. However, the neuropathy associated with vitamin B_{12} deficiency needs a functioning methylation cycle (Weir & Scott 1995). Even though there are plenty of methyl groups being funnelled into the cycle as 5-methyltetrahydrofolate, the cycle cannot operate because of the inactivity of the vitamin B_{12} dependent enzyme methionine synthase (Fig. 1.2). Thus the neuropathy progresses undiagnosed presenting later when more clinically obvious as paraesthesia, paralysis and ataxia. While in its early stages the neuropathy is completely reversible by vitamin B_{12} therapy, at the more advanced stages it is largely irreversible.

Some suggest that treatment with inappropriate ingestion of folic acid by increasing cell turnover in the bone marrow and elsewhere would increase the requirement for protein synthesis and, as a consequence, methionine. This would exacerbate the neuropathy by diverting the scarce supplies of methionine out of the methylation cycle and into protein biosynthesis (Scott & Weir 1981). Dickinson (1995) suggests that an examination of the early literature, where folic acid was inappropriately used to treat PA, indicates that this does not happen. He suggests that the rapid rate at which the neuropathy progresses later in PA has been confused with the so-called explosive development of the neuropathy which, he claims, coincided with, but was not caused by, folic acid therapy. What is not in doubt is that folic acid will at least complicate the diagnosis of PA. The classical presentation for PA is that one-third of patients present with the anaemia, one-third the neuropathy and one-third with both. Thus, potentially, if folic acid is given to patients with PA its diagnosis may be delayed in two-thirds of them.

While neither the Department of Health (1991) nor the CDC (1991) recommendations state exactly how long before conception folic acid should be taken, it is clear that the concentration of the vitamin builds up in plasma over a 3 month period. Recently absorbed folic acid would also be available to the fetus, and the recommendations suggest that in the non-ideal circumstance where a women not taking folic acid suspects she is pregnant, she should immediately begin supplements.

Recently, the US Government decided that all flour sold in the US must be fortified with folic acid and that this legal requirement would be completed by the start of 1998. Because of concerns in masking PA the amount added was low, some would say too low. From food modelling, it is calculated it will deliver a mean increase in the US diet of 100 µg per day. Since the current target for protection against NTDs is 400 µg per day, many feel that this measure will be ineffective. Similar fortification of the UK diet is under consideration. However, recent studies (Ward et al 1997) have shown amounts of 200 µg per day optimally lower plasma homocysteine, the functional marker for folate status. While 100 µg caused suboptimal lowering, it is possible that taken chronically, as in a fortified diet, a low level may also be optimally effective (Daly et al 1997).

OTHER BIRTH DEFECTS

Czeizel (1993, 1996) analysed the data of the intervention trial (Czeizel & Dudas 1992) and found, after reduction of NTD births had been accounted for, that the multivitamin preparation when compared to the multimineral preparation, also significantly lowered the number of major congenital abnormalities, such as urinary tract and cardiovascular defects. Shaw et al (1995a) also concluded that use of multivitamins that contained folic acid reduced cardiotruncal and limb defects.

OROFACIAL CLEFTS

Tolarova and Harris (1995) suggested that women taking multivitamins (containing folic acid) had a decreased risk of having a birth affected by an orofacial cleft. Shaw et al (1995b) also reported that multivitamins containing folic acid reduced the risk of an orofacial cleft by a quarter to a half compared to matched controls. However, Hayes et al (1996) reached a negative conclusion finding no difference in a case/control study. While the presence of some positive association looks interesting, a protective effect of folic acid or indeed multivitamins, on either congenital malformations in general, or orofacial clefts in particular, remains to be confirmed.

SPONTANEOUS ABORTION

Earlier studies (Hibbard 1964, Martin et al 1965, Streiff & Little 1967) reported that folic acid prophylaxis did reduce spontaneous abortions in women. More recently, Wouters et al (1993) found that, out of 102 women with such a history, only five had evidence of a low folate status, however, very few women with an NTD affected fetus had a low folate status in the index pregnancy (Daly et al 1995). Neiger et al (1993) examined a group of women with first trimester bleeding and found that there was no correlation with serum folate levels in those who subsequently had a spontaneous abortion and those who did not.

INTRAUTERINE DEVELOPMENT

Baumslag et al (1970) found that, in children born to poorly nourished black women, the usual outcome of low birth weight could be prevented, in most instances, by maternal folic acid/iron supplements. Such supplements had no effect in well nourished white pregnant women. More recently, Scholl et al (1996) found that a low folate intake or low serum folate at week 28 was associated with a greater risk of preterm delivery and low birth weight.

POST NATAL DEVELOPMENT

In a control study by Worthington et al (1994), supplementation with folic acid/vitamin B_{12} was given to 180 premature infants. Those given vitamin B_{12} alone or combined with folic acid attained higher haemoglobin levels than those untreated ($P < 0.0005$) or treated with folic acid only ($P < 0.01$).

ANTICONVULSANT DRUGS

A variety of drugs, principally the anticonvulsants, are known to reduce both serum folate levels and to cause birth defects but the two may be unrelated (Chanarin 1979). The more recent finding that women on long term treatment with carbamazepine or phenytoin have normal red cell folate levels questions if there is an actual reduction in folate status (Tomson et al 1995). Valproic acid is known to be a potent teratogen both in experimental animals and in humans (Nau 1994). While the use of such anticonvulsants may exert their teratogenic effects through interfering with folate metabolism, it is also suggested that folic acid may interfere with the control of epilepsy or even precipitate it in some patients (Strauss & Berust 1974). However, in two studies where high amounts of folic acid (3–5 mg) for up to a year were given to treat phenytoin-induced gingival hyperplasia, no change in seizure frequency was found (Backman et al 1989, Brown et al 1991). Detailed advice on the management of women of childbearing age on antiepileptic drugs, including the use of folic acid supplements, has been offered by Lindhout and Amtzigt (1994). This presents a dilemma as to whether or not to give prophylaxis with folic acid to women whose epilepsy is controlled by such drugs. The degree to which folic acid has this effect and the amount needed to do this is unclear. By contrast, the benefit in preventing NTDs is unequivocal.

ALCOHOL ABUSE

Chronic alcohol abuse is in general associated with poor folate status probably through diminished dietary intake. There is also some evidence that alcohol directly interferes with folate metabolism (Chanarin 1979). Alcohol, as well as causing the fetal alcohol syndrome, may cause fetal malformation that is folate related (Jones et al 1973).

ORAL CONTRACEPTIVES

Prolonged use of oral contraception does lower folate status (Sauberlich 1995) and pregnancies may be at some risk immediately after cessation of their use.

LACTATION

Through loss of folate in breast milk, lactating women may be at increased risk of becoming folate deficient and extra folate intake is recommended (Picciano 1995).

MULTIPLE PREGNANCIES

Older studies in the literature show clearly that megaloblastic anaemia was more common in pregnancies involving twins (Chanarin 1979). With current practices of prophylaxis with folic acid in pregnancy, this is less often seen but clearly such a pregnancy will put higher than usual demands on folate stores.

GENERAL EFFECTS OF REDUCED FOLATE STATUS DURING PREGNANCY

Homocysteine is known to be an independent risk factor for cardiovascular disease (Scott & Weir 1996) and even very small reductions in folate status cause higher homocysteine levels (Ward et al 1997). Thus, a reduction in folate status which is not prevented by folate prophylaxis, may cause a transient rise in plasma homocysteine. Some evidence links colorectal cancer and cancer of the cervix to reduced folate status (Meenan et al 1997).

Key points for clinical practice

- Women who either are planning a pregnancy or even those who could become pregnant should be advised to take an extra 400 µg of folic acid per day ideally for two or three months before conception.

- While in theory it is possible to get this increased intake by taking foods rich in folate, in practice it is extremely difficult. This is because of the low absorption of the vitamin in most foods, its poor bioavailability and particularly its poor stability.

- By contrast the synthetic forms of the vitamin, folic acid, is very bioavailable and stable and readily available in supplements (tablets) or in foods such as breakfast cereals that are fortified with folic acid.

- Women should be advised to continue to take an extra 400 µg of folic acid per day throughout pregnancy and subsequently during lactation. This is to cover losses of the vitamin during these two periods.

- Expert opinion agrees there is no significant risk to women taking extra folic acid for the times indicated.

References

Backman N, Holm A K, Hanstrom L et al 1989 Folate treatment of diphenylhydantoin-induced gingival hyperplasia. Scand J Dent Res 97: 222–232

Bailey L B 1995 Folate requirements and dietary recommendations. In : Bailey L B (ed) Folate in Health and Disease. Dekker, New York, pp 123–151

Bailey L B, Mahan C S, Dimperio D 1980 Folacin and iron status in low-income pregnant adolescent and mature women. Am J Clin Nutr 33: 1997–2001

Barker D J P 1992 Fetal and infant origins of adult disease. Barker D J P (ed) British Medical Journal, London

Baumslag M. Edelstein. T, Metz J 1970 Reduction of incidence of prematurity by folic acid supplementation in pregnancy. BMJ i: 16–17

Bower C, Stanley F J 1989 Dietary folate as a risk factor for neural tube defects: evidence from a case control study in Western Australia. Med J Aust 150: 613–619

Brown R S, De-Stanisloa P T, Beaver W T, Bottomley W T 1991 The administration of folic acid to institutionalized epileptic adults with phenytoin-induced gingival phyerplasia. A double-blind, randomized, placebo-controlled, parallel study. Oral Surg Oral Med Oral Pathol 71: 565–568

CDC 1991 Recommendations for the use of folic acid to reduce the number of cases of spina bifida and other neural tube defects. MMWR 41: 1–7

Chanarin I 1979 Megaloblastic Anaemias, 2nd Edn. Blackwell, Oxford

Chanarin I 1990 The Megaloblastic Anaemias, 3rd Edn. Blackwell, Oxford

Clark N A C, Fisk N M 1994 Minimal compliance with the Department of Health recommendations: routine folate prophylaxis to prevent fetal neural tube defects. Br J Obstet Gynaecol 19: 709–710

Cuskelly C J, McNulty H, Scott J M 1996 Effect of increasing dietary folate on red-cell folate: implications for prevention of neural tube defects. Lancet 347: 657–659

Czeizel A E 1993 Prevention of congenital abnormalities by periconceptional multivitamin supplementation. BMJ 306: 1645–1648

Czeizel A E 1996 Reduction of urinary tract and cardiovascular defects by multivitamin supplementation. Am J Med Genet 62: 179–183

Czeizel A F, Dudas J 1992 Prevention of the first occurrence of neural-tube defects by periconceptional vitamin supplementation. N Engl J Med 327: 1832–1835

Daly L E, Kirke P M, Molloy A M, Weir D G, Scott J M 1995 Folate levels and neural tube defects. Implications for prevention. JAMA 274: 1698–1702

Daly S, Mills J L, Molloy A M et al 1997 Minimum effective dose of folic acid for food fortification to prevent neural tube defects. Lancet 350: 1660–1669

Department of Health 1991a Report on health and social subjects, number 41. Dietary reference values for food energy and nutrients for the UK. HMSO, London

Department of Health 1991b Report on folic acid and the prevention of neural tube defects, report from expert advisory group. Lancashire Health Publications Unit, Heywood

Dickinson C J 1995 Does folic acid harm people with vitamin B_{12} deficiency? Q J Med 88: 257-364

Ek J 1982 Plasma and red cell folate in mothers and infants in normal pregnancy. Acta Obstet Gynecol Scand 61: 17–20

Elwood J M, Little J, Elwood J H 1992 Epidemiology and control of neural tube defects. Oxford University Press, Oxford

Ganeshaguru K, Hoffbrand A V 1978 The effect of deoxyuridine, vitamin B_{12} folate and alcohol on the uptake of thymidine and on the deoxynucleoside triphosphate concentrations in normal and megaloblastic cells. Br J Haematol 40: 29–41

Hayes C, Werler M M, Willett W C, Mitchell A A 1996 Case control study of periconceptional folic acid supplementation and oral clefts. Am J Epidemiol 143: 1229–1234

Hibbard B M 1964 The role of folic acid in pregnancy with particular reference to anaemia, abruption and abortion. Obstet Gynaecol Br Commonw 71: 529–542

Iyengar L, Apte S V 1972 Nutrient stores in human foetal livers. Br J Nutr 27: 313–317

Jones K L, Smith D W, Ulleland C M, Stressguth A P 1973 Pattern of malformation in offspring of chronic alcoholic mothers. Lancet ii: 1267–1271

Kelly P, McPartlin J, Goggins M, Weir D G, Scott J M 1997 Unmetabolized folic acid in serum: acute studies in subjects consuming fortified food and supplements. Am J Clin Nutr 65: 1790–1795

Laurence K M, James M, Miller M, Tennant G B, Campbell H 1981 Double-blind randomised controlled trial of folate treatment before conception to prevent recurrence of neural-tube defects. BMJ 282: 1509–1511

Lindhout D, Amtzigt J G C 1994 Teratogenic effects of antiepileptic drugs: implications for the management of epilepsy in women of childbearing age. Epilepsia 35 Suppl. 4: S19–S28

McPartlin J, Halligan A, Scott JM, Darling M, Weir DG 1993 Accelerated folate breakdown in pregnancy. Lancet 341: 148–149

McNulty H, McPartlin J, Weir D G, Scott J M 1993 Folate catabolism is increased during pregnancy in rats. J Nutr 123: 1089–1093

McNulty H, McPartlin J M, Weir D G, Scott J M 1995 Folate catabolism is related to growth rate in weanling rats. J Nutr 125: 99–105

Manzoor M, Runzie J 1976 Folate responsive neuropathy : report of ten cases. BMJ i: 1176–1178

Martin R H, Harper T A, Kelso W 1965 Serum folic acid in recurrent abortions. Lancet i: 670–672

Meenan J, O'Hallinan E, Scott J, Weir D G 1997 Epithelial cell folate depletion occurs in neoplastic but not adjacent normal mucosa. Gastroenterology 112: 1163–1168

MRC Vitamin Study Research Group 1991 Prevention of neural tube defects: results of the Medical Research Council Vitamin Study. Lancet 338: 131–137

Nau H, Valproic acid-induced neural tube defects 1994 In: Bock B, Marsh J (eds) Neural tube defects. CIBA Found Symp 181: 144–152

Neiger R, Wise C, Contag S A, Tumber M B, Canick J A 1993 First trimester bleeding and pregnancy outcome with normal and low folate levels. Am J Perinatol 10: 460–462

Picciano M F 1995 Folate nutrition in lactation. In: Bailey L B (ed) Folate in Health and Disease. Dekker, New York, pp 153–169

Sauberlich H E 1995 Folate status of US population groups. In : Bailey L B (ed) Folate in Health and Disease. Dekker, New York, pp 171–194

Scholl T O, Hediger M L, Scholl J I, Khoo C S, Fischer R L 1996 Dietary and serum folate: their influence on the outcome of pregnancy. Am J Clin Nutr 63: 520–525

Scott J M, Kirke P M, Weir D G 1990 The role of nutrition in neural tube defects. Annu Rev Nutr 10: 277–295

Scott J M, Kirke P N, Weir D G 1994 Folate and neural tube defects. In: Bailey L B (ed) Folate in Health and Disease. Dekker, New York, pp 329–360

Scott J M, Weir D G 1981 The methyl folate trap. Lancet ii: 337–340

Scott J M, Weir D G 1994 Folate/vitamin B_{12} interrelationship. Essays Biochem 28: 63–72

Scott J M, Weir D G 1996 Homocysteine and cardiovascular disease. Q J Med 89: 561–563

Senti F R, Pilch S M 1985 Analysis of folate data from Second National Health and Nutrition Examination Survey (NHAMES) J Nutr 115: 1398–1402

Shaw G M, O'Maley C D, Wasserman C R, Tolarova M M, Lammer E J 1995 Maternal periconceptional use of multivitamins and reduced risk of corotruncal heart defects and limb deficiency among offspring. Am J Med Genet 59: 536–545

Shaw G M, Lammer E J, Wasserman C R, O'Malley C D, Tolarova M M 1995b Risks of orofacial clefts in children born to women using multivitamins containing folic acid periconceptionally. Lancet 346: 393–396

Streiff R R, Little A B 1967 Folic acid deficiency and pregnancy. N Engl J Med 276: 766–779

Smithells R W, Sheppard S, Schorah C J et al 1980 Possible prevention of neural tube defects by periconceptional vitamin supplementation. Lancet 1: 339–340

Smithells R W, Ankers C, Carver M E et al 1983 Further experience of vitamin supplementation for prevention of neural tube defect recurrences. Lancet 1: 1027–1031

Strauss R G, Bernstein R 1974 Folic acid and dilantin antagonism in pregnancy. Obstet Gynecol 44: 345–348

Tomson T, Lindbau U, Sundguist A, Berg B 1995 Red cell folate levels in pregnant epileptic women. Eur J Clin Pharmacol 48: 305–308

Tolarova M, Harris J 1995 Reduced recurrence of orofacial clefts after periconceptional supplementation with high dose folic acid and multivitamins. Teratology 51: 71–78

Ward M, McNulty H, McPartlin J J et al 1997 Plasma homocysteine, a risk factor for cardiovascular disease can be effectively reduced by physiological amounts of folic acid. Q J Med 90: 519–524

Wald N 1994 Folic acid and neural tube defects: the current evidence and implications for prevention. CIBA Found Symp 181. Wiley, London

Waters A H, Mollin D L 1993 Observations on the metabolism of folic acid in pernicious anaemia. Br J Haematol 9: 319–329

Weir D G, Scott J M 1995 The biochemical basis of the neuropathy in cobalamin deficiency. Baillière's Clin Haematol 8: 479–497

Wills L 1931 Treatment of 'pernicious anaemia of pregnancy' and 'tropical anaemia' with special reference to yeast extract as curative agent. BMJ i: 1059–1064

Worthington-White D A, Behuke M, Gross S 1994 Premature infants require additional folate and vitamin B_{12} to reduce the severity of the anaemia of prematurity. Am J Clin Nutr 60: 390–395

Wouters M, Boers G, Blom H et al 1993 Hyperhomocysteinemia: a risk factor in women with unexplained recurrent early pregnancy loss. Fertil Steril 60: 820–825

Susan M. Tuck Carl E. Jensen

Effects of major haemoglobinopathies on pregnancy

Haemoglobinopathy is the collective term for the inherited disorders of haemoglobin that are responsible for significant morbidity and mortality world-wide. There is a wide distribution of affected populations, including peoples from the Eastern Mediterranean, Middle East, the Indian subcontinent, South East Asia, Africa and the West Indies. The carrier states for the most important of these haemoglobinopathies, β thalassaemia and sickle cell haemoglobin, are symptomless, with no direct effect on the quality of life or life expectancy. Heterozygous carriers of β thalassaemia usually present no clinical problems except for a mild hypochromic anaemia which is often exacerbated by pregnancy (Perkins 1971). However, the homozygous state of both conditions is becoming important to obstetricians in the UK as increasing numbers of affected females are now living and, with improved haematological and paediatric management, surviving to childbearing age.

Heterozygotes (carriers) for the various haemoglobinopathies should be identified (preferably before pregnancy) and offered genetic counselling and the availability of antenatal fetal testing. This group will not be discussed further in this chapter, which concerns women who themselves have a major haemoglobinopathy.

CLASSIFICATION OF HAEMOGLOBINOPATHIES

1   Inherited abnormalities of the synthesis of globin chains of haemoglobin.

2   The structural haemoglobin variants.

Susan M. Tuck MD MRCGP FRCOG, Consultant Senior Lecturer, University Department of Obstetrics and Gynaecology, The Royal Free Hospital, Pond Street, London NW3 2OG, UK

Carl E. Jensen MMed FCOG(SA) MRCOG, Senior Registrar, Department of Obstetrics and Gynaecology, University College Hospital, Huntley Street, London WC1E 6AU, UK

THE THALASSAEMIAS

The thalassaemias are a group of recessive disorders characterised by a reduced synthesis of one or more of the globin chains of haemoglobin. The most common and clinically important forms of thalassaemia are the α and β thalassaemias. The β chains of women with homozygous β thalassaemia have normal structure but are produced in reduced and sometimes undetectable amounts. In β^0 thalassaemia, no β globin chains are produced by the affected gene, while in β^+ thalassaemia, globin chains are synthesised, but at a reduced rate. As a result of this globin chain imbalance, the thalassaemias have varying degrees of ineffective erythropoiesis and haemolysis contributing to the wide range of clinical severity. The diverse series of clinical disorders which result from the co-inheritance of thalassaemia and a structural haemoglobin variant or from the co-inheritance of more than one type of thalassaemia, constitute the thalassaemia syndromes.

World distribution of thalassaemia

Thalassaemia primarily affects people of Mediterranean, Asian, Arabian and west African ancestry in the malaria-endemic regions. It is believed that malaria has exerted selective pressure for the propagation of the thalassaemia gene because of relative resistance to the malaria parasite exhibited by heterozygotes. (Malaria causes severe illness in homozygotes.) Thalassaemia was originally described in Italians, Greeks, Spaniards and people of Mediterranean origin. However, it is now realised that it is a common disorder with a widespread geographical distribution and is now occasionally identified in persons of northern European origin. β Thalassaemia is one of the most common single gene defects, affecting about 150 million people world-wide. At present there are an estimated 600 people with β thalassaemia major living in the UK. Other names for thalassaemia major are: Cooley's anemia; β-thalassaemia major; homozygous β-thalassaemia; homozygous thalassaemia; and Mediterranean anaemia.

Management of β thalassaemia major

Once the diagnosis of β thalassaemia major is made, the child and its family are destined for a life-long association with their physicians and hospitals. Hence it is preferable for treatment to be delivered by a specialist centre. Conventional treatment consists of regular blood transfusions designed to maintain the haemoglobin concentration near normal. This ensures normal growth and pubertal development without the typical thalassaemic facies. Splenectomy is often indicated to reduce transfusion requirements. Hypersplenism is a characteristic consequence of homozygous β thalassaemia. Splenic sequestration contributes to shortened red blood survival, and splenectomy is generally performed at a young age (Bunn 1987). Unfortunately, hypertransfusion regimens lead to chronic iron overload, despite chelation therapy with desferrioxamine. The massive iron overload results from both the high transfusion requirements and increased intestinal absorption of iron secondary to hypoxia. By the age of 10 or 11 years, transfused patients suffer from the effects of iron overload, which is manifested as hepatic, cardiac and endocrine disturbances. Unless the iron overloading is controlled by iron chelation, death results in the second or third decade, usually from cardiac failure.

An important aspect of the management of thalassaemics is general medical care, including early detection and treatment of infections, immunisation and hormone replacement therapy.

Social and personal concerns: fertility and pregnancy

Increasingly the patients lead a 'normal life', pursue a career, integrate into society and wish to have children. The medical professionals who care for thalassaemics have to recognise this expectation, and need to provide the expertise to fulfil these wishes.

Although young adults with β thalassaemia major have multiple organ effects of iron deposition, the most common endocrine abnormality in these patients is hypogonadotrophic hypogonadism (Landau et al 1987), presenting as either primary or secondary amenorrhoea, with chronic anovulation and decreased oestradiol levels. Male thalassaemics, similarly, frequently have severe oligospermia and azoospermia (Jensen et al 1996). The hypogonadotrophic hypogonadism results from iron deposition in the hypothalamus and pituitary (Canale et al 1984). Other endocrine complications, such as hypothyroidism and diabetes, may also play a role in their reduced fertility. Possible direct ovarian damage due to iron deposition and redox-active iron in follicular fluid has also been postulated (Reubinoff et al 1996). The cause of infertility is, therefore, multifactorial and differs from patient to patient. Many aspects of the disease have to be considered before fertility treatment is embarked upon.

Pregnancy in women with β thalassaemia major has been rarely reported because these patients had a shortened life expectancy until recently, as well as reduced fertility. During the last two decades, because of improved paediatric and haematological management, pregnancy is no longer a rarity. In the 1960s, several authors thought it unlikely that patients with β thalassaemia major could ever reproduce (Bannerman 1961, Zaino & Dolan 1966), but since then there have been a number of successful pregnancies reported in transfusion dependent thalassaemic patients with a total of 15 pregnancies in 10 women in the literature (Walker et al 1969, Perkins 1971, Thomas & Skalioka 1980, Goldfarb et al 1982, Martin 1983, Meadows 1984, Grech et al 1984, Mordel et al 1989, Savona-Ventura & Grech 1991, Savona-Ventura & Bonello 1994). More recently, we have reported 16 pregnancies in 11 women, 10 of whom were transfusion dependent (Jensen et al 1995).

Pregnancy in women with β thalassaemia major is associated with: (i) marked anaemia; (ii) increased transfusion requirements; (iii) concerns about desferrioxamine (see below); and (iv) high caesarean section rate (possibly due to short maternal stature).

Our experience with modern management, in particular giving blood transfusions sufficiently frequently to maintain the minimum pretransfusion haemoglobin concentration above 10 g/dl, has resulted in good maternal and fetal outcomes from pregnancies in women with β thalassaemia major (Jensen et al 1995). However, severe anaemia and hypoxia may affect placental gas exchange, thus altering intrauterine fetal growth and well-being. The relatively high rate of pregnancy loss and prematurity, as well as the intrauterine growth retardation reported in earlier literature (Perkins 1971, Grech et al 1984) may have resulted from these alterations.

Pre-pregnancy assessment and care

In the individual woman, the advisability of embarking on ovulation induction and pregnancy should be assessed carefully. Preconception counselling is vital as they often have other significant medical conditions resulting from tissue iron deposition which need to be stabilised before a pregnancy is contemplated.

Cardiac function

The most common cause of death in patients with β thalassaemia major is cardiac failure due to iron deposition in the myocardium, and cardiac function should be assessed before considering a pregnancy. Cardiomyopathy has a poor prognosis and the physiological changes in pregnancy, including anaemia, increase in plasma volume by 50% and red cell mass by 20–30%, increase in cardiac stroke volume and stroke rate and increase in cardiac output by 20%, may result in cardiac failure. Cardiac function should be assessed either by multi-gated acquisition (MUGA) scan or by echocardiography. It is also important to check cardiac rhythm by an ECG. Significant impairment of cardiac function would make pregnancy strongly inadvisable.

Endocrine disorders

Hypothyroidism The prevalence is about 9% in patients with β thalassaemia major (De Sanctis et al 1989), although some form of thyroid dysfunction has been reported in 75% of Sardinian thalassaemic patients (Masala et al 1984). Women with hypothyroidism are subfertile and have early miscarriages; untreated hypothyroidism in pregnancy has a high fetal wastage and can lead to mental handicap, deafness and cerebral palsy in the child (Ritchie 1986). TSH and T4 should be measured yearly from the age of 10 years in all β thalassaemia patients, and replacement therapy given when this becomes relevant.

Diabetes The prevalence of insulin-dependent diabetes mellitus (IDDM) varies from 4.9–20% in patients with β thalassaemia major, with a further 25% having impaired glucose tolerance (IGT) (Italian Working Group 1995, Jensen et al 1997). Patients with IGT may well become insulin dependent during pregnancy and patients on insulin will need to increase their insulin requirements. As there is an increased incidence of congenital malformations and obstetric complications such as polyhydramnios, preterm labour and pre-eclampsia in IDDM it is important to stabilise the glucose levels prior to conception. Induction of ovulation in these patients is best postponed until a normal glucose level is achieved. An oral glucose tolerance test (OGTT) is recommended yearly from the age of 10 years in all β thalassaemia patients, so that prompt care of diabetes can be instituted.

Genetic counselling

The partner's haemoglobin electrophoresis should be checked and the couples wishes about antenatal testing of the fetus, if relevant, ascertained.

Blood group antibodies

Blood group antibodies, such as anti-Kell or Duffy, may be present due to previous transfusions. This can lead to difficulties with cross matching the blood and, thus, the availability of suitable blood as well as the potential for fetal haemolytic disease. It is, therefore, important to check for antibodies.

Viral screen

Screening for blood-borne viral infections, e.g. hepatitis B and C viruses and HIV, is important in any patient who receives multiple blood transfusions. This is because infection with a blood-borne virus may very occasionally occur despite blood donor screening. Active immunisation against hepatitis B should be offered. We recommend yearly hepatitis B surface antigen, HCV antibody and HIV antibody determination in all regularly transfused patients. This is particularly important in a woman wishing to conceive, both from the maternal health perspective and for the possibility of transmission of infection from mother to child. It would also be prudent to check the woman's rubella antibody status prior to embarking on a pregnancy so that immunisation can be offered if necessary. In addition, screening for varicella-zoster virus antibodies will enable the susceptible pregnant woman to avoid (if possible) contact with shingles or chicken pox and be offered appropriate prophylaxis in the form of zoster immunoglobulin if such contact occurs.

Ferritin

The role of iron-chelating treatment with desferrioxamine before and during pregnancy should be discussed with homozygous β thalassaemia patients. Chelation treatment before pregnancy diminishes tissue iron overload and probably contributes to the improvement in fertility rates, cardiac function and pregnancy outcome (Mordel et al 1989). Monitoring ferritin levels every 3 months gives an approximate indication of the degree of compliance to desferrioxamine treatment and can be a motivating factor prior to embarking on a pregnancy. Generally, as with any sufferers of chronic illness, thalassaemics will, from time to time, find the daily commitment to chelation therapy irksome, particularly since it has to be given parenterally, usually by subcutaneous infusion pump. The aim is to achieve a serum ferritin level of 1000-2000 μg/l (normal reference range: 14–300 μg/l).

> Many of the above issues have a potential interaction with pregnancy and may make fertility treatment inadvisable.

Management of pregnancy

Stop desferrioxamine

It is recommended that desferrioxamine should not be used in pregnancy. Some animal studies have shown skeletal anomalies at doses close to those used in humans. To date no cases of congenital malformations have been reported in the literature in women receiving the drug in early pregnancy. Despite this, termination of pregnancy should be discussed with any women who is worried about the possible risk of congenital malformations. The new-born infant should be considered at risk of iron deficiency secondary to maternal desferrioxamine therapy if the mother continued the drug in late pregnancy.

Stop vitamin C

Vitamin C is given to potentiate the chelation effect of desferrioxamine. This should be stopped during pregnancy as it will increase dietary iron absorption and it has been suggested that this might precipitate cardiac damage (Nienhuis et al 1979).

Folic acid

Folic acid depletion is common in thalassaemia because of marrow over-activity. It is given to thalassaemics, to support their haemopoeisis, and is obviously particularly relevant to continue before and during pregnancy.

Booking visit

At the time of booking, a full clinical examination should be undertaken with specific reference to the cardiovascular and endocrine systems. Blood group and antibody screen should be repeated as well as a baseline liver function test. With continuing transfusion there is always a risk of blood-borne viral infections, therefore, the maternal blood should be rechecked for antibodies to hepatitis B and C and HIV.

Antenatal management

Cardiac status

Cardiac function should be closely monitored throughout, with particular care during the first 12 weeks of pregnancy, during transfusion, at delivery and in the early puerperium. Any significant deterioration should prompt consideration of expediting delivery.

Blood transfusions

It is essential in pregnant thalassaemic patients to maintain the haemoglobin concentration above 10 g/dl. This can be achieved by more frequent, but smaller, volumes of blood transfusions than is usually undertaken for non pregnant thalassaemics. The transfusions must be carefully monitored in view of the potential to precipitate congestive heart failure.

Ferritin

Serum ferritin concentration tends to remain stable despite stopping chelation therapy during pregnancy. This could be a result of a possible haemodilution effect or from fetal consumption of free iron. It is our experience that the serum ferritin concentration does not seem to increase by more than 10% throughout the duration of the pregnancy.

Splenectomy

There is an increased risk of infections in splenectomised patients. Women with thalassaemia major who have had a splenectomy frequently have platelet counts in excess of $500 \times 10^9/l$. High platelet counts superimposed on the changes that occur in the clotting system during pregnancy may predispose to venous thrombosis. This increased thrombotic risk may possibly be diminished by the use of low dose aspirin.

Fetal surveillance

Serial ultrasound scans for fetal growth are recommended in view of the isolated reports of IUGR in the literature. However, as mentioned above, this has not been our experience, possibly due to our policy of keeping the pretransfusion haemoglobin concentration above 10 g/dl. throughout pregnancy.

Labour

Induction of labour

There are generally no specific haematological indications for induction of labour and normal obstetric principles should apply. Prostaglandin induction can be safely used, but care must be taken with oxytocin infusions not to overload an already compromised cardiovascular system.

Pain relief

There are no contra-indications to the use of any of the usual analgesic modalities. Care must be taken when preloading the cardiovascular system prior to an epidural not to precipitate cardiac failure.

Mode of delivery

Vaginal delivery should be encouraged, however, a high caesarean section rate was noted in our series (Jensen et al 1995). There are two possible reasons: cephalopelvic disproportion due to the short maternal stature characteristic of patients prior to the adoption of hypertransfusion regimens combined with well grown fetuses in pregnancies managed with high haemoglobin maintenance, or fetal distress due to hypoxaemia possibly as a result of placental iron deposition.

Although delayed onset of menarche, amenorrhoea, anovulation and infertility are the usual events in patients with β thalassaemia major, their management by intensive transfusion regimens and desferrioxamine therapy together with appropriate use of ovulation induction therapy has made successful pregnancies an increasing possibility.

Puerperium

Breast feeding

There is concern about the possible excretion of desferrioxamine in breast milk. However, it is poorly absorbed from the human gut and, therefore, unlikely to have a harmful effect on the infant. Breast feeding should therefore be encouraged.

Chelation

Desferrioxamine should be recommenced within the first week of the puerperium.

Contraception or HRT

Given the major medical problems and shortened life expectancy which these women have, it is of paramount importance to discuss contraception with them. There is no contra-indication to the use of any type of contraception, although some authorities feel that the increased thrombotic risk of splenectomised women would contra-indicate the use of oral contraceptives in these individuals. Those who have developed secondary amenorrhoea should be given oestrogen replacement therapy.

HAEMOGLOBIN VARIANTS

Sickle cell disease (SCD)

Sickle cell disease includes a group of inherited disorders characterised by a defect(s) in haemoglobin structure which predominantly present with vaso-occlusive symptoms and complications of haemolysis. The most commonly encountered conditions are sickle cell anaemia (HbSS), sickle cell haemoglobin C disease (HbSC) and sickle cell β-thalassaemia (HbSβthal).

World distribution of sickle cell syndromes

Sickle cell disease is the most common known hereditary blood disorder. It is not limited to people of Afro-Caribbean ethnic origin, but is widely distributed among peoples of southern Italy, northern Greece, southern Turkey, Saudi Arabia, India, Equatorial Africa and parts of South America. In the UK, people with SCD are predominantly Afro-Caribbean and West African in origin, but some are also from the Mediterranean, Middle East and Asia. At present, there are an estimated 5000 people with a SCD living in the UK (Streetly et al 1993). Affected babies can be diagnosed at birth, and at least 150 babies with SCD are born in the UK annually (Brozovic & Davies 1987).

Management of sickle cell disease

The diagnosis of SCD should be made as early as possible, so that appropriate medical care and support can be instituted. The clinical picture is highly variable and, therefore, management should be supervised by a specialist centre. One of the most important features of the condition is acute painful episodes of tissue infarction, occurring at any and sometimes multiple sites, with unpredictable timing. The acute episodes and their consequences result in significant limitations to activities and lifestyle (Midence & Elander 1994). Conventional treatment consists of prophylaxis against infections or prompt diagnosis and treatment of infections, management of painful crises by hydration, oxygen and narcotic pain relief. Blood transfusions are used for symptomatic anaemia or for the treatment of some of the vaso-occlusive complications, such as strokes, acute chest syndrome, acute splenic sequestration or priapism.

An important aspect in the management of SCD is education of the family and the patient about the disease.

Social and personal concerns: fertility and pregnancy

At one time, few people with SCD survived to adulthood. However, as with thalassaemia, women with sickle cell disease are now reaching child-bearing age due to modern management protocols, a better understanding of the disease processes and more effective measures against infections and other complications.

There is very little good evidence that fertility in young women with SCD is affected, but pregnancy is potentially problematical. However, in male patients with SCD, lower semen volume, sperm counts and sperm motility have all been observed (Davies 1988).

The first major review of pregnancy in sickle cell anaemia was reported in 1941 (Kobak et al 1941). More recently, pregnancy has been regularly reported (Charache et al 1980, Powars et al 1986, El-Shafei et al 1992). Pregnant women with sickle cell disease are at increased risk of antenatal and postnatal complications. Pregnancy complications are more frequent in the third trimester, at delivery or in the immediate puerperium. The maternal mortality rate in the UK is of the order of 1–2%.

Pregnancy in women with HbSS is associated with: (i) marked anaemia; (ii) infections – chest, pyelonephritis, puerperal sepsis; (iii) sickling crises; and (iv) proteinuric hypertension. Fetal problems are: (i) an increased miscarriage rate; (ii) intrauterine growth restriction; and (iii) prematurity.

Perinatal mortality for sickle cell pregnancies in the UK is more than 7 times that of comparable pregnancies (Howard et al 1995). The chronic maternal anaemia could account for the increased rates of fetal growth retardation (Charache & Niebyl 1985), or a degree of sickling and poor perfusion in the placenta may play a part (Howard et al 1995).

The clinical course of HbSS women is not adversely affected by their pregnancies (Smith et al 1996), but the complications of the sickle cell disease (acute chest syndrome, infection and pre-eclampsia) can precipitate delivery, either spontaneously or by medical intervention (Howard et al 1995).

Pre-pregnancy assessment and care

Women with SCD must be appropriately counselled on the advisability of pregnancy and potential motherhood. This needs to take into account any chronic handicaps as a result of previous sickling episodes, e.g. impaired vision, impaired mobility, and the frequency of episodes of acute illness. As with any chronic, incurable, life-threatening illness (including thalassaemia), SCD sufferers may feel a strong urge to achieve parenthood. However, their children may be faced with the loss of a parent at a relatively young age.

Genetic counselling

The partner's haemoglobin electrophoresis should be checked and the wishes of the couple regarding antenatal testing of the fetus, if relevant, ascertained.

Blood group antibodies

The relatively frequent occurrence of atypical antibodies in SCD patients repeatedly transfused from a blood bank almost exclusively supplied by white donors can be a serious problem (Tuck et al 1982). The presence of antibodies can cause difficulties in finding compatible blood for future transfusions, and may cause fetal haemolytic disease.

Viral infections

For those women with SCD receiving multiple blood transfusions, the same considerations apply as for thalassaemics (see above).

Ferritin

A few individuals on hypertransfusion regimens will have high ferritin concentrations and the related considerations already discussed in the context of thalassaemia with regard to chelation therapy and iron overload will apply. It may be necessary to establish central venous access in order to perform exchange blood transfusions, if peripheral veins have become fibrosed from previous repeated cannulation.

Management of pregnancy

Regular antenatal care by an obstetrician and haematologist experienced in the management of SCD is essential.

Booking visit

A full clinical examination should be undertaken with specific reference to complications of SCD, such as proliferative retinopathy, leg ulcers, renal and hepatic impairment. Blood group and antibody screen should be rechecked as well as baseline renal and liver function tests. Antibodies to hepatitis B, C and HIV should be rechecked. A mid-stream urine sample should be sent to the laboratory for microscopy and culture.

Antenatal management

This should entail a joint approach between obstetrician and haematologist with close communication and clear management plans. Infections and painful crises should be treated promptly, and the patient should have clear instructions on whom to contact to arrange hospital admission, when necessary.

The use of prophylactic blood transfusion programmes and exchange blood transfusions to improve the outcome of pregnancy is controversial. Some authors recommend prophylactic transfusions to improve fetal outcome (Morrison et al 1991), whilst others advise transfusion only for obstetric or haematological indications (Koshy et al 1988). A recent retrospective study found few sickling complications in patients who had received prophylactic blood transfusions from 26 weeks' gestation, compared with untransfused patients (Howard et al 1995).

Regular urinalysis should be performed due to the high incidence of acute pyelonephritis and renal sickling (Tuck et al 1983).

Episodes of bone pain are more frequent in the third trimester and the puerperium. The mechanism for this increase is unclear, but hormonal, coagulation changes and the effects of prostaglandins have been proposed (Midence & Elander 1994). Acute chest syndrome is characterised by the sudden onset of pleuritic chest pain and dyspnoea and has been reported in up to 35% of pregnant women (Omu et al 1982). Management of these sickling crises should be as for the non pregnant individual, including the treatment of infections, hydration, oxygen and analgesia.

Proteinuric hypertension has been reported in SCD since 1941 (Kobak et al 1941) and since then many reports have noted a higher incidence than in the general population. Chronic hypertension and mild pre-eclampsia were found to be less common, but severe pre-eclampsia significantly more common among patients with HbSS than controls (Tuck et al 1983). Regular and frequent blood pressure recordings should be obtained in the third trimester of pregnancy so that early and appropriate management can be instituted.

Serial ultrasound scans for fetal growth are recommended in view of the increased risk of IUGR. Patients should be warned about the symptoms and signs of preterm labour.

Labour

Induction of labour

There are no specific indications in SCD for induction of labour, which should be considered, as relevant, for the usual obstetric reasons. Prostaglandin induction and oxytocin infusions can be safely used.

Pain relief

There are no contra-indications to any of the usual analgesic modalities presently available. SCD sufferers are used to episodes of very severe pain and can, therefore, often tolerate normal labour pains better than can the general population. However, their frequent need of narcotic analgesia for sickling episodes may mean that therapeutic doses required are higher than generally used.

Mode of delivery

In general, normal vaginal delivery should be encouraged, although caesarean section may be necessary for disproportion due to pelvic bone deformity. Continuous fetal monitoring should be used in view of the impaired placental function common in SCD. Careful attention to optimal hydration and oxygenation, and the avoidance of infection and acidosis during labour, are essential to reduce the risk of precipitating sickling crises.

Puerperium

Infections

Post-partum fever is common and may result from endometritis or post-delivery wound infection. Antibiotics should be routinely administered. Women should be managed on a high dependency ward for the first few days. Since SCD patients are often not fully mobile at this stage, prophylactic measures against thrombo-embolism should be considered.

Breast feeding

There is no specific contra-indication to breast feeding in SCD. However, if the mother is on high doses of narcotic analgesia because of repeated acute sickling episodes the neonate may need special care with regard to drug withdrawal.

Contraception

Pregnancy planning advice must be given to all sexually active patients with SCD due to the substantial risks accompanying pregnancy. All methods of contraception may be considered, although a possible risk of crises and thrombotic episodes when using the oral combined contraceptive pill must be balanced against the risk of a less reliable form of contraception (Howard et al 1993). The current policy in a Jamaican clinic is to advise tubal ligation for permanent contraception, and intrauterine devices, medroxyprogesterone acetate, and oral contraceptives, in that order, as reversible methods (Serjeant 1992). Since women with SCD often have need of courses of broad spectrum antibiotics, they should be given the relevant advice about using additional contraception at these times if the are taking an oral contraceptive pill.

Although pregnancy in patients with SCD should be considered at high risk of complications, the previous practice of recommending avoidance of pregnancy or abortion to women with SCD, based on the severity of these risks is no longer appropriate (Smith et al 1996).

Key points for clinical practice

- Consider the social aspects of childbearing in the context of severe chronic illness.

- Genetic counselling should be discussed and offered if appropriate.

- Careful assessment of disease sequelae relevant to pregnancy planning.

- Transmission from mother to child of blood-borne viral infections must be considered.

- Pre-pregnancy and pregnancy care should entail a joint approach between an obstetrician and haematologist.

- The high risk of complications in pregnancy requires a detailed management plan and good communications.

- Good rapport and mutual confidence with the patient must be established.

- Contraceptive advice and ongoing care after delivery is essential.

References

Bannerman R M 1961 Thalassaemia: a survey of some aspects. Grune and Stratton, New York

Brozovic M, Davies S C 1987 Management of sickle cell disease. Postgrad Med J 63: 605–609

Bunn H F 1987 Disorders of hemoglobin: thalassemia. In: Isselbacher K J, Adams R D, Braunwald E, Petersdorf R G, Wilson J D (eds) Harrison's principles of internal medicine, 11th edn. McGraw-Hill, New York, pp 1518–1527

Charache S, Scott J, Niebyl J, Bond D 1980 Management of sickle cell disease in pregnant patients. Obstet Gynecol 55: 407–410

Charache S, Niebyl J R 1985 Pregnancy in sickle cell disease. Clin Haematol 14: 729–746

Davies S C 1988 Obstetric implications of sickle cell disease. Midwife, Health Visitor Community Nurse 24: 361–363

De Sanctis V, Vullo C, Katz M, Wonke B, Hoffbrand A V, Bagni B 1989 Endocrine complications in thalassaemia major. In: Bruckner CD, Gale RP, Lucarelli G, eds. Advances and controversies in thalassaemia therapy: bone marrow transplantation and other approaches. Alan R. Liss, Urbrino, pp 77–83

El-Shafei A M, Dhaliwal J K, Sandhu A K 1992 Pregnancy in sickle cell disease in Bahrain. Br J Obstet Gynaecol 99: 101–104

Goldfarb A W, Hochner-Celnikier D, Beller U 1982 A successful pregnancy in transfusion dependent homozygous beta-thalassaemia: a case report. Int J Gynaecol Obstet 20: 319–322

Grech E S, Silva L J P, Savona-Ventura C 1984 Homozygous beta-thalassaemia and pregnancy. Aust NZ J Obstet Gynaecol 24: 45–48

Howard R J, Lillis C, Tuck S M 1993 Contraceptives, counselling, and pregnancy in women with sickle cell disease. BMJ 306: 1735–1737

Howard R J, Tuck S M, Pearson T C 1995 Pregnancy in sickle cell disease in the UK: results of a multicentre survey of the effect of prophylactic blood transfusion on maternal and fetal outcome. Br J Obstet Gynaecol 102: 947–951

Howard R J, Tuck S M, Pearson T C 1995 Optimal haematocrit and haemoglobin S levels in pregnant women with sickle cell disease. Clin Lab Haematol 17: 157–161

Italian Working Group on Endocrine Complications in Non-Endocrine Diseases 1995 Multicentre study on prevalence of endocrine complications in thalassaemia major. Clin Endocrinol 42: 581–586

Jensen C E, Tuck S M, Wonke B 1995 Fertility in β thalassaemia major: a report of 16 pregnancies, preconceptual evaluation and a review of the literature. Br J Obstet Gynaecol 102: 625–629

Jensen C E, Abdel-Gadir A, Cox C, Tuck S M, Wonke B 1996 Sperm concentrations and quality in β-thalassaemia major. Int J Androl 19: 362–364

Jensen C E, Tuck S M, Old J et al 1997 Incidence of endocrine complications and clinical disease severity related to genotype analysis and iron overload in patients with β-thalassaemia. Eur J Haematol 59: 76–81

Kobak A J, Stein P J, Daro A 1941 Sickle-cell anemia in pregnancy. A review of the literature and report of six cases. Am J Obstet Gynecol 41: 811–821

Koshy M, Burd L, Wallace D, Moawad A, Baron J 1988 Prophylactic red-cell transfusions in pregnant patients with sickle cell disease. N Engl J Med 319: 1447–1452

Masala A, Meloni T, Gallisia D, Rovasio P P, Rassu S, Milia A F 1984 Endocrine functioning in multitransfused prepubertal patients with homozygous β thalassaemia. J Clin Endocrinol Metab 58: 667–670

Martin K 1983 Successful pregnancy in beta-thalassaemia major. Aust Paediatr 19: 182–183

Meadows K 1984 A successful pregnancy outcome in transfusion dependent thalassaemia major. Aust NZ J Obstet Gynaecol 24: 43–44

Midence K, Elander J 1994 Sickle cell disease. A psychosocial approach. Radcliffe Medical Press, Oxford

Mordel N, Birkenfeld A, Goldfarb A N, Rachmilewitz E A 1989 Successful full-term pregnancy in homozygous thalassaemia major: case report and review of the literature. Obstet Gynecol 73: 837–840

Morrison J C, Morrison F S, Floyd R C, Roberts W E, Wayne Hess L, Weiser W L 1991 Use of continuous flow erythrocytapheresis in pregnant patients with sickle cell disease. J Clin Apheresis 6: 224–229

Nienhuis A W, Benz E J, Propper R et al 1979 Thalassaemia major molecular and clinical aspects. Ann Intern Med 91: 883–897

Omu A E, Tabowei O, Okpere E E 1982 The effect of sickle cell anaemia on obstetric performance in a Nigerian community. Trop Geogr Med 34: 47–50

Perkins R P 1971 Inherited disorders of hemoglobin synthesis and pregnancy. Am J Obstet Gynecol 111: 120–151

Powars D R, Sandhu M, Niland-Weiss J, Johnson C, Bruce S, Manning P R 1986 Pregnancy in sickle cell disease. Obstet Gynecol 62: 217–228

Ritchie J W K. 1986 Diabetes and other endocrine diseases complicating pregnancy. In: Whitfield C R (ed) Dewhurst's textbook of obstetrics and gynaecology for postgraduates, 4th edn. Blackwell Scientific Publications, Oxford, pp 284–298

Reubinoff B E, Har-EL R, Kitrossky N et al 1996 Increased levels of redox-active iron in follicular fluid: a possible cause of free radical-mediated infertility in β-thalassemia major. Am J Obstet Gynecol 174: 914–918

Savona-Ventura C, Grech E 1991 Pregnancy complications in homozygous thalassaemia patients. J Obstet Gynaecol 11: 175–176

Savona-Ventura C, Bonello F 1994 Beta-thalassemia syndromes and pregnancy. Obstet Gynecol Survey 49: 129–137

Serjeant G R 1992 Pregnancy and contraception. In: Serjeant G R (ed) Sickle cell disease, 2nd edn. Oxford University Press, Oxford, pp 353–363

Smith J A, Espeland M, Bellevue R, Bonds D, Brown A K, Koshy M 1996 Pregnancy in sickle cell disease: experience of the cooperative study of sickle cell disease. Obstet Gynecol 87: 199–204

Streetly A, Dick M, Layton M 1993 Sickle cell disease: the case for coordinated information. BMJ 306: 1491–1492

Thomas R M, Skalicka A E 1980 Successful pregnancy in transfusion-dependent thalassaemia. Arch Dis Child 55: 572–574

Tuck S M, Studd J W W, White J M 1982 Sickle cell disease in pregnancy complicated by anti-U antibodies. Br J Obstet Gynaecol 89: 91–92

Tuck S M, Studd J W W, White J M 1983 Pregnancy in sickle cell disease in the UK. Br J Obstet Gynaecol 90: 112–117

Walker E H, Whelton M J, Beaven G H 1969 Successful pregnancy in a patient with thalassaemia major. J Obstet Gynaecol Br Comnwlth 76: 549–553

Zaino E C, Dolan W S C 1966 Thalassaemia minor and pregnancy in a non-Mediterranean. Am J Obstet Gynecol 96: 295–297

Isobel D. Walker

CHAPTER 3

Inherited coagulation disorders and thrombophilia and pregnancy

As obstetric care has developed and previously major causes of maternal mortality and morbidity, such as sepsis and eclampsia have become less frequent and better managed, disorders of haemostasis – bleeding and thrombosis – have become the most important causes of maternal morbidity and death.

Obstetricians have always been cogniscent of the risk of sudden acquired bleeding problems complicating delivery but there has, until relatively recently, been less awareness of the increased thrombotic risk associated with even a normal pregnancy. During the past 10 years, enormous advances have been made in our understanding of the chemistry of haemostasis and of the many important interactions between those factors which promote blood clot formation and those which inhibit or limit blood clotting. With this information and understanding of the basic chemistry has come a realisation that genetic variation of components of haemostasis are not uncommon and variants, particularly of blood clotting factors or of natural anticoagulants, may result in clinical problems for affected individuals.

HAEMOSTASIS AND NORMAL PREGNANCY

Pregnancy is normally associated with significant changes in virtually all aspects of the haemostatic mechanism – vessels, platelets, coagulation factors, natural anticoagulants and the fibrinolytic system – altering the concentrations of procoagulant and anticoagulant, profibrinolytic and antifibrinolytic components such that towards the end of pregnancy the overall 'balance' of the haemostatic system is shifted towards apparent hypercoagulability.

In a recently completed study of the changes in the concentrations of haemostasis components in healthy women during normal pregnancy, we noted an increase in all coagulation factors with the exception of factor XIC,

Dr Isobel D. Walker MD FRCP FRCPath, Consultant Haematologist, Department of Haematology, Glasgow Royal Infirmary, 3rd Floor Macewen Building, Castle Street, Glasgow G4 0SF, UK

Table 3.1 Mean values, 95% ranges and % changes for coagulation factors in normal pregnancy

	6–11 weeks (n = 41)			36–40 weeks (n = 23)			3 days post partum (n = 87)		
	Mean	(Range)		Mean	(Range)	% change*	Mean	(Range)	% change*
PT (s)	15	(14–16)		15	(12–17)	–	14	(12–16)	–
APTT (s)	42	(33–51)		40	(33–48)	–	38	(32–45)	–
Fibrinogen (g/l)	3.6	(2.4–4.8)		4.2	(3.2–5.3)	+ 17%	4.5	(3.1–5.8)	+ 25%
FVIIIC (IU/dl)**	107	(62–220)		76	(50–320)	+ 65%	192	(54–331)	+ 79%
vWf Ag (IU/dl)**	118	(52–248)		221	(98–464)	+ 87%	226	(102–545)	+ 92%
RiCof activity (IU/dl)**	117	(47–258)		240	(100–544)	+ 105%	247	(97–630)	+ 111%
FVC (U/dl)	99	(39–159)		129	(65–194)	+ 30%	141	(71–211)	+ 42%
FIIC (IU/dl)	153	(107–200)		162	(107–217)	+ 6%	169	(108–231)	+ 10%
FVIIC (IU/dl)**	94	(48–180)		164	(96–270)	+ 74%	238	(90–398)	+ 153%
FIXC (IU/dl)	100	(49–151)		114	(79–150)	+ 14%	136	(65–207)	+ 36%
FXC (IU/dl)	125	(88–162)		152	(113–191)	+ 22%	162	(69–254)	+ 30%
FXIC (IU/dl)	102	(50–154)		92	(36–181)	– 10%	96	(46–146)	– 6%
FXIIC (U/dl)	137	(70–204)		179	(62–296)	+ 31%	174	(86–262)	+ 27%

*Relative to 6–11 weeks, **data which required log transformation for calculation of normal range.
PT = prothrombin time; APTT = activated partial thromboplastin time; vWf Ag = von Willebrand factor antigen; RiCof = ristocetin cofactor.

when blood samples collected at 6–11 weeks gestation were compared with those collected at 36–40 weeks (Clark et al 1997). The greatest changes were noted in factor VIII complex – mean factor VIIIC having increased 65% above the first trimester baseline at term and von Willebrand factor antigen and ristocetin cofactor levels rising, respectively, 87% and 105% above the first trimester baseline. For each of these components of the factor VIII complex, the rise was sustained at 3 days post partum (Table 3.1).

Factor VIIC also showed a substantial rise – the term sample having a factor VIIC level 74% above the first trimester baseline and the 3 day postnatal level having risen even further. None of the other vitamin K dependent clotting factors (prothrombin, factor IXC or factor XC) showed such significant increases. In particular, factor IXC demonstrated only a 14% increase above baseline at term. The only clotting factor which fell during pregnancy was factor XIC. These findings are similar to previously published reports.

Mean antithrombin activity was slightly higher in the women at term than in the first trimester women, but there was no difference in protein C activity at term compared with early pregnancy. However, there was a significant increase in protein C activity in the 3 day post natal sample. Although unexplained, this rise in protein C activity is consistent with a rise in protein C antigen levels previously reported in post partum patients and, like the increase in factor VIIC, is related to changes in plasma lipid levels (Table 3.2).

A fall not only in free protein S antigen, but also in the total protein S antigen was noted. Although total protein S antigen levels had begun to rise again slightly towards the baseline by 3 days post partum, the free protein S antigen levels remained reduced at this stage. Wide variation in both total and free protein S antigen levels throughout pregnancy results in an extremely wide reference range for both total and free antigen.

Table 3.2 Mean values, 95% ranges and % changes for natural anticoagulants and APC resistance (APC:SR) tests in normal pregnancy

	6–11 weeks (n = 41)		36–40 weeks (n = 23)			3 days post partum (n = 87)		
	Mean	(Range)	Mean	(Range)	% change*	Mean	(Range)	% change*
AT activity (IU/dl)	96	(70–122)	102	(70–133)	6%	108	(77–137)	+ 13%
PC activity (IU/dl)	95	(65–125)	94	(52–136)	– 1%	118	(78–157)	+ 24%
PS total antigen (U/dl)	80	(34–126)	58	(27–90)	– 28%	69	(37–85)	– 14%
PS antigen free (U/dl)	81	(47–115)	57	15–95	– 30%	58	(29–87)	– 27%
APC:SR	3.12	(1.94–4.30)	2.63	(1.77–3.49)	– 16%	2.76	(2.14–3.38))	– 12%
mAPC:SR**	2.39	(1.91–2.87)	2.24	(1.68–2.80)	– 6%	2.39	(1.99–2.79)	0%

*Relative to 6–11 weeks, **after predilution in factor V deficient plasma.

There are also major changes in the balance of the fibrinolytic system during pregnancy. The concentration of plasminogen increases significantly along with the antigen concentrations of the plasminogen activators, tissue plasminogen activator (t-PA) and urinary type plasminogen activator (uPA). At the same time, the concentration and activity of plasminogen activator inhibitor-1 (PAI-1) increases almost 5-fold and an additional plasminogen activator inhibitor (PAI-2), not generally detectable in the blood of non pregnant women, is produced by the placenta. The concentration of PAI-2 antigen and activity increases as gestation progresses. These two plasminogen activator inhibitors successively depress fibrinolytic activity during pregnancy although, even at term, there is some remaining fibrinolytic potential evident in some women by the presence in plasma of measurable levels of fibrin degradation products (D-dimers). Following placental separation, maternal plasma fibrinolytic activity increases rapidly.

INHERITED COAGULATION DISORDERS

Haemophilias

Although families with an apparently increased tendency to bleed have been recognised for many centuries, modern knowledge of inherited bleeding disorders dates only from early in the 19th Century when the term 'haemophilia' was coined. For the past 50 years or so, it has been realised that haemophilia is not a single entity. The most common type, haemophilia A, is due to deficiency of clotting factor VIII and the second most frequent variety, haemophilia B, is due to deficiency of clotting factor IX.

The prevalence of haemophilia has been reported to be 13 18 per 100 000 males (Rosendaal et al 1991), the ratio between haemophilia A and haemophilia B being of the order of 4:1. Both the gene for factor VIII and the gene for factor IX are located on the long arm of the X-chromosome. The gene for factor VIII is one of the largest known human genes.

Female carriers of these X-linked recessive disorders usually inherit their abnormal gene from one or other parent – a haemophilic father or a mother who is herself a carrier. Since they have a second normal gene the majority of female carriers of haemophilia do not have significant bleeding problems and, indeed, many will remain undetected unless specifically sought. Troublesome bleeding may, however, occur in the minority of carriers in whom clotting factor activity is less than 40 IU/dl, particularly if the level is very low (5–10 IU/dl). Matings between affected males and carrier females are very unusual. Thus homozygosity or compound heterozygosity for factor VIII or factor IX deficiency is distinctly rare. However, unexpectedly low clotting factor activity may be the result of extreme Lyonization or of the co-inheritance of a variant von Willebrand factor allele or, very rarely, of the co-inheritance of another chromosomal abnormality which affects the X-chromosome such as Turner's syndrome.

von Willebrand's disease

von Willebrand's disease is the most common clinically significant heritable abnormality of coagulation which affects women. The prevalence of von

Table 3.3 Simplified classification of von Willebrand's disease

Type	Bleeding time	FVIIIC	vWf antigen	RiCof activity	Multimers
I	N or P	R	R	R	All present
IIA	P	N or R	N or R	R	Large + intermediate absent
IIB	P	N or R	N or R	R	Large absent
III	P	R or ND	R or ND	ND	ND

N = normal; P = prolonged; R = reduced; ND = not detectable.

Willebrand's disease in the general population has been put as high as 1 in 100 (Rodeghierio et al 1987). von Willebrand factor synthesis is controlled by a gene situated on the short arm of chromosome 12. von Willebrand's disease is, therefore, autosomally inherited and both dominant and recessive forms are described. von Willebrand factor is essential for normal platelet function and patients with von Willebrand's disease frequently, although not invariably, have a prolonged bleeding time. Since von Willebrand factor acts as the 'carrier' for clotting factor VIII in the circulation, patients with von Willebrand's disease frequently have reduced plasma factor VIIIC activity and may have a prolonged activated partial thromboplastin time. von Willebrand's disease is classified into three major types (Table 3.3).

In approximately 70–75% of patients with von Willebrand's disease, the full range of von Willebrand factor multimers, including the highest molecular weight forms, remain detectable in the patient's plasma but are present at reduced concentrations. Type I von Willebrand's disease is usually dominant but, in some patients, the inheritance is autosomal recessive and the heterozygotes are asymptomatic. Non pregnant patients with type I von Willebrand's disease usually have levels of von Willebrand factor antigen of between 10 and 40 U/dl – equivalent to that of the factor VIIIC activity in their plasma and roughly equivalent to their plasma von Willebrand factor ristocetin cofactor activity. In general, patients with type I von Willebrand's disease respond to injection of desamino-8-D-arginine vasopressin (DDAVP) with a rise in the plasma concentration of all von Willebrand factor multimers and a resultant shortening of their bleeding time. In general, patients with type I von Willebrand's disease have a mild bleeding tendency only.

Type II von Willebrand's disease is characterised by a loss of high molecular weight (HMW) von Willebrand factor multimers. In these patients, the von Willebrand factor is qualitatively impaired and the bleeding time is usually prolonged. The von Willebrand ristocetin cofactor activity is usually significantly lower than the von Willebrand factor antigen level. Factor VIIIC activity is equal to or may be greater than the von Willebrand factor antigen level and even in non pregnant patients the factor VIIIC and von Willebrand factor antigen levels may be within the normal ranges or only slightly reduced.

A number of sub types of type II von Willebrand's disease are well recognised. In type IIA HMW forms of von Willebrand factor are lost and the patient's plasma contains predominantly low molecular weight multimers. Treatment of these patients with DDAVP results in an increase in the smaller multimers, but not in the larger ones and, thus, the bleeding time is not usually corrected completely. In type IIB von Willebrand's disease, there is again a loss of the large multimers, but in these patients intermediate and small forms are present and there is increased interaction between their platelets and von Willebrand factor in the presence of ristocetin – the abnormal von Willebrand factor appearing to have increased reactivity with platelet glycoprotein 1b (GP1b). Patients with type IIB von Willebrand's disease frequently have mild or moderate thrombocytopenia. If these patients are given DDAVP, large multimers of von Willebrand factor may appear transiently in their plasma, but the bleeding time is not corrected fully and the platelet count may drop further. Infusion of DDAVP should therefore be avoided in patients with type IIB von Willebrand's disease. A number of other sub variants of type II von Willebrand's disease are recognised. In the majority of the sub variants of type II von Willebrand's disease the inheritance is dominant. However autosomal recessive type IIA and type IIB von Willebrand's disease have been described. Bleeding in type II von Willebrand's disease (particularly type IIA von Willebrand's disease) tends to be more severe and the episodes occur more frequently than in patients with type I von Willebrand's disease.

Type III von Willebrand's disease is clinically the most severe. These patients have very low levels of factor VIIIC (1–10 IU/dl) and undetectable or very low levels (< 5 U/dl) of von Willebrand factor antigen. No multimers can be demonstrated in their plasma. Treatment with DDAVP has no effect in this type of von Willebrand's disease where patients have haemophilia like symptoms, such as joint bleeds, in addition to mucosal bleeding. It is likely that the majority of type III von Willebrand's disease patients are homozygotes of recessively inherited von Willebrand's disease but some may be compound heterozygotes. The prevalence of type III von Willebrand's disease is low in the UK (approximately 1 in 10^6) but is higher in cultures where consanguinity is common. Usually the parents are clinically unaffected and have von Willebrand factor levels at or just below the lower limits of normality. Obviously it is essential to investigate the parents of any child found to have type III von Willebrand's disease so that they may be counselled with respect to the management of future pregnancies and the availability of prenatal diagnosis.

Like women who have no evidence of heritable bleeding problems, haemophilia carriers and the majority of women with von Willebrand's disease show a rise in the components of factor VIII complex during pregnancy. In general, haemophilia A carriers and patients with type I von Willebrand's disease do not bleed excessively during pregnancy. On the other hand, type II and type III von Willebrand's disease patients do have an increased tendency to bleed particularly post partum. In type IIA von Willebrand's disease not all patients show a significant increase in the HMW multimers of von Willebrand factor antigen during pregnancy and type IIB von Willebrand's disease patients may develop worsening thrombocytopenia during their pregnancy. Type III von Willebrand's disease patients show little or no increase in the factor VIII complex levels and remain at significant risk of bleeding antepartum, during delivery and post partum.

The vitamin K dependent coagulation factors have many properties in common, but they do not all behave similarly during pregnancy and although factors VIIC and XC show moderate increases, the levels of prothrombin and factor IXC remain unchanged or rise very slightly only. Carriers of haemophilia B may, therefore, have factor IXC levels which remain substantially beneath normal even at term (Greer et al 1991, Clark et al 1997).

Other inherited coagulation defects

A wide variety of other inherited defects of clotting factors has been described. In general, these are uncommon, but recently attention has been drawn to the problems which women with FXI deficiency may encounter in association with pregnancy. Factor XI deficiency is an autosomal disorder most prevalent amongst Ashkenazi Jews but also found in other families of European extraction. Bleeding is most frequent amongst individuals with significantly reduced factor XIC activity but the likelihood of bleeding cannot be predicted totally based on factor XIC levels and in particular women with XIC levels of around 50% of normal have reported troublesome menorrhagia or have presented with post partum bleeds.

All families with heritable bleeding disorders – whether they are due to specific clotting factor defects or due to inherited platelet abnormalities should be registered with a Haemophilia Centre.

Counselling and family planning

Historically, the clientele of Haemophilia Units was predominantly male but nowadays Comprehensive Care Haemophilia Centres see the counselling and care of the female carriers of the X-linked haemophilias and women with autosomally transmitted bleeding disorders including von Willebrand's disease, factor XI deficiency and the rarer inherited deficiencies of other clotting factors, as an integral part of their service. It is essential that families with heritable bleeding problems understand the genetics of their disorder and have easy and open access to informed advice and counselling, including advice on contraception and family planning.

Males with haemophilia A or B do not transmit their disorder to their sons, but all of their daughters are obligate carriers. Statistically, 50% of the male children of female carriers of haemophilia will have haemophilia and a similar percentage (50%) of the daughters of female haemophilia carriers will themselves carry the abnormal haemophilia gene. Because von Willebrand's disease is autosomally transmitted both males and females are affected and 50% of the offspring of an affected man or woman will themselves be affected. Many of the rarer inherited clotting factor deficiencies are also autosomally transmitted and either parent may transmit a defective gene to children of either sex.

Haemophilia Centres actively seek to educate families and to promote the importance of carrier testing. Ideally this testing should be performed just ahead of puberty when the girl is old enough to understand the implications but before she is sexually active and certainly before her first pregnancy. This requires that the parents of possible carrier females should themselves be counselled and advised about the requirement to encourage their daughters to present for early investigation. In the past families with haemophilia have felt stigmatised and undoubtedly in some families negative attitudes still prevail, particularly amongst older women. As a result, many young female relatives of haemophiliacs present only when they have already committed themselves and are already pregnant or in a relationship that is likely to lead to pregnancy. Advances in molecular haematology have made possible accurate DNA based carrier diagnosis particularly for haemophilia B, but also in many families with haemophilia A. As a result, carrier detection can in some women be done during pregnancy. This, however, is not ideal and should be avoided if possible. It must remain a priority to encourage potential carriers to present for testing well ahead of the time at which they first become pregnant.

In general, von Willebrand's disease is a milder disorder than haemophilia and thus counselling of affected women is less stressful. Nonetheless, family planning advice and genetic counselling are important for couples in which either partner is affected with a heritable coagulation disorder. Counselling may allay fears about the risks to affected women during pregnancy and delivery and fears that their offspring might have a more serious bleeding disorder.

Haemophilia Centres should encourage female carriers of haemophilia and women with von Willebrand's disease or other autosomally transmitted bleeding disorder to attend for regular review even if they are asymptomatic. These review visits allow informal counselling and can be used to promote positive attitudes to carrier testing, family planning and prenatal diagnosis.

Prenatal diagnosis

With the availability of fetal genotype analysis by mutation detection or by linked polymorphism, chorionic villus sampling (CVS) has become the main method of prenatal diagnosis and diagnosis of clotting factor deficiency in fetal blood obtained by cordocentesis is used only in circumstances where mother's DNA analysis is non informative or there is inadequate information about the family. Accurate prenatal diagnosis increases the available options for carrier women and is important in the management of pregnancy. However, the uptake of prenatal diagnosis remains relatively low. In a recently reported study haemophilia carriers opted for prenatal diagnosis in only 17 of 48 (35%) pregnancies (Kadir et al 1997). These findings are in keeping with a previously published survey of attitudes towards prenatal diagnosis amongst 549 non pregnant potential and obligate carriers of haemophilia (Varecamp et al 1990) where almost all considered carrier testing to be of value but only 31% of the study group favoured prenatal diagnosis with the implication of possible pregnancy termination if the fetus was affected. In those women who said they would not favour prenatal diagnosis the main reason offered was that they did not consider haemophilia to be a disorder serious enough to justify termination of pregnancy. Careful counselling on the availability, benefits and risks of prenatal diagnostic testing should be offered to couples before they embark on a first pregnancy.

Preconception counselling

Prior to starting their family, individuals affected by or carrying heritable bleeding disorders should have the opportunity to discuss again with their haematologist, and if possible also an obstetrician, the options for prenatal diagnosis and other aspects of the management of pregnancy. This is obviously most important and most easily achieved where the patient is an affected or carrier female, but couples where the potential father has a heritable bleeding disorder should also be offered pre-pregnancy counselling.

Women who may require blood product therapy and who are not already immune should be immunised against hepatitis B. If possible immunisation should be completed prior to conceiving but if the patient is already pregnant, although it is not ideal, immunisation against hepatitis B is safe during pregnancy. Because of reports of outbreaks of hepatitis A in some haemophiliacs, immunisation against hepatitis A is also currently offered to non immune patients who might require blood products. If not already documented, the possibility of confirming a woman's carrier status by genetic testing with DNA probes should be reviewed.

Management during pregnancy

Pregnancy should be managed by an obstetric team experienced in the management of families with heritable bleeding disorders and in close liaison with the local Haemophilia Centre. Maternal coagulation factor activity and, if appropriate, the levels of von Willebrand factor antigen and activity should be checked at booking. Clotting factor activity and the levels of von Willebrand factor do not show a significant increase until the second trimester and, in the case of factor IX, may show no significant rise. Invasive procedures during pregnancy which might result in maternal, fetal or placental bleeding must, therefore, be considered carefully and on an individual basis. Patients and their partners should understand that even CVS for prenatal diagnosis may result in bleeding and CVS should be performed only after full discussion not only of the perceived benefits but also of the risks.

Both polymerase chain reaction (PCR) and fluorescent *in situ* hybridisation (FISH) have been used to sex human pre-implantation embryos, resulting from in vitro fertilisation, for X-linked disorders. The use of FISH to identify and transfer only female embryos in a haemophilia carrier has been reported.

In carriers or potential carriers of haemophilia where prenatal diagnostic tests have not been performed (and this remains the majority), fetal gender can be assessed by ultrasound visualisation of the fetal external genitalia from about 18–20 weeks (Plattner et al 1983) and with advances in transvaginal sonography fetal gender can be determined as early as the first trimester (Bornshtein et al 1990). If, due to fetal position, visualisation of the genital area is difficult ultrasound examination should be repeated.

Maternal coagulation factor activity and, if appropriate, von Willebrand factor levels should be rechecked at 28 weeks gestation and again at 34 weeks gestation. Surgery, invasive procedures, miscarriage or other accidental bleeding must precipitate immediate re-assessment of the patient's coagulation factor activity and, if appropriate, von Willebrand factor levels.

Management of delivery

Monitoring of coagulation factor and, if necessary, von Willebrand factor levels in the third trimester allows opportunities for re-evaluation of the management of delivery. For some women, a planned delivery may be advisable if there is any concern that the levels of clotting factor or von Willebrand factor may be inadequate for haemostasis. In the absence of obstetric contra-indication, vaginal delivery at term is usually preferred (Ljung et al 1994) but for all women with heritable bleeding disorders early recourse to caesarean section should be considered if labour fails to progress steadily. In particular, early recourse to caesarean section is recommended for carriers of haemophilia with a known affected male fetus or where there is a lack of information that the fetus is either female or an unaffected male.

Labour and delivery are critical periods for the fetus. Those with inherited bleeding disorders may suffer serious scalp haemorrhage, including scalp abrasions and cephalhaematoma from the birth process itself, instrumental delivery or invasive monitoring techniques. The incidence of intracranial haemorrhage in haemophilic newborn infants has been reported to be between 1 and 4% (Eyster et al 1978, Bray & Luban 1989). Since fetal scalp electrodes and scalp vein sampling can cause massive haematomas, it would seem prudent to avoid them if the fetus may have von Willebrand's disease or one of the rarer autosomally transmissible coagulation defects or in haemophilia carriers where the fetus is known to be male (unless he is known to be unaffected) or its sex is unknown. Likewise, ventouse extraction should be avoided in a potentially affected fetus. Ventouse has been shown to constitute a significant risk factor – in one study 10 of 12 infants with sub galeal and cephalhaematoma were delivered by vacuum extraction (Ljung et al 1994). Although ventouse extraction should be avoided, low forceps delivery may be considered less traumatic than caesarean section when the head is deeply engaged in the pelvis and delivery can be achieved as an easy outlet procedure providing it is performed by an experienced obstetrician. Mid cavity forceps and forceps involving rotation of the head should be avoided if possible.

Analgesia

Because it is important to avoid intramuscular injections in patients with defective haemostasis, analgesia to cover delivery has to be given subcutaneously or intravenously. There is a lack of consensus on the safety of epidural anaesthesia to cover delivery in patients with heritable bleeding disorders or carriers of haemophilia. It has, however, been suggested that providing the coagulation screen is normal, the Simplate bleeding time less than 10 min and the platelet count greater than $100 \times 10^9/l$, there should normally be no contra-indication to inserting an epidural catheter (Letsky 1991). In a recent report, the Haemophilia Centre at the Royal Free Hospital, London, indicated that it is their policy to use a regional block providing coagulation factor levels are greater than 50 IU/dl (Kadir et al 1997). Before the catheter is withdrawn, a repeat coagulation screen would seem prudent. In cases of elective surgery, spinal anaesthesia may be a safer option (Milaskiewicz et al 1990).

Factor replacement

Pregnancy induces a rise in factor VIIIC levels in normal women, in carriers of haemophilia A and in women with type I von Willebrand's disease. Practically, it is useful to recheck coagulation factor activity at around 34 weeks gestation in haemophilia carriers and in women with von Willebrand's disease or other inherited bleeding disorders to allow planning for delivery. During labour, the maternal coagulation screen and appropriate factor assays should be rechecked if possible. Women with factor VIIIC levels (or activity levels of other appropriate clotting factors) of less than 50 IU/dl should have an intravenous line inserted.

In haemophilia A carriers, providing the factor VIIIC activity exceeds 40 IU/dl, excessive bleeding during uncomplicated vaginal delivery is unusual and factor replacement therapy is seldom required. However, the rise is factor VIIIC in haemophilia A carriers is variable and not all patients raise their factor VIIIC levels even to 40 IU/dl (Greer et al 1991). If caesarean section is planned or an operative or instrumental delivery become necessary, factor VIIIC activity should be in excess of 50 IU/dl. In some women this may require infusion of a factor VIII concentrate. Plasma derived concentrates of factor VIII carry a small risk of transmitting parvo virus B19 (Sanagostino et al 1994). Parvo virus B19 may cause severe fetal infection and hydrops. Therefore, recombinant factor VIII rather than plasma derived factor VIII should be used during pregnancy.

Factor IXC activity shows little change during pregnancy and female carriers of haemophilia B not infrequently reach term with factor IXC levels inadequate for haemostasis during delivery. As with carriers of haemophilia A, carriers of haemophilia B should be reviewed at 28 weeks and at 34 weeks gestation to allow their factor IXC levels to be checked and, on admission in labour, factor IXC levels should be rechecked if possible. Women with factor IXC levels of less than 50 IU/dl should have an intravenous line established. For vaginal delivery, factor IXC activity should be raised to 40 IU/dl and for caesarean section or instrumental delivery to 50 IU/dl. Recombinant factor IX has recently been licensed in the UK and wherever possible should be used. If recombinant factor IX is not available, a high purity plasma derived factor IX concentrate should be used and factor IX concentrates containing factors II, VII and X avoided as they are potentially thrombogenic.

Frequently women with type IIA or type III von Willebrand's disease and occasionally those with type IIB von Willebrand's disease require factor replacement to raise their factor VIIIC and von Willebrand factor complex levels for delivery. As with carriers of haemophilia, it is important to review women with von Willebrand's disease in the third trimester, around 34 weeks, to allow planning of delivery. Factor VIIIC and von Willebrand factor activity levels in excess of 40 IU/dl are required for vaginal delivery and levels of above 50 IU/dl for caesarean section or instrumental delivery. Where women have lower levels, prophylactic infusion of a factor VIII concentrate containing significant amounts of larger von Willebrand factor multimers should be commenced at the onset of labour.

Factor XI concentrate is available and may be used if necessary to cover delivery in women with factor XI deficiency. However, if no concentrate is available for women with rarer defects, fresh frozen plasma may have to be used. It is essential that management of pregnancy and delivery of all women with heritable bleeding problems is carried out with close and effective liaison between the obstetric team and a Haemophilia Centre.

DDAVP infusion

DDAVP is a synthetic analogue of antidiuretic hormone. Administration results in an increase in factor VIIIC and von Willebrand factor in carriers of haemophilia A and in some patients with type I or type IIA von Willebrand's disease. In non pregnant patients, DDAVP is frequently used to cover dental work or minor surgery, but there have been no controlled studies of its use during pregnancy and its safety and efficacy in obstetrics have not been confirmed. For this reason, some haematologists and obstetricians prefer to avoid DDAVP during ongoing pregnancy. It has, however, been shown to be useful immediately prior to or after delivery or following abortion or termination where a moderate rise in factor VIIIC and von Willebrand factor complex is required. Care must be taken since DDAVP has been shown to cause water retention and hyponatraemia following surgery (Lowe et al 1977) and maternal water retention provoking a grand mal seizure has been reported with repeated therapy (Chediak et al 1986). If DDAVP is used, blood urea and electrolytes should be monitored and excessive fluid input (e.g. dextrose infusions) avoided.

DDAVP should be avoided in patients with type IIB von Willebrand's disease because of the risk of causing platelet aggregation and thrombocytopenia due to binding of abnormal intermediate sized von Willebrand factor multimers to the platelets.

The response to DDAVP is greater in normal pregnant women than in normal non pregnant women (4-fold versus 2-fold). DDAVP has no significant effect on factor IXC levels.

Post partum management

With careful management, excessive bleeding during delivery is relatively uncommon in most carriers of haemophilia and in women with the common type I von Willebrand's disease and the type IIA variant, but women with inherited bleeding disorders are at risk of post partum haemorrhage. Greer et al (1991) reported 5 post partum haemorrhages and one large perineal haematoma in 43 pregnancies in haemophilia carriers – similar to the incidence of primary and secondary post partum haemorrhage reported by Kadir et al 1997 – respectively, 22% and 11%. The patients who are at greatest risk are those who have clotting factor activity levels of less than 50 IU/dl and those who have variant (non type I) forms of von Willebrand's disease. It has been suggested that the increased risk of bleeding after delivery in these women is due to rapidly falling levels of clotting factors and von Willebrand factor after delivery. In type IIA von Willebrand's disease, although the levels of factor VIIIC and von Willebrand factor antigen may rise during pregnancy, the large multimers of von Willebrand factor antigen do not appear in the blood and von Willebrand factor activity therefore remains low. It is important that patients with variant (non type I) von Willebrand's disease are assessed not only with respect to their factor VIIIC activity but also in terms of their plasma von Willebrand factor activity and if factor replacement is required they are given products which contain the larger von Willebrand factor multimers. To minimise the risk of bleeding in these patients both factor VIIIC and von Willebrand factor activity have to be raised above 40–50 U/dl.

In all patients with heritable bleeding disorders it is important to ensure that clotting factor activity and von Willebrand factor activity is maintained above 40–50 U/dl for at least 4–5 days after delivery to minimise the risk of post partum haemorrhage.

Care of the neonate

A blood sample should be collected from the neonate at delivery but, because some haemostatic factors are physiologically relatively reduced in neonates, it may be difficult to exclude some disorders including mild to moderate haemophilia B or von Willebrand's disease at birth and repeat examination 3–6 months later may be necessary. Intramuscular injections must be avoided in neonates of either sex with proven or possible heritable bleeding disorders including von Willebrand's disease and in male children of haemophilia carriers (unless the baby is known to be unaffected). Prophylactic vitamin K_1 should be given orally to these children and their General Practitioner informed and asked to ensure that routine immunisations are given either subcutaneously or intradermally. Immunisation against hepatitis B should be considered. The parents of affected babies should be given follow-up counselling and the babies themselves should be registered with and reviewed regularly at a Haemophilia Centre.

Other pregnancy complications

It is difficult to obtain information about the risk of miscarriage in women with heritable bleeding disorders. An international registry established to report on reproductive health in women with variant von Willebrand's disease recorded 15 of 69 pregnancies (22%) in women with type II and type III von Willebrand's disease and in variant type I von Willebrand's disease unresponsive to DDAVP ended in spontaneous abortion (Foster 1995). The authors of this survey record that, on reviewing the literature, they found reports of 71 pregnancies in von Willebrand's disease where the fetal outcome was specified – and, of the 71 pregnancies, 3 resulted in spontaneous abortion and 1 resulted in an intrauterine death suggesting a fetal loss rate of 5–6%. The author suggests that the fetal loss rate in women with all types of von Willebrand's disease is higher than the overall incidence of spontaneous abortion in the general obstetric population. Kadir et al (1997) report that of 82 pregnancies in 32 carriers of haemophilia, 22 resulted in spontaneous abortion and 10 were terminated for social reasons.

CONGENITAL THROMBOPHILIC DEFECTS

The pathogenesis of venous thromboembolism (VTE) is complex and the precise mechanisms whereby acquired risk factors, including pregnancy, interact with genetic factors remain incompletely elucidated. It is, however, becoming increasingly clear that, in general, it is the supervention of acquired thrombotic risk on an underlying genetic predisposition which precipitates clinical events and, furthermore, the genetic predisposition is most frequently not the result of a single gene defect, but more commonly a multigene disorder. Whilst great emphasis has recently been placed on the diagnosis of heritable abnormalities of haemostasis which predispose to thrombosis, practically it remains immensely important in assessing an individual patient's thrombotic risk that not only these heritable abnormalities are considered but acquired thrombotic risk factors are also recognised.

Pregnancy and venous thrombosis

It is not clear exactly how large a risk of thrombosis pregnancy and the puerperium themselves confer. In a retrospective study of 72 201 deliveries in two Glasgow hospitals between 1985 and 1996, 62 objectively proven venous thrombotic events occurred (51 deep vein thromboses + 11 pulmonary emboli). The incidence of deep vein thrombosis was 0.71 per 1000 deliveries with 0.5 per 1000 occurring in the antenatal period. The incidence of pulmonary embolism was 0.15 per 1000 deliveries with 0.07 per 1000 occurring antenatally (McColl et al 1997). Taking into account the average duration of pregnancy, the incidence of VTE antenatally is, therefore, 0.78 per 1000 pregnant women years. This is approximately ten times the reported incidence of VTE in non-pregnant non-pill using women in the UK in the same age range (Rosendaal 1997a,b). Although the actual number of venous thrombotic events occurring post partum was smaller, since the post partum period studied was considerably shorter (6 weeks), the incidence of post partum VTE of 2.5 per 1000 women years is higher than the incidence antepartum and the risk of venous thrombosis is around 3.5-fold higher after delivery than during pregnancy.

In this study, a further 49 superficial venous thrombotic events were recorded with an overall incidence of 0.68 per 1000 deliveries. Most of these superficial venous thrombotic events occurred post partum (0.54 per 1000 deliveries). If the total number of events – objectively proven venous thromboembolism plus superficial venous thrombotic events are considered together, then the overall incidence of antenatal thrombotic events was 0.97 per 1000 pregnant women years and the total number of post partum events was 7.19 per 1000 women years.

Heritable thrombophilias

Although there is no internationally agreed definition of thrombophilia, the term is generally used to describe 'familial or acquired abnormalities of haemostasis likely to predispose to thrombosis'. The heritable defects which are currently accepted as proven to be associated with familial venous thromboembolism are antithrombin deficiency, protein C deficiency, protein S deficiency, Factor V (FV) Leiden, dysfibrinogenaemia (rarely) and the recently described mutation in the prothrombin gene (factor 20210A). In addition, there are a number of thrombotic risk factors which appear to have a combined genetic and acquired origin. These include high factor VIII levels, high fibrinogen levels and hyperhomocysteinemia.

The heritable thrombophilic defects are much more prevalent than was originally recognised. Estimates for the prevalences of antithrombin, protein C

Table 3.4 Approximate prevalences of heritable thrombophilic defects in Caucasians; in the general population and in patients presenting with VTE (venous thromboembolism) – consecutive unselected patients and patients selected because they have a family history of VTE

	General population	Unselected patients with first VTE	Selected patients with familial VTE
Antithrombin deficiency	0.02%	1%	4–5%
Protein C deficiency	0.3%	3%	6–8%
Protein S deficiency	?	1%	3–6%
Factor V Leiden	3–7%	20%	50%
Prothrombin 20210A	1–2%	6%	18%

and protein S deficiency and for the FV Leiden mutation and the 20210A mutation in factor II have been derived from 3 sources – healthy individuals (including blood donor studies), unselected patients with venous thrombosis and patients who present with venous thrombotic events and who, in addition, belong to families with a familial thrombotic tendency. These prevalences are shown in Table 3.4.

Two different approaches have been used to assess the risk of venous thrombosis for individuals with heritable thrombophilic defects – family studies based on families in which the heritability of the thrombophilic defect has been shown by including only families with one or more individuals with the defect, apart from the proband, who are both symptomatic for thrombosis and have the defect and population based studies (case control) in which patients with thrombosis are compared with healthy individuals with regard to the prevalence of thrombophilic abnormalities. The results from family studies are based on families identified because they had a conspicuous frequency of thrombosis. Strictly speaking, therefore, the results of these family studies really only apply to families detected in a similar way. Population based studies, on the other hand, give estimates of relative risk and indicate how much higher the risk of thrombosis is for an individual with a particular defect compared to the risk for an individual without that defect. It is essential that extreme caution is exercised and the results of family studies are not applied to unselected individuals nor the results of population based studies used to assess risk in individuals from thrombophilic families.

Antithrombin deficiency

Antithrombin is the most important physiological inhibitor of thrombin and of the activated clotting factors of the intrinsic coagulation system. The identification of antithrombin deficient patients is relatively simple using well standardised functional assays. Two major types of heritable antithrombin deficiency are recognised. Type I defects are characterised by quantitative reduction of qualitative (functionally) normal antithrombin. Type II antithrombin deficiency is due to the production of a qualitatively abnormal protein – often due to a mutation which results in a single amino acid substitution. In type II defects, although functional antithrombin activity is reduced, the protein antigen level is higher and may even be within the normal range. The incidence of venous thromboembolism is higher in type I defects and in type II defects where the mutation affects the active serine protease inhibiting site than in type II defects which affect the heparin binding site. During uncomplicated pregnancy, antithrombin levels remain within the normal (non pregnant) range. Antithrombin deficiency appears to be clinically more severe than deficiencies of protein C or protein S with about 50% of affected patients suffering a first thrombotic event before the age of 25 years.

Protein C deficiency

Protein C circulates in the plasma as an inactive zymogen which once activated by thrombin to activated protein C (APC) with its cofactor protein S inactivates the activated clotting cascade cofactors factors Va and VIIIa. Unlike antithrombin deficiency, where the level of antithrombin activity and the site of the mutation on the antithrombin gene appear to be important in predicting the risk of thrombosis, there is no clear correlation between the level of functional protein C activity or the mutation site and the risk of venous thrombosis. Interpretation of protein C activity results is complicated by the overlap which exists between individuals with normal protein C genes and those heterozygous for protein C variants (Allaart et al 1993) Some authors have suggested that protein C antigen levels may rise towards the end of pregnancy and in the puerperium but no consistent change in protein C activity during pregnancy has been reported. Family studies have shown that family members who are protein C deficient have an 8–10-fold increased risk of venous thrombosis and approximately 50% of affected individuals in thrombophilic families will have had a venous thrombotic event by the age of 40 years (Allaart et al 1993, Bovill et al 1989). In a population based study, the relative risk of thrombosis for unselected patients with a first DVT with protein C deficiency was 6.5 – very similar to the result from family studies.

Protein S deficiency

Protein S is a necessary cofactor for the anticoagulant function of APC. Like protein C it is vitamin K dependent. In the circulation, 60% of protein S is bound to C4b binding protein (a regulatory protein of the complement pathway) and the remaining 40% is free. Only free protein S acts as a cofactor for APC in the proteolytic cleavage of factor Va and factor VIIIa. Technical problems with the detection of protein S deficiency persist and, to date, there is no clear published estimate of the prevalence of protein S deficiency in the general population. Both free and total protein S antigen levels, as well as protein S activity, are significantly reduced during pregnancy (Fernandez et al 1989, Clark et al 1997). Because of the lack of data about the prevalence of protein S deficiency, the risk of thrombosis associated with protein S defects has not been quantitated. Although there are many published reports of increased incidence of thrombosis in families with protein S deficiency, a population based case control study failed to demonstrate the relationship between protein S deficiency and venous thrombosis (Koster et al 1995a). Whilst it remains likely that, in some kindred, defects in protein S are associated with thrombotic risk, the evidence that protein S deficiency substantially increases thrombotic risk is less convincing than for protein C deficiency.

Activated protein C (APC) resistance and factor V Leiden

The term activated protein C resistance (APC) is used to describe the phenomenon whereby plasma fails to be anticoagulated by the addition of activated protein C in vitro, even in the presence of normal protein S function. Many groups have confirmed that APC resistance is a common finding in patients with venous thrombosis (Dahlback et al 1993).

Where resistance to APC is familial, the defect is associated with a mutation in the gene for clotting factor V (1691G→A). This mutation destroys one of the APC cleavage sites in activated factor V by replacement of Arg506 by Gln(factor V R506Q) (Bertina et al 1994). This is the so-called factor V Leiden mutation. In Caucasian populations, APC resistance is much more common than any of the other heritable thrombophilic defects (prevalence 3–7%).

In family studies, the risk of venous thrombosis is clearly higher in affected (APC resistant) members than in those who are unaffected (Svensson & Dahlback 1994) and by the age of 50 years about a quarter of the affected relatives had suffered a thrombotic event. Although these family studies have suggested that the risk of thrombosis associated with the FV Leiden mutation might be lower than that associated with protein C deficiency, this may be the result of selection bias in the protein C deficient families (Lensen et al 1996). In population based case control studies, the relative risk of venous thrombosis associated with APC resistance was reported to be 7 – not significantly different from the relative risk of 6.5 associated with protein C deficiency (Koster et al 1995a).

Screening for APC resistance is most commonly performed using an APTT based test. Using this original test, 45% of pregnant women at term have an APC sensitivity ratio beneath the 95th percentile for the normal range for non pregnant women of similar age (Mathonnet et al 1996). This original unmodified test is, therefore, not a suitable screen for the FV Leiden mutation during pregnancy. A modified APC resistance test, which includes sample predilution in factor V deficient plasma, has been developed (Jorquera et al 1994, Trossaert et al 1994). Using this modified APC resistance test, the gestation dependent APC resistance observed with the original test is no longer noted (Clark et al 1997). This modified APC resistance test can, therefore, be used during pregnancy as a screening test for FV Leiden.

Until recently, the FV Leiden mutation was the only genetic defect shown to be associated with APC resistance. However, this mutation does not explain 100% of cases of familial APC resistance and the variable expression of APC resistance in FV Leiden heterozygotes has been puzzling. A specific factor V gene haplotype (HR2) has recently been shown to occur more frequently in individuals with APC resistance ratios beneath the 15th percentile than in those with higher ratios or in normal controls. Thus the factor V gene marked by the HR2 haplotype contributes to the APC resistance phenotype both in FV Leiden carriers and in non carrier patients (Bernardi et al 1997).

Prothrombin gene 20210A

Recently, a mutation in the gene for prothrombin (factor II 20210A) has been described in patients with venous thrombosis (Poort et al 1996). This polymorphism is closely related to plasma prothrombin levels which are, in turn, associated with thrombotic risk. The relative risk of thrombosis associated with this mutation has been estimated to be between 3 and 6 – similar to or less than those associated with protein C deficiency and the FV Leiden mutation.

Heritable thrombophilia is a multigene defect

Originally, it was believed that familial thrombosis was an autosomal dominant trait caused by a dominant gene defect with a reduced penetrance for the disease. This view of familial thrombophilia as a monogenic disorder has, however, been increasingly challenged over the past 10 years, until now the general view is that familial thrombophilia is a multiple gene disorder. The practical result of this changing view of heritable thrombophilia has been the requirement to try to identify subjects who have the highest risk of developing thrombosis – those carrying multiple defects – and to question previous guidelines on the investigation and management of patients with these thrombophilic defects, not least the management of patients with thrombophilic defects during pregnancy. It is essential that, when an individual with a heritable thrombophilic defect is identified, they are fully investigated and assessed for other genetic and acquired thrombotic risk factors.

Complex thrombophilic defects

Already it has become clear that in symptomatic families more than a single genetic abnormality may be found – combined defects are frequently reported including combinations of FV Leiden with antithrombin deficiency, protein C deficiency or protein S deficiency.

Factor VIIIC activity

Elevated factor VIIIC levels (in excess of 150 IU/dl) are associated with a 6-fold increased risk of venous thrombosis compared to factor VIIIC levels below 100 IU/dl (Koster et al 1995b). Increased factor VIIIC are, in part, genetic and, in part, acquired. At term and in the early puerperium, factor VIIIC levels are generally above 150 IU/dl – but some women have levels well in excess of this.

Hyperhomocysteinemia

Two case control studies have demonstrated a 2.5-fold increased risk for venous thrombosis in individuals with homocysteine levels exceeding 18.5 µmol/l and a 3–4-fold increased risk associated with levels exceeding 20 µmol/l (Den Heijer et al 1996, Simioni et al 1996). Hyperhomocysteinemia is a complex abnormality frequently resulting from an interplay of acquired and genetic defects. Classic homocysteinuria due to heterozygosity for cystathionine beta synthase is uncommon (Mudd et al 1985) but the recently described methylene-tetrahydrofolate-reductase (MTHFR) variant which leads to mildly increased levels of homocysteine is common (Kluijtmans et al 1996). Environmental causes of hyperhomocysteinaemia include reduced vitamin B6, vitamin B12 or folic acid levels (Ubbink et al 1993). The mechanism of the relationship between hyperhomocysteinemia and venous thrombosis is not clarified but it has been suggested that the elevated homocysteine levels which result from carriership of the MTHFR thermolabile variant are not sufficient in themselves to cause thrombosis (Rosendaal 1997a). In the meantime, hyperhomocysteinemia cannot be disregarded in the aetiology of venous thrombosis since it would appear that 5–10% of Europeans have homocysteine levels over 18.5 μmol/l (Den Heijer et al 1996, Simioni et al 1996).

Heritable thrombophilic defects and antiphospholipid antibodies

Antiphospholipid antibodies are a common cause of thrombosis and may be found in combination with heritable thrombophilic defects – in particular (because of its high prevalence) with FV Leiden. The simultaneous presence of antiphospholipid antibodies and a heritable thrombophilic defect may lead to a severe thrombotic tendency. It has been suggested that there may be a synergistic effect between the presence of anticardiolipin antibodies or lupus anticoagulant and the FV Leiden mutation (Bokarewa et al 1995).

Heritable thrombophilic defects, pregnancy and thrombotic risk

Early estimates suggested that, in the absence of anticoagulant prophylaxis, the incidence of pregnancy related thrombosis in antithrombin deficient women may exceed 60% (Conard et al 1987, Hellgren et al 1992). In 1990, Conard et al revised their previously published estimates and reported that the overall incidence of thrombosis associated with pregnancy in antithrombin deficient women was around 44% – the incidence of events occurring during pregnancy being 18% and not significantly more than the incidence (33%) in the puerperium. Roughly similar estimates of the overall incidence of pregnancy associated VTE in antithrombin deficient women have been reported by other groups – 37% of pregnancies in an Italian study (De Stefano et al 1994), 32.3% in a study in the UK (Hough et al 1996) and 40% in a study reporting patients in Austria, Germany and Switzerland (Pabinger et al 1996). It must be emphasised that all of these studies were retrospective and each of them is subject to bias since the patients selected came from symptomatic kindred. Nonetheless, it has to be accepted that for this particular patient group – women with antithrombin deficiency belonging to symptomatic families – the risk of thrombosis complicating pregnancy is high.

The incidence of pregnancy associated thrombosis in women with protein C or protein S deficiency appears to be considerably lower than that for antithrombin deficient women. In 1990, Conard et al reported that the incidence of thrombosis occurring antenatally in protein C and protein S deficient women (respectively, 7% and 0%) is significantly less than the incidence of post partum thrombotic events – 19% in protein C deficient and 17% in protein S deficient women. Other workers have confirmed the lower incidence of pregnancy associated thrombosis in protein C and protein S deficiency (De Stefano et al 1994, Hough et al 1996, Pabinger et al 1996) and Pabinger et al confirmed that the risk of thrombosis in protein S deficient females is higher post partum than during pregnancy. As in the studies of antithrombin deficient women, these studies of protein C and protein S

Inherited bleeding and thrombotic disorders

deficient women were all retrospective and subject to bias because the women included came from symptomatic kindred.

In a recently published paper, Friedreich et al 1996 report that the incidence of venous thrombosis in the affected female members of 69 symptomatic families with antithrombin, protein C or protein S deficiency, after exclusion of the probands, was overall 4.1%. Although this study demonstrates that women with heritable thrombophilic defects are at substantially increased risk of pregnancy associated thrombosis, this risk estimate is significantly less than previous estimates. One event occurred in 33 pregnancies in antithrombin deficient women (3%) – during the third trimester. One occurred in 60 pregnancies in protein C deficient women (1.7%) – this also occurred during the third trimester. Five events were recorded in 76 pregnancies in the protein S deficient group (6.6%) – only 2 of these events, however, were objectively diagnosed (2.9%). All 5 of the events recorded in the protein S deficient group occurred in the puerperium.

Our own group initially suggested that familial APC resistance may be associated with thrombosis in pregnancy (Cook et al 1994). Shortly thereafter, a study from Sweden reported that 60% of women who had had pregnancy associated venous thrombosis had evidence of APC resistance (Hellgren et al 1995). This very high prevalence of APC resistance in Swedish women who have had thrombosis associated with pregnancy was confirmed in a study which demonstrated that 46% of 70 women with a history of pregnancy associated thrombosis had the FV Leiden mutation (Bokarewa et al 1996).

However, in a study of 43 women with the FV Leiden mutation from symptomatic families, the overall incidence of thrombosis during pregnancy and the puerperium was reported as 14% which is similar to that in protein C or protein S deficient women (Hough et al 1996) and in our own group's investigation of 50 unselected women with objectively proven pregnancy associated venous thrombosis only 4 (8%) were found to have the FV Leiden mutation (McColl et al 1997).

Heritable thrombophilia, fetal loss and other pregnancy complications

It has been demonstrated that there is an increased risk of fetal loss in women with deficiencies of antithrombin, protein C or protein S. The risk appears to be greatest for women with antithrombin deficiency and in women who have more than one identifiable thrombophilic abnormality (Preston et al 1996). There was no apparent increase in the overall risk of fetal loss for women with FV Leiden in this study but, in agreement with other workers who have reported an increased risk of late pregnancy loss in women with APC resistance (Rai et al 1996), a trend towards increased risk of third trimester loss was noted.

Several studies have suggested that women with APC resistance are at increased risk of pregnancy associated hypertension and pre-eclampsia (Lindoff et al 1997).

Assessment of thrombotic risk

It cannot be stressed too strongly that in assessing the thrombotic risk associated with pregnancy, acquired risk factors, as well as genetic predisposition, must be taken into account. Patient age, parity and weight have each been shown to be associated with pregnancy and puerperal venous thrombotic risk. As in non pregnant patients, immobilisation and serious medical disorders increase thrombotic risk and in the post partum period the risk of venous thrombosis is increased in women who have had caesarean section (particularly emergency caesarean section) or a difficult instrumental delivery. In the study reported by McColl et al (1997), acquired thrombotic risk factors were shown to be important both in women who had no evidence of heritable thrombophilic defect and in those who had evidence of congenital thrombophilia.

Screening for congenital thrombophilia

At present it would seem prudent to include the following tests in a screen for heritable thrombophilic defects – antithrombin activity, protein C activity, protein S antigen (total and free), screen for FV Leiden and testing for the prothrombin 20210A variant. As already mentioned, if FV Leiden mutation detection is not available then, during pregnancy and the puerperium, a modified APC resistance test must be used since the original APC resistance test is affected by the increasing factor VIIIC levels during pregnancy. In addition, it is advised that a coagulation screen, including an activated partial thromboplastin time, prothrombin time and thrombin clotting time (to detect dysfibrinogenaemia) is included and lupus anticoagulant screening and assays for IgG and IgM anticardiolipin performed. Full assessment of an individual patient's thrombotic risk must also take into account factor VIIIC and fibrinogen activities (Table 3.5). Most laboratories currently do not include homocysteine assays as part of their routine because these assays are technically difficult.

Inevitably, with the developing interest in the potential role of genetic thrombophilic defects in venous thrombosis and other complications of pregnancy, obstetricians and haematologists have come under pressure to screen increasing numbers of women for these abnormalities. It must be re-emphasised, however, that familial thrombosis is a multigene defect and that the studies published on the risk of pregnancy complication in women with heritable thrombophilia are all retrospective and report on the risk of problems in women from symptomatic families. There are no large prospective studies of pregnancy complication and outcome in women with abnormalities in their antithrombin or protein C-protein S systems or studies of women from asymptomatic kindred. Random screening would identify large numbers of women with laboratory evidence of thrombophilic defects – the vast majority of whom would have a single gene defect and would belong to asymptomatic families. Apart from being an extremely costly exercise this would result in many worried patients whose obstetricians and haematologists were unable to advise on their management on any rational basis. Thus it would seem advisable that, at present, screening for heritable thrombophilic defects should be limited to women who give a personal or family history of venous thromboembolism and, in addition, to consider screening women who have a history of pregnancy associated hypertension, pre-eclampsia, intrauterine growth retardation or recurrent fetal loss.

Table 3.5 Venous thromboembolism (VTE) risk assessment for women with a family history of VTE or a personal history of previous VTE or vascular complications of pregnancy

---

Clinical evaluation
- ❏   Personal or family history of VTE
- ❏   Age, parity, weight
- ❏   General medical examination
- ❏   Method of delivery

Routine laboratory tests
- ❏   Full blood and platelet count
- ❏   Coagulation screen – APTT, PT, TCT
- ❏   Fibrinogen assay

Inherited thrombophilia screen
- ❏   Antithrombin activity
- ❏   Protein C activity
- ❏   Protein S antigen – total and free
- ❏   Factor V Leiden screen
- ❏   Prothrombin 20210 G→A

Acquired thrombophilia laboratory tests
- ❏   Lupus anticoagulant screen
- ❏   IgG and IgM anticardiolipin assays
- ❏   Factor VIIIC assay

APTT = activated partial thromboplastin time; PT = prothrombin time; TCT = thrombin clotting time.

Preconception

It is essential that thrombophilia clinics looking after young women have close liaison with an obstetric unit with a special interest in the prevention of venous thrombosis and familiar with the management of thrombophilic women. In symptomatic families with familial thrombophilia, girls should be offered thrombophilia screening before they reach puberty to allow time to introduce discussion on contraception before they become sexually active. Affected women should be encouraged to plan their pregnancies and should be given information about the perceived risk of pregnancy associated venous thrombosis and allowed the opportunity to discuss plans for managing their future pregnancies.

It is generally accepted that it is not justifiable even in symptomatic kindred to put affected, but asymptomatic, family members onto prophylactic anticoagulants. So the majority of young women with heritable thrombophilic defects will not be using anticoagulant prophylaxis when they first become pregnant.

Women who are already symptomatic and who are on long term oral anticoagulant prophylaxis must understand the risks of fetal complications associated with maternal coumarin ingestion. It is our practice to avoid coumarins during pregnancy wherever possible and to suggest to women with heritable thrombophilia that, if anticoagulation is necessary during pregnancy, a heparin would be preferable. Those women likely to require heparin during pregnancy are counselled about the potential risk of osteopenia associated with heparin usage. All sexually active women with heritable thrombophilic defects attending our Thrombophilia Clinic are strongly encouraged to report any expected menstrual period which is overdue by 3 days or more as soon as possible. Immediate pregnancy testing is offered and, if the pregnancy test is positive, ultrasound confirmation of pregnancy is sought, if possible, by 5–6 weeks gestation. For women on long term warfarin prophylaxis who are planning a pregnancy, a number of possible approaches may be considered. For a few it may be reasonable to discontinue oral anticoagulation and institute self administered heparin once the couple have agreed that they wish a baby. This approach has the potential disadvantage of exposing a patient to several or many months of heparin therapy before pregnancy is achieved and we reserve it for use only in women who have already demonstrated the fertility of their partnerships and who are unwilling to accept the possibility of any risk to their fetuses from continuing coumarin for even a very limited time after conception. A second and more convenient approach is to continue coumarin until conception is confirmed and only then to replace the oral anticoagulant with heparin. This second approach requires the full co-operation and understanding of the patient, her thrombophilia clinic and the obstetric unit to ensure that there will be no delay in diagnosing and confirming pregnancy. With careful counselling and good liaison this approach is practicable and in the author's experience acceptable to the majority of patients.

Prenatal diagnosis

Prenatal diagnosis can only be considered appropriate in the rare cases where the fetus may be expected to be homozygous or compound heterozygous for coagulation inhibitor (antithrombin, protein C or protein S) deficiency. To date, prenatal diagnosis has been performed in a few instances only in an attempt to avoid severe thrombophilia – for example homozygous protein C deficiency (Millar et al 1994), homozygous protein S deficiency (Formstone et al 1993) or homozygous type II antithrombin deficiency (Lane et al 1996).

Management during pregnancy

Empirically, women with heritable thrombophilic defects may be considered to be at high, moderate or low thrombotic risk antenatally depending on their defect(s) and on the presence or absence of additional acquired risk factors.

Women who have already had a previous thrombotic episode and who are on long term anticoagulant prophylaxis and women who have type I antithrombin deficiency or a type II reactive site antithrombin defect, whether or not they have already had a thrombotic episode, should be considered at high risk of antenatal venous thrombosis and it is our practice to continue anticoagulation throughout pregnancy in these women changing to heparin or introducing heparin as soon as pregnancy is confirmed. Although low molecular weight heparins are still not licensed for use in pregnant women in the UK, there is increasing experience of their safety and efficacy during pregnancy and it is now our practice to use a low molecular weight heparin rather than unfractionated heparin for antenatal thromboprophylaxis. For women at high thrombotic risk we divide the total daily dose into two 12 hourly doses to give a peak anti-Xa activity of between 0.35 and 0.5 U/ml 2 h after injection. In our experience, enoxaparin 4000 IU 12 hourly or dalteparin 5000 IU 12 hourly is adequate for most patients. Plasma anti-Xa activity is rechecked approximately monthly as pregnancy progresses.

Women who have a previous history of venous thromboembolism, but who are not on long term anticoagulant prophylaxis and women who have protein C or protein S deficiency and a clear family history of venous thrombosis or who have some added acquired thrombotic risk factor (in addition to pregnancy) may be considered to be at moderately increased risk of antenatal thrombosis. These women, along with some women with FV Leiden with clear family histories of venous thrombosis are also usually offered thromboprophylaxis during pregnancy but in lower dose. In our practice, we usually use a single daily dose of a low molecular weight heparin (4000 units of enoxaparin or 5000 units of dalteparin) for women at moderate risk of antenatal thrombosis. We do not routinely monitor the response to these lower prophylactic doses.

Guidance on when prophylaxis should be commenced antenatally in this group of patients (at moderate risk) is empirical. For those who have already had a venous thrombotic event, prophylaxis is introduced roughly 4–6 weeks ahead of the gestation stage at which the previous event occurred, if that previous event occurred during an earlier pregnancy. If, on the other hand, the previous thrombotic event was not pregnancy associated, then thromboprophylaxis is usually introduced late in the second or early in the third trimester. Women considered to be at moderate risk of antenatal thrombosis but with no previous thrombotic history would also generally be offered thromboprophylaxis from late second or early third trimester. There is evidence that protein S deficiency may not significantly increase the risk of antepartum thrombosis. It may, therefore, be reasonable to delay thromboprophylaxis until late in the third trimester or until after delivery in protein S deficient women with no previous history of thrombosis providing they have no other evident thrombotic risk factors.

Currently, we consider women who have FV Leiden and no past or clear family history of venous thrombosis to be at relatively low risk of antenatal venous thrombosis (compared with women with antithrombin, protein C or protein S deficiency or who have a personal or family history of thrombosis). These women are sometimes identified effectively by chance when they are screened pre-oral contraceptive pill on poor clinical indications. At present, we do not offer these women antenatal thromboprophylaxis if they have no other evident thrombotic risk, but many of them are given anticoagulant thromboprophylaxis for 6 weeks following their delivery.

At present, we have no protocol for the management of women with the prothrombin gene mutation presenting for pregnancy management and each would be assessed and managed on an individual basis depending on their clinical history and examination and on the results of detailed thrombophilia screening looking for other inherited or acquired defects.

Management of delivery

As term approaches, heparin or a low molecular weight heparin are the only safe anticoagulants for use in women requiring antenatal prophylaxis.

Normalisation of plasma antithrombin activity levels to cover delivery may be achieved in antithrombin deficient women by infusion of antithrombin concentrates. Recommended regimens suggest raising plasma antithrombin activity to 80–120% on the day of delivery to allow heparin dose reduction or discontinuation (Walker 1991). In otherwise healthy pregnant women, infusion of 0.65–0.70 U antithrombin concentrate per kg maternal weight may be expected to raise plasma antithrombin activity by 1 IU/dl. Other workers question whether antithrombin replacement offers any advantage in preventing venous thrombosis and have advocated the use of carefully adjusted heparin only (Leclerc et al 1986).

It has been reported that pregnant women receiving subcutaneous unfractionated heparin present a management problem at term because they may be at increased risk of bleeding if a prolonged activated partial thromboplastin time persists for longer than anticipated (Anderson et al 1991). These authors recommended that subcutaneous heparin therapy should be discontinued 24 h prior to elective induction or labour or immediately spontaneous labour is confirmed. It is our policy, in general, to allow women to go into labour spontaneously if possible and to instruct them that they should discontinue their heparin immediately they are convinced that they are established in labour. These women should be delivered in hospital and their requirement for anticoagulation is re-evaluated immediately on admission.

Analgesia

As in women with heritable bleeding disorders, it is recommended that women with heritable thrombophilic defects who have been on antenatal unfractionated heparin may be considered for epidural anaesthesia providing their coagulation screen is normal, their platelet count is in excess of $100 \times 10^9/l$ and their bleeding time normal. It should be noted that low molecular weight heparins do not produce prolongation of the activated partial thromboplastin time to the same extent as unfractionated heparin. Monitoring of the effect of a low molecular weight heparin requires anti Xa assay – which in many hospitals is not routinely available 24 h per day. In practice, many anaesthetists are willing to consider epidural anaesthesia in most women providing no heparin or low molecular weight heparin has been administered within the preceding 4–6 h – and the coagulation screen is normal and the platelet count greater than $100 \times 10^9/l$.

Post partum follow-up

All women with heritable thrombophilic defects from symptomatic kindred should be offered anticoagulant prophylaxis for 3 months following their delivery whether or not they have received anticoagulant prophylaxis antenatally. Providing the patient is not bleeding excessively, unfractionated heparin or a low molecular weight heparin may be introduced or re-introduced approximately 12 h after completion of delivery. Generally, oral anticoagulants may be commenced on the first or second post partum day and heparin withdrawn when the International Normalised Ratio (INR) has been in the recommended therapeutic range for 3 days.

Any woman who suffers venous thromboembolism during pregnancy or after delivery or following abortion or pregnancy termination should be referred for thrombophilia screening. This recommendation becomes stronger if she has suffered recurrent events or if she has a family history of venous thrombosis.

Management of the newborn

Parents should understand that all of the heritable thrombophilic defects described above are transmitted autosomally and that statistically each of their children – male or female – has a 50% chance of being affected. Obviously diagnosis by DNA analysis is possible for neonates from families with FV Leiden or the prothrombin gene variant. Antithrombin deficiency is also relatively easy to diagnose in the neonate. However, protein C or protein S deficiency may pose diagnostic problems. It is unusual for healthy children to suffer venous thrombosis unless some acquired thrombotic trigger supervenes. With this reassurance many parents will accept that it may be practically easiest to delay thrombophilia screening of their child until he or she is around 10–12 years of age and can co-operate in the investigation. It must, however, be made clear to parents who accept this option that it is important that they inform any medical attendant who looks after their child during illness or injury that they may have a thrombophilic defect and suggest that if necessary at that point in time testing may become appropriate earlier than originally planned.

Management of pregnancy complications other than venous thromboembolism

In management of other pregnancy complications, early reports have suggested that there may be a place for prophylactic anticoagulation during pregnancy in women who have thrombophilic defects and have suffered recurrent fetal loss, but it is too early to report on the management of women with heritable thrombophilia and with a history of other pregnancy complications such as pre-eclampsia or intrauterine growth retardation.

Key points for clinical practice

- The management of pregnancy in women with heritable bleeding or thrombotic disorders demands a multidisciplinary approach with obstetric and haematology teams working closely together and liaising with General Practitioners, anaesthetists and neonatologists.

Inherited coagulation disorders

- Girls from families with heritable bleeding disorders should be encouraged to seek investigation around the time of puberty to allow detection of factor deficiency or carrier status before they become sexually active. Women who may be exposed to blood products should be immunised against hepatitis B.

(continued on next page)

Key points for clinical practice (continued)

- Male fetuses with haemophilia and fetuses of either sex with auto-somal bleeding disorders are at risk of severe intracranial bleeding during delivery. Prenatal diagnosis wherever feasible should, therefore, be encouraged. In families with haemophilia where prenatal diagnosis is unacceptable or not possible fetal gender determination is important.

- During pregnancy maternal clotting factor activity should be checked at booking, at 28 weeks and at 34 weeks.

- On admission in labour, the maternal clotting factor levels should be rechecked. When clotting factor activity is less than 50 IU/dl an intra-venous line should be established and prophylactic treatment given if the factor level is less 40 IU/dl and an uncomplicated delivery is anticipated or less than 50 IU/dl if an operative or instrument delivery becomes necessary.

- Invasive fetal monitoring techniques and instrumental deliveries should be avoided unless the fetus is known to be unaffected.

- Epidural anaesthesia is not contra-indicated in patients with normal coagulation screens providing their clotting factor level is greater than 50 IU/dl, their platelet count greater than $100 \times 10^9/l$ and their bleeding time normal.

- It is important that the neonate is investigated as quickly as possible after birth but until such time as they have clearly been shown to be unaffected they should be treated as being at high risk of bleeding.

Heritable thrombophilia

- The heritable defects which are at present accepted as proven to be associated with familial venous thrombosis are deficiency of anti-thrombin, protein C or protein S, the factor V Leiden mutation and the recently described mutation in the prothrombin gene. In women from symptomatic kindred, these defects appear to be associated with an increased risk of pregnancy associated venous thrombosis and possibly an increased risk of fetal loss.

- Heritable thrombophilic defects are common. There is growing evidence that congenital thrombophilia is a multigene defect and that the abnormalities so far described represent only part of the genetic thrombotic predisposition in symptomatic families. Currently, therefore, it seems reasonable to focus resources on women with heritable thrombophilic defects who are themselves already symptomatic or who come from symptomatic families.

- Pregnancies should be planned and each pregnancy in each patient managed individually.

- In general, women with antithrombin deficiency from symptomatic families require adjusted dose anticoagulant prophylaxis throughout pregnancy and for at least 3 months post partum, whereas those with protein C deficiency, protein S deficiency, factor V Leiden or the prothrombin gene mutation may require third trimester plus post partum prophylaxis or post partum anticoagulant prophylaxis only.

References

Allaart C F, Poort S R, Rosendaal F R et al 1993 Increased risk of venous thrombosis in carriers of hereditary protein C deficiency defect. Lancet 341: 134–138

Anderson D R, Ginsberg J S, Burrows R, Brill-Edwards P 1991 Subcutaneous heparin therapy during pregnancy: a need for concern at the time of delivery. Thromb Haemost 65: 248–250

Bernardi F, Faioni E M, Castoldi E et al 1997 A factor V genetic component other than the Leiden mutation is associated with APC resistance. Thromb Haemost (Suppl) 165: Abstract

Bertina R M, Koeleman B P C, Koster T et al 1994 Mutation in blood coagulation factor V association with resistance to activated protein C. Nature 369: 64–67

Bokarewa M I, Blomback M, Bremme K 1995 Phospholipid antibodies in resistance to activated protein C in women with thrombophilia. Blood Coagul Fibrinolysis 6: 417–422

Bokarewa M I, Bremme K, Blomback M 1996 Arg 506 to Gln mutation in factor V and risk of thrombosis during pregnancy. Br J Haematol 92: 473–478

Bornshtein N, Rottern S, Yoffe N, Blumenfeld Z, Brandes J M 1990 Early determination of fetal sex using transvaginal sonography: technique and pitfalls. J Clin Ultrasound 18: 302–306

Bovill E G, Bauer K A, Dickermann J D, Callas P, West B 1989 The clinical spectrum of heterozygous protein C deficiency in a large New England kindred. Blood 73: 712–717

Bray G L, Luban N L 1989 Haemophilia presenting with intracranial haemorrhage. Am J Dis Child 141: 1215–1217

Chediak J R, Albon G M, Maxey B 1986 von Willebrand's disease and pregnancy: management during delivery and outcome of offspring. Am J Obstet Gynecol 155: 618–624

Clark P, Brennand J, Conkie J A, McCall F, Greer I A, Walker I D 1997 Haemostasis in normal pregnancy. Thromb Haemost (submitted)

Conard J, Horellou M H, van Dreden P, Samama M M 1987 Pregnancy and congenital deficiency in antithrombin III or protein C. Thromb Haemost 58: 38

Conard J, Horellou M H, van Dreden P, Lecompte T, Samama M M 1990 Thrombosis and pregnancy in congenital deficiencies of antithrombin III, protein C or protein S: study of 78 women. Thromb Haemost 63: 319–320

Cook G, Walker I D, McCall F, Conkie J A, Greer I A 1994 Familial thrombophilia and activated protein C resistance: thrombotic risk in pregnancy? Br J Haematol 87: 873–875

Dahlback B, Carlsson M, Svensson P J 1993 Familial thrombophilia due to a previously unrecognised mechanism characterised by poor anticoagulant response to activated protein C: prediction of a cofactor activated protein C. Proc Natl Acad Sci USA 90: 1004–1008

De Stefano V, Leone G, Masterangelo S et al 1994 Thrombosis during pregnancy and surgery in patients with congenital deficiency of antithrombin III, protein C-protein S. Thromb Haemost 71: 799–800

Den Heijer M, Koster T, Blom H I et al 1996 Hyperhomocysteinemia as a risk factor for deep vein thrombosis. N Engl J Med 334: 759–762

Eyster M E, Gill F M, Blatt P M, Hilgartner M W, Ballard J O, Kinney T R 1978 Central nervous system bleeding in haemophiliacs. Blood 51: 1179–1188

Fernandez J A, Estelles A, Gilabert J et al 1989 Functional and immunologic protein S in normal pregnant women and in full term newborns. Thromb Haemost 61: 474–478

Formstone C I, Voke J, Tuddenham E G D et al 1993 Prenatal exclusion of severe protein S deficiency by indirect RFLP analysis. Thromb Haemost 69: 931

Foster P A 1995 The reproductive health of women with von Willebrand disease unresponsive to DDAVP: results of an international survey. Thromb Haemost 74: 784–790

Friedreich P W, Sanson B-J, Simioni P et al 1966 Frequency of pregnancy-related venous thromboembolism in anticoagulant factor-deficient women: implications for prophylaxis. Ann Intern Med 125: 955–960

Greer I A, Lowe G D O, Walker J J, Forbes C D 1991 Haemorrhagic problems in obstetrics and gynaecology in patients with congenital coagulopathies. Br J Obstet Gynaecol 98: 909–918

Hellgren M, Tengborn L, Abildgaard U 1992 Pregnancy in women with congenital antithrombin III deficiency: experience of treatment with heparin and antithrombin. Gynaecol Obstet Invest 14: 127–141

Hellgren M, Svensson P, Dahlback B 1995 Resistance to activated protein C as a basis for venous thromboembolism associated with pregnancy and oral contraceptives. Am J Obstet Gynecol 173: 210–213

Hough R E, Makris M, Preston F E 1996 Pregnancy in women with thrombophilia: incidence of thrombosis and pregnancy outcome. Br J Haematol 93 (Suppl 2): 136

Jorquera J I, Montoro J M, Fernandez M A, Aznar J A, Aznar J 1994 Modified test for activated protein C resistance. Lancet 344: 1162–1163

Kadir R A, Economides D L, Braithwaite J, Goldman E, Lee C A 1997 The obstetric experience of carriers of haemophilia. Br J Obstet Gynaecol 104: 803–810

Kluijtmans L A J, van den Heuvel L P W J, Boers G H J et al 1996 Molecular genetic analysis in mild hyperhomocysteinaemia: a common mutation in the 5,10-methylene tetrahydrofolate reductase gene is a genetic risk factor for cardiovascular disease. Am J Hum Genet 58: 35–41

Koster T, Rosendaal F R, Briet E et al 1995a Protein C deficiency in a controlled series of unselected outpatients: an infrequent but clear risk factor for venous thrombosis (Leiden thrombophilia study). Blood 85: 2756–2761

Koster T, Blann A D, Briet E et al 1995b Role of clotting factor VIII and effect of von Willebrand factor on occurrence of deep vein thrombosis. Lancet 345: 152–155

Lane D A, Auberger J, Ireland H, Roscher A A, Thein S L 1996 Prenatal diagnosis in combined antithrombin in factor V mutation. Br J Haematol 94: 753–755

Leclerc J R, Geerts W, Panju A, Nguyen P, Hirsh J 1986 Management of antithrombin deficiency during pregnancy without administration of antithrombin III. Thromb Res 41: 567- 573

Lensen R P M, Rosendaal F R, Koster T et al 1996 Apparent different thrombotic tendency in patients with FV Leiden and protein C deficiency due to selection of patients. Blood 88: 4205–4208

Letsky E A 1991 Haemostasis and epidural anaesthesia. Int J Obstet Anaesth 1: 51–54

Lindoff C, Ingemarsson I, Martinsson G, Segelmark M, Thysell H, Astedt B 1997 Pre-eclampsia is associated with a reduced response to activated protein C. Am J Obstet Gynecol 176: 457–460

Ljung R, Lindgren A C, Petrini P, Tengborn L 1994 Normal vaginal delivery is to be recommended for haemophilia carrier gravidae. Acta Paediatr 83: 609–611

Lowe G D O, Pettigrew A, Middleton S, Forbes C D, Prentice C R M 1977 DDAVP in haemophilia. Lancet ii: 614

Mathonnet F, De Mazancourt P, Bastenaire B et al 1996 Activated protein C sensitivity ratio in pregnant women at delivery. Br J Haematol 92: 244–246

McColl M D, Ramsay J E, Tait R C et al 1997 Risk factors for pregnancy associated venous thromboembolism. Thromb Haemost 74: 1183–1188

Milaskiewicz R M, Holdcroft A, Letsky E A 1990 Epidural anaesthesia and von Willebrand's disease. Anaesthesia 45: 462–464

Millar D S, Allgrove J, Rodeck C, Kakkar V V, Cooper D N 1994 A homozygous deletion/insertion mutation in the protein C (PROC) gene causing neonatal purpura fulminans: prenatal diagnosis in an at risk pregnancy. Blood Coagul Fibrinolysis 5: 647–649

Mudd S H, Levy H L, Skovby F 1985 The natural history of homocysteinuria due to cystatoine beta-synthase deficiency. Am J Hum Genet 37: 1–31

Pabinger I, Schneider, Gesellschaft fur Thrombose-und Haemostase forschung (GTH) Study Group on Natural Inhibitors 1996 Thrombotic risk in hereditary antithrombin III, protein C and protein S deficiency. Arterioscler Thromb Vasc Biol 16: 742–748

Plattner G, Renner W, Went J, Beaudette L, Vain J 1983 Fetal sex determination by ultrasound scanning in the second and third trimesters. Obstet Gynecol 61: 454–458

Poort S R, Rosendaal F R, Reitsma P H, Bertina R M 1996 A common genetic variation in the 3'- untranslated region of the prothrombin gene is associated with elevated plasma prothrombin levels and an increase in venous thrombosis. Blood 88: 3698–3703

Preston F E, Rosendaal F R, Walker I D et al 1996 Increased fetal loss in women with heritable thrombophilia: European Prospective Cohort on Thrombophilia (EPCOT). Lancet 348: 913–916

Rai R, Regan L, Hadley E 1996 Second trimester pregnancy loss associated with activated protein C resistance. Br J Haematol 92: 489–490

Rodeghiero F, Castaman G, Dini E 1987 Epidemiological investigation of the prevalence of von Willebrand's disease. Blood 69: 454–459

Rosendaal F R, Smit C, Briet E 1991 Haemophilia treatment in historical perspective: a review of medical and social developments. Ann Haematol 62: 5–15

Rosendaal F R 1997a Risk factors for venous thrombosis: prevalence, risk and interaction. Semin Haematol 34: 171–187

Rosendaal F R 1997b Thrombosis in the young: epidemiology and risk factors. A focus of venous thrombosis. Thromb Haemost 78 (Suppl 1): 1–6

Sanagostino E, Mannucci P M, Gringeri A, Azzi A, Morfin M 1994 Eliminating parvo virus B19 from blood products. Lancet 343: 798

Simioni P, Prandoni P, Burlina A et al 1996 Hyperhomocysteinemia and deep vein thrombosis: A case control study. Thromb Haemost 76: 883–886

Svensson P J, Dahlback B 1994 Resistance to activated protein C is a basis for venous thrombosis. N Engl J Med 330: 517–522

Trossaert M, Conard J, Horellou M H et al 1994 Modified APC resistance assay for patients on oral anticoagulants. Lancet 344: 1709

Ubbink J B, Vermaak W J, van der Merwe A, Becker P J 1993 Vitamin B12, vitamin B6 and folate nutritional status in men with hyperhomocysteinemia. Am J Clin Nutr 57: 47–53

Varecamp I, Suurmeijer T P, Brocker-Vriends 1990 Carrier testing and prenatal diagnosis for haemophilia: experiences and attitudes of 549 potential and obligate carriers. Am J Med Genet 37: 142–154

Walker I D 1991 Management of thrombophilia in pregnancy. Blood Rev 5: 227–233

John C.P. Kingdom Rekha Bajoria

CHAPTER 4

Fetal assessment and management of labour in twin pregnancy

Recent advances in ultrasound and recognition of the importance of chorionicity have reshaped many aspects of antenatal care in twin pregnancy. More widespread use of assisted conception technology has increased the incidence of multiple pregnancy and multifetal reduction has created a new category of twin pregnancy. Alongside these developments have been concerns about the safety of attempted vaginal delivery given the rising incidence of caesarean section for the second twin. This review will focus on these issues and offer guidelines for antenatal assessment and intrapartum management.

PRENATAL DIAGNOSIS ISSUES

Diagnosis and determination of chorionicity

The case for offering all pregnant women an ultrasound examination at the 'booking' visit, typically 10–13 weeks of gestation, is now strong. The advantages include: accurate dating, detection of uterine and adnexal pathology; diagnosis of non-viable and ectopic pregnancy; and the diagnosis of multiple pregnancy. The counter-argument to diagnosis of twin gestation in the first trimester is the 'over-diagnosis' of multiple pregnancy and the psychological problems that could ensue (Landy 1986). For the ongoing twin gestation, determination of chorionicity and measurement of nuchal translucency at this gestation are especially important.

The accuracy of chorionicity determination is inversely related to gestational age as illustrated in Table 4.1 (Bajoria & Kingdom 1997). During the

John C.P. Kingdom MD MRCP MRCOG DCH, (*Formerly* Senior Lecturer, Department of Obstetrics and Gynaecology, University College London Medical School, London WC1E 6HX, UK)
Associate Professor University of Toronto, Department of Obstetrics and Gynaecology, Mount Sinai Hospital, 600 University Avenue, Toronto M5G 1X5, Canada

Rekha Bajoria PhD MRCOG, Senior Lecturer, Department of Obstetrics and Gynaecology, St Mary's Hospital, University of Manchester Medical School, Whitworth Park, Manchester M13 0JH, UK

Table 4.1 Positive predictive values* of ultrasonographic parameters in the prediction of chorionicity

	Monochorionicity	Dichorionicity
Placenta	Single (42%)	Separate (97.7%)
Fetal sex	Concordant (40%)	Discordant (100%)
Dividing membrane	Absent-MCMA (100%)	
No of layers	Two layers (94.4%)	Four layers (100%)
Thickness	Thickness < 2 mm (82%–39%)	Thickness > 2 mm (95%)
Twin peak sign	Not present (44%)	Present (97.3%)
Use of all criteria	(92%)	97%
Monochorionic placenta = monozygous		
Dichorionic placenta with discordant sex = dizygous		

*Positive predictive value are given in parenthesis. For specific references see Bajoria and Kingdom (1997).

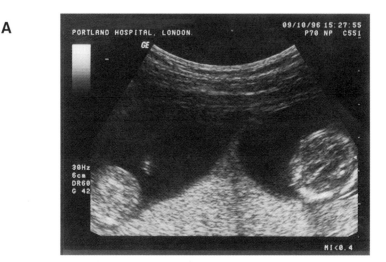

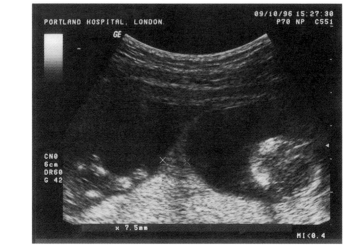

Fig. 4.1 Demonstration of the 'twin-peak' sign in a dichorionic gestation by transabdominal ultrasound at 12 weeks of gestation *(courtesy of Dr Eric Jauniaux).*

first trimester and early second trimester, dichorionic gestations can be recognised by the 'twin peak' sign as illustrated in Figure 4.1; this sign is not always apparent by the 20 week scan because the fused intervening chorion laeve degenerates. Likewise, the easy identification of two yolk sacs during the early first trimester confirms a dichorionic gestation, but this structure regresses thereafter. Following fetal viability, a confident diagnosis of dichorionicity is normally only possible if the genders differ. In third the trimester, colour flow Doppler and newer techniques, like harmonic imaging with use of ultrasound contrast agent, may be useful to ascertain chorionicity in selected complex twin pregnancies (Denbow et al 1997).

Aneuploidy and structural abnormalities

Maternal serum screening for Down's syndrome during the second trimester is invalid in twin pregnancy because the analyte values are a summation of both fetoplacental units (Neueux et al 1996). By contrast, determination of nuchal translucency at the 10–13 week stage appears to be a valid screening method, especially in dichorionic gestation (Sebir et al 1996). Caution is advised in interpreting discordant nuchal translucency measurements in monochorionic twins since this observation may herald the development of chronic twin–twin transfusion syndrome (TTTS) – see below.

Provided the placental discs are not fused, chorionic villous sampling (CVS) can, in experienced hands, be offered for prenatal diagnosis of aneuploidy from 11 + 0 weeks of gestation. In the context of an increased nuchal translucency or a structural abnormality such as exomphalos, an abnormal direct preparation may be acceptable for selective termination, but the need to consider selective termination as early as possible means that fluorescent *in situ* hybridisation (FISH) analysis will assume increasing importance in this context. Amniocentesis can be considered from 14–15 weeks of gestation, and concerns about volume of amniotic fluid removed may be obviated by advances in FISH technology (Steinborn et al 1996). Opinions differ on the optimal technique for twin amniocentesis in dichorionic twins: in the 'double-puncture' method, each sac is entered separately which avoids puncturing the intervening membrane. Instillation of a dye into the first sac is not necessary provided the procedure is done under continuous ultrasound control. Monochorionic twins are virtually always cytogenetically concordant such that single-sampling will suffice, the exception being the possibility of co-existent XO, though normally this would be associated with an increased nuchal translucency (Kaplowitz et al 1991).

Structural abnormalities are commoner in twin gestations, and many of these can de detected at the end of the first trimester (Souka & Nicolaides 1997); for example, anencephaly, body wall defects such as exomphalos, and the rarer abnormalities related to monochorionic twinning as shown in Figure 4.2. Early diagnosis of lethal abnormalities is important in the context of twin pregnancy because any associated risk of polyhydramnios in later gestation could initiate preterm delivery of the normal co-twin.

The normal method of selective termination in dichorionic gestation is by injection of KCl into the fetal heart. Recent data illustrate the much lower rates of complication (bleeding, ruptured membranes and co-twin loss) if this can be accomplished before 16 weeks of gestation (Lynch et al 1996). The risk of

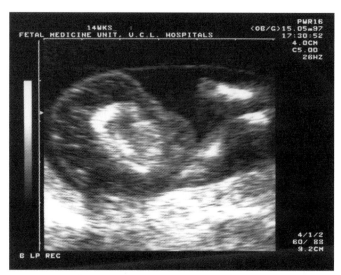

Fig. 4.2 Demonstration of acardiac twin at 12 weeks' gestation – the acardiac twin is located in the sac on the right. Selective fetocide was accomplished one week later by unipolar diathermy to the umbilical cord *(courtesy of Dr Eric Jauniaux).*

feto–fetal transfusion and ischaemic brain damage to the co-twin means alternative techniques are required for selective fetocide in monochorionic gestation. These include: unipolar diathermy to the umbilical vessels (Rodeck & Jauniaux, submitted for publication); injection of thrombogenic materials (Bebbington et al 1995); and endoscopic ligation of the umbilical cord (Deprest et al 1996). Clearly, the complexity of the screening and diagnosis issues in twin gestation, together with a need for expert skills in invasive procedures, indicate that the whole process should ideally be conducted within a regional referral fetal medicine unit.

FETAL ASSESSMENT AFTER 20 WEEKS

The major threat to survival of the normally formed twin gestation fetus is preterm delivery. However, a range of obstetric problems can initiate preterm birth, albeit only a proportion are amenable to measures which can prolong gestation (Kingdom & Morrison 1995, Goldenberg et al 1996).

Cervical incompetence

The much larger volume of a twin gestation challenges the integrity of the cervix such that effacement and dilation may occur as early as 20 weeks of gestation (Michaels et al 1991, Neilson & Crowther 1993). Frustratingly, this process is typically asymptomatic, or the relatively mild degree of accompanying backache and abdominal discomfort is attributed to the general discomfort of pregnancy. Elective bedrest or routine cervical cerclage are not effective measures for the prevention of preterm delivery (Neilson & Crowther 1993) and thus selective measures need to be adopted. Home uterine activity monitoring may provide an early warning (Knuppel et al 1990) but subsequent bedrest is not an effective treatment. More recently, attention has been focused on serial transvaginal assessment of the cervix (Fig 4.3) following from earlier clinical work demonstrating the value of serial digital examination in the prediction of preterm birth (Neilson & Crowther 1993). Ultrasound has the advantage of being able to assess the integrity of the internal os (Kushnir et al 1995), which may be more important than the length of the cervical canal since the latter is affected by parity (Iams et al 1995). An earlier publication utilising transabdominal ultrasound followed by selective transvaginal rescue cervical cerclage reduced the incidence of preterm birth and very low birthweight (Michaels et al 1991); reports of ongoing studies using transvaginal ultrasound and cerclage in twins are awaited with interest. However, in order to have an impact on perinatal mortality, an effective strategy of cervical surveillance (with a view to selective cerclage) would demand fortnightly scans between 18–30 weeks of gestation – a significant demand for many hard-pressed ultrasound departments.

A

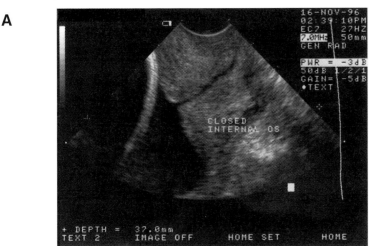

B

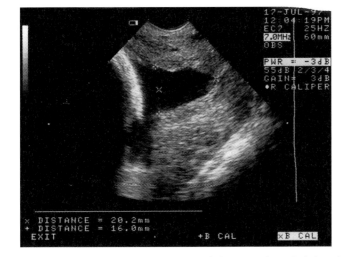

Fig. 4.3 Transvaginal ultrasound demonstration of the normal cervix (**A**) and herniation of the membranes through the internal os at 24 weeks of gestation (**B**). Note the internal os is dilated to 16 mm and the apex of the herniation extends 22 mm into the cervical canal.

Fetal growth

Dichorionic gestation

Discordant fetal growth is a common complication of twins, affecting over 15% of cases, and is the rational for routine serial ultrasound examination. In dichorionic twins, both the location of the placenta and the genetic composition of each twin will vary, though the metabolic demands of two fetuses means that a diagnosis of intrauterine growth restriction (IUGR) is more common in dichorionic twins than singleton gestations (Rydhstrom 1994).

In an uncomplicated dichorionic pregnancy, the first growth assessment should be performed at 28 weeks of gestation when amniotic fluid volume and umbilical artery Doppler are determined for each fetus, in addition to fetal biometry. Umbilical artery Doppler is a reliable tool for the recognition of early-onset IUGR (Kingdom et al 1997a). A high impedance waveform, together with reduced amniotic fluid volume, would be an indication for tests of fetal hypoxia (fetal breathing, middle cerebral artery Doppler, computerised cardiotocography) followed by a plan of serial monitoring, administration of dexamethasone and discussions about the merits of subsequent elective preterm delivery (Devoe & Ware 1995). There is some evidence to suggest that the phenomenon of IUGR with absent end-diastolic flow velocity (AEDFV) in the umbilical artery is tolerated for longer, often for 2–3 weeks (Devoe & Ware 1995), than in a singleton pregnancy. One must be careful when counselling couples where this observation has been made, yet remember that AEDFV may he a 'marker' of a chromosome abnormality, hence a further detailed scan should be performed.

In rare instances, the severity of IUGR would preclude this option (Kingdom et al 1997b) and lack of placental vascular anastomoses means that fetal demise would not jeopardise the health of the normal co-twin. More commonly, the observation of normal umbilical artery Doppler and amniotic fluid volume allows minor differences in estimates of fetal weight to be dismissed as normal biological variation, such that reassessment on a 4 weekly basis to 36 weeks, followed by an amniotic fluid index and CTG at 38 weeks, is a safe and cost effective strategy. This also allows more rational focusing of attention on monochorionic pregnancies.

Monochorionic gestation

The rational behind more intensive ultrasound monitoring of monochorionic gestations is the notion that chronic twin-to-twin transfusion syndrome (TTTS) can be recognised before the development of potentially fatal or handicapping complications. These include: polyhydramnios and preterm delivery; compromise or death of the 'donor' twin from severe oligohydramnios and IUGR; 'recipient' morbidity from cardiac dysfunction (Zosmer et al 1994). The motivation to scan these pregnancies on a 2 weekly basis from as early as 18 weeks of gestation is to try and avoid the dismal prognosis of the most severe forms of chronic TTTS seen in referral fetal medicine units. Such a policy has been in place at Queen Charlotte's Hospital, London since 1992 and the publication of prospective data is awaited with interest.

The management of polyhydramnios resulting from chronic TTTS is normally amnioreduction (Elliott et al 1994), though endoscopic surgery in the form of laser ablation to communicating artery-to-vein anastomoses has been proposed (Ville et al 1995). The latter treatment may result in death of the donor and, since the treatment occludes anastomotic vessels, this is thought to protect the recipient from ischaemic brain damage. However the risk of ischaemic brain injury in the recipient following death of the donor is probably much less than the empirical figure of 25%, because blood is unlikely to pass in a reverse direction along a 'veno-arterial' connection (Bajoria, unpublished data). The debate over management can only be clarified by a multicentre trial where cases randomised to laser therapy are managed in a single centre and compared with amnioreduction performed locally.

Multifetal pregnancy reduction

The much greater risks of preterm delivery, death and neurological handicap amongst triplets, and higher order births, in comparison with twins has led to the development of multifetal pregnancy reduction to a twin gestation. This is a contentious issue for two reasons: firstly, the gestational age-specific morbidity rates for preterm infants are falling with improvements in intensive care (Luke 1996); secondly, the increased understanding of the role of cervical monitoring and selective cerclage to prevent extreme preterm birth. These points must be set against the significant maternal morbidity of triplet and higher gestations. The technique of reduction is the same as for selective termination, i.e. transabdominal injection of KCl into the most accessible fetus, normally at 10–12 weeks of gestation paying attention to the implications of chorionicity. Recent follow-up studies of twin gestations reduced from higher order births suggest a higher incidence of perinatal complications than in standard twins (Bernasko et al 1997).

Death of co-twin

Reports of the prevalence of co-twin death range from 0.5–6.8% depending on the degree of selection and the proportion of monochorionic gestations. In these circumstances, there is an increased risk of neurological morbidity in the surviving co-twin, especially if the gestation is monochorionic because communicating placental vessels allow a rapid transfusion of blood from the survivor across the 'watershed' artery-to-artery and vein-to-vein compensatory vessels which are characteristic of normal monochorionic gestation. Since there is a paucity of these compensatory vessels in pregnancies complicated by chronic TTTS (Bajoria et al 1995), these two forms of TTTS tend not to overlap. Sudden movement of blood across compensatory vascular communications is known as the 'acute' form of TTTS. Since this acute feto–fetal transfusion may also occur in labour, there is increasing interest in the use of colour or power Doppler to map the communicating vessels in monochorionic gestation as part of the risk assessment (Haberman et al 1997). Since feto–fetal transfusion is an acute process following co-twin death, so is the time course of ischaemic brain injury (risk about 25% overall) or even death. It therefore follows that elective preterm delivery following co-twin death confers no advantage to the survivor (Murphy 1995). Communicating vessels are extremely rare in dichorionic gestations (Benirschke et al 1995) but may account for the small additional risk of handicap in the surviving co-twin.

Monoamniotic and acardiac twins

Monoamniotic and acardiac twin gestations are rare complications of mono-chorionic gestation, occurring in 1/10,000 and 1/35,000 pregnancies, respectively. Monoamniotic gestation is reliably established in the late first and early second trimesters, but can easily be 'over-diagnosed' as pregnancy advances, particularly in the context of discordant amniotic fluid volumes. The high perinatal mortality and morbidity in this group is not related to TTTS, but to cord entanglement and the high incidence of major structural abnormalities including conjoint twinning. Early prenatal diagnosis of the latter group allows the option of vaginal termination of pregnancy, but it is possible to give a prognosis for postnatal survival following surgery depending on the site and nature of the twinning. Delivery is usually by elective classical caesarean section. Attempts to predict and prevent death from cord entanglement from monitoring the extent of knotting and the umbilical artery Doppler have been disappointing, though reducing fetal mobility by inducing oligohydramnios in the second trimester, when the entanglement mainly occurs, has been tried with some success (Peek et al 1997). Planned delivery by elective caesarean section is generally advised, though reports of successful vaginal delivery (of unrecog-nised cases) indicate that vaginal delivery is not absolutely contra-indicated (Dubecq et al 1996).

Acardiac twinning results in the twin reversed arterial perfusion (TRAP) sequence where fetal tissue parts, which may be recognisable as part of a fetus, grow in tandem with the normal fetus and are perfused in the reverse direction along the umbilical cord. Hence, the normally formed twin may be referred to as the 'pump twin'. The risk to pump twin (of death from cardiac failure or

Table 4.2 Obstetric indications for caesarean section in twin gestation

Accepted indications for caesarean section
Non-cephalic presentation of twin 1 (23%)
IUGR in dichorionic twins (< 5%)
Twin 2 significantly larger (> 500 g) than twin 1 – including antepartum death of 1st twin (1–2%)
Placenta praevia (1–2%)
Fetal abnormality precluding safe vaginal delivery (1%)
Chronic TTTS in monochorionic twins (< 1%)
Monoamniotic twins (< 1%)
Contentious indications for caesarean section
Maternal request (? 5–10%)
Unfavourable cervix at 39 weeks in nulliparas
Death of 2nd twin co-twin
Uncomplicated monochorionic twins
Previous caesarean section

*Houlihan and Knuppel (1996).

preterm delivery from associated polyhydramnios) is related to the size and growth of the acardic fetus. Spontaneous cord occlusion may occur if acardiac fetus is small, though some form of invasive procedure may be worthwhile where the acardiac fetus is larger – to protect the normal fetus from ischaemic brain injury or cardiac failure. Unipolar diathermy to thrombose the vessels has been used at University College Hospital (Fig. 4.2) and other occlusive devices (Sepulveda et al 1995, Quintero et al 1996), or even selective delivery by hysterotomy, have been used (Fries et al 1992).

Extreme preterm delivery of one twin

In rare instances, particularly if the gestation is known to be dichorionic, spontaneous delivery of the first fetus before 28 weeks of gestation does not imply a need to expedite delivery of the second. In the absence of overt chorion-amnionitis, pre-eclampsia or fetal compromise, a combination of antibiotics, tocolysis and rescue cervical cerclage may prolong the inter-twin delivery interval by a clinically-significant degree. In a 7 year cohort of 1806 multiple births, Kurzel and colleagues (1995) found a 4.7% incidence of 1st twin delivery between 18–26 weeks, of which a quarter were considered potential candidates for this treatment, but it does have the capacity to cause more harm than good, e.g. prolongation of gestation to survive with major handicap.

TIMING AND MODE OF DELIVERY

Induction of labour (IOL) for twin gestation and a cephalic presentation for the first twin is common practice by 38 weeks of gestation. However, there is no good evidence to support the practice of IOL before 40 weeks of gestation in an uncomplicated dichorionic twin gestation with normal fetal growth velocity and amniotic fluid volumes. IOL is not necessarily a straightforward intervention, with attendant risks of caesarean section for failed induction, fetal heart rate abnormalities following oxytocin augmentation, and an increased risk of postpartum haemorrhage. This increased risk of emergency caesarean section during labour, including caesarean section for the second twin (Bider et al 1995), has led to a rising trend in favour of elective caesarean section for twin gestation.

The obstetric indications for elective caesarean section, together with their relative importance, in twin gestation are shown in Table 4.2. The two common indications for elective caesarean section are non-vertex presentation of twin 1 and maternal request. The latter indication is increasing where a high proportion of twins is a consequence of infertility treatment in older couples. Given the background rate of emergency caesarean section in spontaneous singleton nulliparous labour of 16% in 1996 at UCH, the desire of nulliparous women to avoid the morbidity of emergency caesarean section following induction of labour in twin gestation is understandable.

Caesarean section for preterm labour with a non-vertex 2nd twin remains controversial. Although the mature second twin will come to no harm from a breech extraction in experienced hands, this is not necessarily true for the fetus with an estimated fetal weight < 1500 g. A comprehensive review of 19 studies

Recent Advances in Obstetrics and Gynaecology 20

on this subject was unable to clarify the need for caesarean section (Houlihan & Knuppel 1996), largely because the studies reported were retrospective and the majority from deliveries before widespread use of ultrasound and continuous CTG monitoring in the mid-1980s. The largest modern series of 416 pairs, from deliveries between 1985–1990 (Creig et al 1992) did not support caesarean section for non-vertex second twins > 500 g and demonstrated the safety and applicability of external cephalic version. The key point is confidence with ultrasound and a willingness to perform ECV or breech extraction (Chervenak et al 1985), and thus the seniority of obstetric staff at delivery will determine the likely success of attempted vaginal delivery (Sharma et al 1990).

The University of California at Los Angeles reported their experience of 210 twin gestations with previous caesarean deliveries (39 with ≥ 2 previous operations), representing 11.3% of all twins delivered during this time (Miller et al 1996). A trial of labour of labour was conducted in 118, in 10 of which there had been ≥ 2 previous operations. An unspecified number had been induced, with no details of the methods chosen, though 8 underwent caesarean section following a failed attempt at induction. Both twins delivered successfully in 64 cases (70%), and caesarean section of the 2nd twin following vaginal delivery of the 1st occurred in 13 women. There were no uterine ruptures and the option of vaginal delivery reduced overall maternal morbidity and hospital stay.

Concern for successful vaginal delivery of twin 2 is sometimes expressed if the EFW is > 500 g above that of twin 1. Where twin 2 is non-vertex, an attempt at ECV and vertex delivery was not successful where twin 2 was > 500 g heavier than twin 1 exposing the fetus to the risk of head entrapment during breech extraction (Chervenak et al 1983).

Technique of caesarean section

Epidural anaesthesia is commonly employed for elective caesarean section in the absence of placenta praevia. By contrast with general anaesthesia, the latter method results in preservation of uterine tone which may, in turn, cause problems with delivery of the second twin. Examples include: IUGR of the 2nd twin, chronic TTTS resulting in a 'stuck-twin" in the fundus, uterine distortion by fibroids. Under these circumstances, the second twin may become entrapped in the fundus, especially if the membranes are ruptured early to attempt a breech extraction. Significant fetal morbidity, to an already compromised fetus, can occur before it is realised that a classical or lateral extension to the uterine incision is required. This situation is avoided by one or more of the following measures:

1. Always plan the strategy for delivery of the twins before scrubbing – ultrasound can be very helpful to warn of potential difficulties.

2. Consider an elective classical uterine incision – blood loss is likely to be less than if a 'J-shape' extension is made into the territory of the uterine artery.

3. Consider administration of intravenous nitroglycerin to temporarily relax the uterus for delivery of twin 2. This is given as a bolus (100–150 mcg) following reflection of the bladder (Mayer & Weeks 1992) and, though not often used in the UK, is a popular strategy in Continental Europe. Reduction

in maternal blood pressure is reported to be minimal because of fluid pre-loading, but caution is advised if the patient is hypotensive or has tachycardia.

Management of labour at University College Hospital, London

Epidural anaesthesia is recommended for twin delivery, so as to facilitate either external or internal manipulation of twin 2 into a longitudinal lie and/or perform breech extraction where indicated. Where epidural anaesthesia is contra-indicated, declined by the woman, or she presents in advanced labour, then an anaesthetist should be present throughout the 2nd and 3rd stages of labour, since any indication for general anaesthesia is likely to be immediate.

1. On admission, the woman should be reviewed by the registrar who should re-evaluate the safety of attempted vaginal delivery since the last clinic visit. Routine serial ultrasound reports will alert to the problems of discordant growth, malpresentation, placenta praevia, etc. Intravenous access is obtained together with a full blood count and either group and save or cross-match depending on the perceived risk of subsequent blood loss. Oral ranitidine should be given 6 hourly and epidural anaesthesia should be discussed once established labour has been diagnosed. Management should then be discussed with the senior registrar or consultant on-call.

2. Labour should ideally be managed in a large room which can be converted for caesarean section and accommodate staff and equipment. In the advanced first stage a scalp clip is recommended for twin 1 to simplify abdominal monitoring to twin 2. Management of the second stage of labour is the same as for a singleton gestation, but delivery should be conducted in the presence of obstetric and anaesthetic staff. The key role for the senior obstetrician is to palpate the abdomen immediately following delivery of twin 1 and we advocate the use of ultrasound during this time to ensure presentation is correctly assessed and the fetal heart of twin 2 is reliably recorded.

3. In the UK, the practice of ECV for breech presentation of the 2nd twin is not encouraged since it confers little advantage to the fetus, may result in complications and, of course, may fail, tempting the obstetrician into a caesarean section. Complications include: (i) spontaneous rupture of the membranes and transverse lie necessitating caesarean section; and (ii) fetal bradycardia due to version may necessitate caesarean section.
   Where rapid delivery of the 2nd twin is indicated, for example due to fetal bradycardia, vaginal bleeding or cord prolapse, the fastest (and, therefore, safest) method is normally by breech extraction. This is why skilled obstetricians are comfortable with the 2nd twin presenting as a breech, which exposes the weakness of the argument in favour of routine external cephalic version for the 2nd twin presenting as a breech (Chervenak et al 1983, Chauhan et al 1995).

4. Next commence an intravenous oxytocin infusion at 4 mIU/min if not previously used, or double the dose used prior to delivery of the 1st twin. Immediate augmentation shortens the inter-twin delivery interval by preventing the commonly-observed 'lull' in uterine activity following delivery of twin 1. As such, efficient descent of the presenting part, surrounded by intact forewaters, is achieved, thereby, preventing the cervix from closing. Once the presenting part is felt below the ischial spines, the woman should be encouraged to push again with each contraction. In these circumstances the presenting part and intact forewaters act together to ensure the cervix remains 'fully-dilated'. It follows that the membranes should not be ruptured routinely in these circumstances, particularly with a breech presentation, so as to avoid the pitfalls of either a 'high-head' or an unnecessary breech extraction. The key to success is to have the oxytocin ready to commence upon delivery of twin 1 and to have confidence in monitoring the fetal heart for up to 30 min to ensure deep descent of the presenting part during pushing before amniotomy.

5. Where operative delivery is required for the cephalic second twin, this is commonly associated with malposition and a high station. For this reason, the ventouse is far safer than forceps delivery and the risk of failed delivery is remote because this follows successful delivery of twin 1. A small silastic or metal (Malstrom) cup is preferred such that application at a higher station, than in a singleton delivery, will not include maternal soft tissue. In the unlikely event of a failed attempt at delivery by vacuum, forceps delivery may be attempted by an experienced obstetrician provided descent has been achieved and he/she is certain of the position. Ultrasound location of the fetal back may assist recognition of persistent occipito-posterior position to allow confident application of the blades.

6. The acceptable interval between vaginal delivery of twins remains actively debated. Before epidural analgesia and widespread electronic fetal heart rate monitoring, it was common to push the presenting part into the pelvis after 5 min and perform amniotomy, resorting to operative vaginal delivery after a further 10 min if spontaneous delivery was not imminent (Donald 1979). In view of the real concerns about 2nd twin mortality, such a practice led to impressive results. These arguments do not apply in modern obstetrics when epidural analgesia (which slows the second stage), and continuous fetal heart rate monitoring (for rapid recognition of fetal compromise) is the norm. Early routine recourse to oxytocin to achieve 'pharmacological' descent of the second twin will result in few women remaining undelivered after 30 min. Delay beyond this time is acceptable, provided progress is being made towards successful vaginal delivery, bleeding is minimal, and the CTG is normal. This is more often the case where the second twin is cephalic than breech since experienced obstetricians will expedite a breech delivery yet by contrast will generally prefer to let maternal effort advance the vertex before attempting operative delivery.

The risk of atonic primary post-partum haemorrhage is considerably increased with twin delivery. Upon delivery of the second twin, the oxytocin infusion should be accelerated and intramuscular syntometrine given. Where bleeding is excessive, manual removal of the placenta and uterine massage should be accompanied by administration of intravenous ergometrine (0.5 mg diluted in 10 ml 0.9% saline) over 5 min (unless contra-indicated by pre-eclampsia). The oxytocin infusion should continue for 4 h following delivery and the placental discs inspected for completeness before repair of any episiotomy and/or vaginal tears. Following successful completion of the 3rd stage, it is sensible to continue observations, in a high-dependency setting for 12 h, normally within the labour and delivery suite.

Key points for clinical practice

- A policy of offering all women a routine ultrasound examination scan at the end of the first trimester will facilitate the diagnosis of twins, thereby allowing a more accurate diagnosis of chorionicity. Screening for aneuploidy by nuchal translucency and early detection of discordant structural abnormalities are additional advantages.

- Given the complex issues surrounding prenatal diagnosis in twin gestations, this activity should ideally be undertaken in a regional fetal medicine unit.

- A specialist antenatal clinic for women expecting twin gestations offers several advantages, including preparation for parenthood, which can be linked to an ultrasound service and the advice of an interested obstetrician.

- More intensive monitoring of monochorionic pregnancies after 18–20 weeks of gestation, for the detection of chronic twin–twin transfusion syndrome or discordant fetal growth, may be justified.

- Clear guidelines on the management of labour, together with good support for junior staff, are essential to ensure that this is a safe exercise.

References

Bajoria R, Wigglesworth J, Fisk N M 1995 Angioarchitecture of monochorionic placentas in relation to the twin-twin transfusion syndrome. Am J Obstet Gynecol 172: 856–863

Bajoria R, Kingdom J C P 1997 The case for routine determination of chorionicity in multiple pregnancy. Prenat Diagn 13: 1207–1225

Bebbington M W, Wilson R D, Machan L, Wittmann B K 1995 Selective feticide in twin transfusion syndrome using ultrasound-guided insertion of thrombogenic coils. Fetal Diagn Ther 10: 32–36

Benirschke K, Kaufmann P 1995 Multiple pregnancy. In: Pathology of the human placenta, 3rd Edn. Springer-Verlag, New York, pp 719–826

Bernasko J, Lynch L, Lapinski R, Berkowitz R L 1997 Twin pregnancies conceived by assisted reproductive techniques: maternal and neonatal outcomes. Obstet Gynecol 89: 368–372

Bider D, Korach J, Hourvitz A, Dulitzky M, Goldenberg M, Mashiach S 1995 Combined vaginal-abdominal delivery of twins. J Reprod Med 40: 131–134

Chauhan S P, Roberts W E, McLaren R A, Roach H, Morrison J C, Martin Jr J N 1995 Delivery of the nonvertex second twin: breech extraction versus external cephalic version. Am J Obstet Gynecol 173: 1015–1020

Chervenak F A, Johnson R E, Berkowitz R L, Hobbins J C 1983 Intraparium external version of the second twin. Obstet Gynecol 62: 160–165

Chervenak F A, Johnson R E, Youcha S, Hobbins J C, Berkowitz R L 1985 Intrapartum management of twin gestation. Obstet Gynecol 65: 119–124

Denbow M L, Blomley M J, Cosgrove D O, Fisk N M 1997 Ultrasound microbubble contrast angiography in monochorionic twin fetuses [letter]. Lancet 349: 773

Deprest J A, Evrard V A, Van Schoubroeck D, Vandenberghe K 1996 Endoscopic cord ligation in selective feticide [letter]. Lancet 348: 890–891

Devoe L D, Ware D J 1995 Antenatal assessment of twin gestation. Semin Perinatol 19: 413–423

Donald I 1979 Practical obstetric problems. Loyd-Luke, London

Dubecq F, Dufour P, Vinatier D et al 1996 Monoamniotic twin pregnancies. Review of the literature, and a case report with vaginal delivery. Eur J Obstet Gynecol Reprod Biol 66: 183–186

Elliott J P, Sawyer A T, Radin T G et al 1994 Large-volume therapeutic amniocentesis in the treatment of hydrarimios. Obstet Gynecol 84: 1025–1027

Fries M H, Goldberg J D, Golbus M S 1992 Treatment of acardiac–acephalus twin gestation by hysterotomy and selective delivery. Obstet Gynecol 79: 601–604

Goldenberg R L, Iams J D, Miodovnik M et al 1996 The preterm prediction study: risk factors in twin gestations. National Institute of Child Health and Human Development Maternal-Fetal Medicine Units Network. Am J Obstet Gynecol 175: 1047–1053

Greig P C, Veike J C, Morgan T, Henderson L 1992 The effect of presentation and mode of delivery on neonatal outcome in the second twin. Am J Obstet Gynecol 167: 901–906

Haberman S, Haratz-Ubinstein N, Baxi L, Helle D 1997 Power Doppler sonography in monochorionic twins: a preliminary study. J Matern Fetal Invest 7: 84–88

Houlihan C, Knuppel R A 1996 Intrapartum management of multiple gestations. Clin Perinatol 23: 91–116

Iams J D, Johnson F F, Sonek J, Sachs L, Gebauer C, Samuels P 1995 Cervical competence as a continuum: a study of ultrasonographic cervical length and obstetric performance. Am J Obstet Gynecol 172: 1097–1103

Kaplowitz P B, Bodurtha J, Brown J, Spence J E 1991 Monozygotic twins discordant for Ullrich-Turner syndrome. Am J Med Genet 41: 78–82

Kingdom J C P, Morrison J J 1995 Prediction, prevention and management of preterm labour in multiple pregnancy. In: Ward R H, Whittle M (eds) Multiple pregnancy. RCOG Press, London, pp 148–163

Kingdom J C P, Burrell S J, Kaufmann P 1997a Pathology and clinical implications of abnormal umbilical artery Doppler waveforms. Ultrasound Obstet Gynaecol 9: 271–286

Kingdom J C P, Rodeck C H, Kaufmann P 1997b Umbilical artery Doppler – more harm than good. Br J Obstet Gynaecol 104: 393–396

Knuppel R A, Lake M F, Watson D L et al 1990 Preventing preterm birth in twin gestation: home uterine activity monitoring and perinatal nursing support. Obstet Gynecol 76: 24S–27S

Kurzel R B, Kovacs B W, Goodwin T M, Gazit G, Everton LR 1995 Delivery of previable twins: when to attempt delay of delivery of the second twin. Am J Obstet Gynecol 172: 413 (Abstract)

Kushnir O, Izquierdo L A, Smith J F, Blankstein J, Curet L B 1995 Transvaginal monographic measurement of cervical length. Evaluation of twin pregnancies. J Reprod Med 40: 380–382

Landy H J 1986 The vanishing twin: ultrasonographic assessment of fetal disappearance in the first trimester. Am J Obstet Gynecol 155: 14–19

Luke B 1996 Reducing fetal deaths in multiple births: optimal birthweights and gestational ages for infants of twin and triplet births. Acta Genet Med Gemellol (Roma) 45: 333–348

Lynch L, Berkowitz R L, Stone J, Alvarez M, Lapinski R 1996 Preterm delivery after selective termination in twin pregnancies. Obstet Gynecol 87: 366–369

Mayer D C, Weeks S K 1992 Antepartum uterine relaxation with nitroglycerin at caesarean delivery. Can J Anaesth 39: 166–169

Michaels W H, Schreiber F R, Padgett R J, Ager J, Pieper D 1991 Ultrasound surveillance of the cervix in twin gestations: management of cervical incompetency. Obstet Gynecol 78: 739–744

Miller D A, Mullin P, Hou D, Paul R H 1996 Vaginal birth after cesarean section in twin gestation. Am J Obstet Gynecol 175: 194-198

Murphy K W 1995 Intrauterine death in a twin: implications for the survivor. In: Ward R H, Whittle M (eds) Multiple pregnancy. RCOG Press, London, pp 218–231

Neilson J P, Crowther C A 1993 Preterm labour in multiple pregnancies. Fetal Matern Med Rev 5: 105–119

Neueux L M, Palomaki G E, Knight G J, Haddow J E 1996 Multiple marker for Down syndrome in twin pregnancies. Prenat Diagn 16: 29–34

Peek M J, McCarthy A, Kyle P, Sepulveda W, Fisk N M 1997 Medical amnioreduction with sulindac to reduce cord complications in monoamniotic twins. Am J Obstet Gynecol 176: 334–336

Quintero R A, Romero R, Reich H et al 1996 In utero percutaneous umbilical cord ligation in the management of complicated monochorionic multiple gestations. Ultrasound Obstet Gynecol 8: 16–22

Rydhstrom H 1994 Discordant birthweight and late fetal death in like-sexed and unlike-sexed twin pairs: a population-based study. Br J Obstet Gynaecol 101: 765–769

Sebir N J, Snijders R J M, Hughes K, Sepulveda W, Nicolaides K H 1996 Screening for trisomy 21 in twin pregnancies by maternal age and nuchal translucency thickness at 10–14 weeks of gestation. Br J Obstet Gynaecol 103: 999–1003

Sepulveda W, Bower S, Hassan J, Fisk N M 1995 Ablation of acardiac twin by alcohol injection into the intra-abdominal umbilical artery. Obstet Gynecol 86: 680–681

Sharma J S, Spillane H, Mukoyoka J, Tange L, Obhrai M S 1990 Caesarean section for the birth of the second twin after vaginal delivery of the first twin. Br J Obstet Gynaecol 97: 234–236

Souka AP, Nicolaides KH 1997 Diagnosis of fetal abnormnalities at the 10–14 week scan. Ultrasound Obstet Gynaecol 10: 429–442

Steinborn A, Roddiger S, Born H J, Baier P, Halberstadt E 1996 Prenatal chromosome analysis using the FISH technique allows fetal aneuploidy detection within a few hours. Z Geburtshilfe Neonatol 200: 186–190

Ville Y, Hyett J, Hecher K et al 1995 Preliminary experience with endoscopic laser surgery for severe twin-twin transfusion syndrome. N Engl J Med 332: 224–227

Zosmer N, Bajoria R, Weiner E, Rigby M, Vaughan J, Fisk N M 1994 Clinical and echographic features of in utero cardiac dysfunction in the recipient twin in twin-twin transfusion syndrome. Br Heart J 72: 74–79

Patricia Crowley

Antenatal corticosteroids prior to preterm delivery

While studying the effect of corticosteroids on the initiation of parturition in the ewe, Liggins (1969) observed that lambs exposed to prenatal corticosteroids appeared viable at an earlier gestational age than might have been expected. Subsequently, a randomised, placebo controlled trial of betamethasone administration in women who were expected to give birth preterm found a statistically significant reduction in the frequency of respiratory distress in babies born before 32 weeks gestation and a 5-fold reduction in neonatal mortality among preterm babies born after corticosteroids compared with placebo administration (Liggins & Howie 1972). In the 22 years since this initial study, numerous investigations have suggested that antenatal corticosteroid administration reduces neonatal morbidity in preterm infants. However, obstetricians were slow to incorporate this ability to manipulate fetal maturity pharmacologically into clinical practice. A 1980 survey of self-reported practice among fellows and members of the Royal College of Obstetricians and Gynaecologists resident in the UK showed that 42% used this treatment 'frequently', 40% 'sometimes' and 18% 'never' (Lewis et al 1980). In a similar study of practice in northern Belgium and The Netherlands, Keirse (1984) found that only 32.5% of respondents used the treatment 'routinely'.

The recorded use of antenatal corticosteroids during the randomised controlled trials of surfactant therapy for neonatal respiratory distress syndrome suggests that corticosteroid usage continued to be low on both sides of the Atlantic up to the late 1980s and early 1990s. Only 12% of babies from the UK Ten Centre trial (Ten Centre Study Group 1987) and 20% of those enrolled in the US Exosurf trial (Corbet et al 1991) received corticosteroids administered antenatally. Antenatal corticosteroid therapy finally came of age in 1995 with the publication of the National Institutes of Health Consensus Statement on Effects of Corticosteroids for Fetal Maturation on Perinatal

Dr Patricia Crowley MRCOG FRCP(I), Senior Lecturer and Consultant, Department of Obstetrics and Gynaecology, Trinity College Dublin, Coombe Women's Hospital, Dublin 8, Ireland

Outcomes (NIH 1995). This statement concludes: 'antenatal corticosteroids therapy is indicated for women at risk of premature delivery with few exceptions and will result in a substantial decrease in neonatal morbidity and mortality, as well as substantial savings in health care costs'.

MODE OF ACTION OF ANTENATAL CORTICOSTEROIDS

Prenatal corticosteroid therapy is thought to mimic the physiological effects of a surge in endogenous fetal and neonatal corticosteroids that occurs *in utero* prior to spontaneous delivery at term and postnatally following preterm birth. Following the administration of corticosteroids, there is a generalised acceleration of the rate of tissue differentiation without any alteration in the normal sequence of development. Because respiratory distress syndrome is the most immediate cause of mortality and morbidity in the majority of preterm infants and because of the amenability of lung tissue to explant culture, the pulmonary effects of antenatal corticosteroids have been the main focus of interest in the past. This pre-occupation with the pulmonary effects of cortico-steroids may have restricted the use of antenatal corticosteroids. Evaluation of the efficacy of corticosteroid therapy has focussed excessively on respiratory distress syndrome. Corticosteroids may have been inappropriately withheld both when lung maturity was assumed to have been already achieved, and when it was thought to be unattainable because of extreme prematurity. Roberton (1984), for example, suggested that corticosteroids benefit only white male infants and that even for them the benefit is mainly among those born between 30 and 32 weeks' gestation. The need for continued use of antenatal corticosteroid therapy was again questioned when postnatal surfactant therapy became available (Silver et al 1996). A broader view of the effect of antenatal corticosteroids is more appropriate and may prevent similar errors occurring in the future.

Pulmonary effects

The best known effect of antenatal corticosteroid therapy is a receptor mediated effect on all components of the surfactant system including phospholipids, lipogenic enzymes and sufactant-associated proteins. However, structural development is also affected, resulting in an increase both in lung compliance and in maximum volume that is independent of surfactant. Protein leak from vessels to airways is reduced and clearance of lung liquid at delivery is accelerated (Ballard & Ballard 1995).

Extrapulmonary effects

Glucocorticoids have been shown to accelerate cytodifferentiation and protein and enzyme synthesis in a variety of tissues including liver, pancreas, kidney, intestine, adrenal, skin and myocardium. The accelerated maturation of the fetal intestine may account for the reduced incidence of necrotising enterocolitis observed in corticosteroid-treated neonates. Accelerated maturation of fetal skin may result in reduced insensible water loss. Effects on the myocardium, and on catecholamine responsiveness may explain the reduced incidence of intra-ventricular haemorrhage seen in extremely preterm infants that appeared to be independent of any effect on respiratory distress syndrome (Garite et al 1992).

EVIDENCE OF EFFICACY

The efficacy of antenatal corticosteroid therapy has been evaluated in a systematic review (Crowley 1997). A systematic review is one in which evidence, usually from randomised trials, has been systematically identified, appraised and summarised according to predetermined criteria in order to reduce bias. The results can then be subjected to meta-analysis, a statistical technique which summarises the results of several studies into a single estimate, giving more weight to results from larger studies, enabling a more precise estimate of the effects of interventions. In order to exclude bias, the literature should be searched using a prespecified search strategy to identify and select relevant randomised trials. These trials must be critically evaluated using predetermined criteria for quality as evidenced by measures taken to avoid bias. Prespecified outcome data must be extracted from the trials and quantitatively synthesised. Finally, the reviewer can draw conclusions about the effectiveness of the intervention. All these processes must be explicitly described in order for the reader to draw any conclusions about the validity of the review.

Systematic review of antenatal corticosteroid therapy

A systematic review of randomised controlled trials of antenatal corticosteroids therapy was conducted according to standard methods for literature searching (Chalmers et al 1989) and statistical analysis (Yusuf et al 1985).The search yielded 15 trials which reported clinically relevant outcomes (Block et al 1977; Carlan et al 1994; Cararach et al 1990; Collaborative Group 1981; Doran et al 1980; Gamsu et al 1989; Garite et al 1992; Howie & Liggins1977; Kari et al 1994; Morales et al 1986; Morrison et al 1978; Papageorgiou et al 1979; Parsons et al 1988; Schutte et al 1980; Tauesch et al 1979; Teramo et al 1980; Schmidt et al 1984).

Neonatal mortality

Table 5.1 and Figure 5.1 summarise the effects of antenatal corticosteroid therapy on the odds of neonatal death. Antenatal corticosteroid therapy is associated with a reduction in neonatal mortality (typical odds ratio 0.60, 95% CI 0.48–0.76). The magnitude of this effect is greatest in trials conducted before 1980 when the case-fatality rate for respiratory distress syndrome was higher. The reduction in neonatal mortality is mainly due to a significant reduction in two important causes of neonatal death – respiratory distress syndrome and intraventricular haemorrhage.

Respiratory distress syndrome

Table 5.2 and Figure 5.2 indicate that, overall, the risk of neonatal respiratory distress syndrome is reduced by about 50% (typical odds ratio 0.53 (95% CI

Table 5.1 Effect of antenatal corticosteroids on neonatal mortality – numerical data

	Treated	Control	Weight %	Odds ratio	[95% Confidence intervals]
Neonatal death (all babies)					
Amsterdam 1980	3/64	12/58	4.4		0.23 [0.08, 0.67]
Auckland 1972	36/532	60/538	29.3		0.58 [0.38, 0.89]
Block 1977	1/69	5/61	1.9		0.22 [0.04, 1.12]
Doran 1980	4/81	11/63	4.5		0.26 [0.09, 0.77]
Gamsu 1989	14/131	20/137	10.0		0.70 [0.34, 1.44]
Garite 1992	9/40	11/42	5.1		0.82 [0.30, 2.24]
Kari 1994	6/95	9/94	4.7		0.64 [0.22, 1.84]
Morales 1986	7/121	13/124	6.2		0.54 [0.22, 1.33]
Morrison 1978	3/67	7/59	3.1		0.37 [0.10, 1.33]
Papageorgiou 1979	1/71	7/75	2.6		0.22 [0.05, 0.91]
Parsons 1988	0/23	1/22	0.3		0.13 [0.00, 6.52]
Schmidt 1984	5/49	4/31	2.6		0.77 [0.19, 3.15]
Tauesch 1979	8/56	10/71	5.1		1.02 [0.37, 2.76]
US Steroid Trial	32/371	34/372	20.2		0.94 [0.57, 1.56]
Subtotal (95% CI)	129/1770	204/1747	100.0		0.60 [0.48, 0.75]
Chi-square 14.70 (df = 13) Z = 4.42					
Neonatal death in babies treated before 1980					
Amsterdam 1980	3/64	12/58	7.3		0.23 [0.08, 0.67]
Auckland 1972	36/532	50/538	48.1		0.58 [0.38, 0.89]
Block 1977	1/69	5/61	3.2		0.22 [0.04, 1.12]
Doran 1980	4/81	11/63	7.3		0.26 [0.09, 0.77]
Gamsu 1989	14/131	20/137	16.4		0.70 [0.34, 1.44]
Morrison 1978	3/67	7/59	5.1		0.37 [0.10, 1.33]
Papageorgiou 1979	1/71	7/75	4.2		0.22 [0.05, 0.91]
Tauesch 1979	8/56	10/71	8.4		1.02 [0.37, 2.76]
Subtotal (95% CI)		70/1071	132/1062	100.0	0.51 [0.38, 0.68]
Chi-square 9.20 (df = 7) Z = 4.60					
Neonatal death in babies treated after 1980					
Garite 1992	9/40	11/42	13.1		0.82 [0.30, 2.24]
Kari 1994	6/95	9/94	11.9		0.64 [0.22, 1.84]
Morales 1986	7/121	13/124	15.8		0.54 [0.22, 1.33]
Parsons 1988	0/23	1/22	0.9		0.13 [0.00, 6.52]
Schmidt 1984	5/49	4/31	6.6		0.77 [0.19, 3.15]
US Steroid Trial	32/371	34/372	51.7		0.94 [0.57, 1.56]
Subtotal (95% CI)		59/699	72/685	100.0	0.78 [0.54, 1.12]
Chi-square 2.12 (df = 5) Z = 1.33					

0.44–0.63). A secondary analysis, stratified by time interval between trial entry and delivery indicates that babies delivered between 24 h and 7 days after corticosteroid administration show a more marked benefit (typical odds ratio of respiratory distress syndrome 0.38, 95% CI 0.25–0.57). The odds ratios for respiratory distress syndrome in those delivered less than 24 h (0.70, 95% CI 0.43–1.16) after trial entry suggests a trend towards a treatment effect which does not attain statistical significance at the 5% level. Babies delivered more than 7 days after trial entry experienced a low level of respiratory distress syndrome and so the point estimate (0.41) for the odds ratio for respiratory distress is surrounded by wide confidence intervals (95% CI 0.18–0.98).

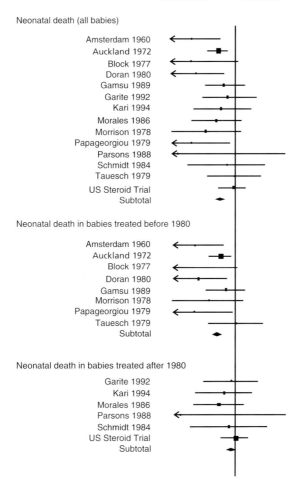

Fig 5.1 Effect of antenatal corticosteroids on neonatal mortality – graphical data representing odds ratios and 95% confidence intervals.

Contrary to opinions expressed in previous reviews of this subject (Roberton 1982), the beneficial effect of corticosteroids is not confined to babies delivered between 30 and 34 weeks' gestation. Seven trials supply data allowing a secondary analysis of the risk of respiratory distress syndrome in babies born at less than 30 weeks' gestation. This shows an unambiguous reduction in the risk of respiratory distress syndrome in this high-risk group (typical odds ratio 0.48, 95% CI 0.30–0.77). Only 35 babies, from 8 trials, developed respiratory distress syndrome after 34 weeks' gestation, so the typical odds ratio of 0.65 is surrounded by wide confidence limits (0.33–1.29) and is thus compatible with either a beneficial effect or a chance variation.

Effect of gender

There is no evidence from the few trials available that the gender of the infant determines the likelihood of benefit from antenatal corticosteroids. The typical

Table 5.2 Effect of antenatal corticosteroids on respiratory distress syndrome – numerical data

	Treated	Control	Weight %	Odds ratio	[95% Confidence intervals]
Respiratory distress syndrome (all babies)					
Amsterdam 1980	11/64	17/58	4.3		0.51 [0.22, 1.18]
Auckland 1972	49/532	84/538	23.1		0.56 [0.39, 0.80]
Block 1977	5/69	12/61	2.9		0.34 [0.12, 0.94]
Cararach 1990	1/12	0/6	0.2		4.48 [0.07, 286.51]
Carlan 1991	1/11	4/13	0.08		0.28 [0.04, 1.97]
Doran 1980	4/81	10/63	2.5		0.29 [0.10, 0.88
Gamsu 1989	7/131	16/237	4.2		0.45 [0.19, 1.05]
Garite 1992	21/40	28/42	4.0		0.56 [0.23, 1.34]
Kari 1994	35/95	45/94	9.2		0.64 [0.36, 1.13]
Morales 1986	30/121	63/124	11.5		0.33 [0.20, 0.56]
Morrison 1978	6/67	14/59	3.3		0.33 [0.13, 0.87]
Papageorgiou 1979	7/71	23/75	4.7		0.28 [0.13, 0.63]
Parsons 1988	3/23	3/22	1.1		0.95 [0.17, 5.21]
Schmidt 1984	17/49	10/31	3.4		1.11 [0.43, 2.87]
Silver 1995	43/54	34/42	3.0		0.92 [0.34, 2.52]
Tauesch 1979	7/56	14/71	3.4		0.60 [0.23, 1.52]
Teramo 1980	3/38	3/42	1.1		1.11 [0.21, 5.83]
US Steroid Trial	42/371	59/372	17.3		0.68 [0.45, 1.03]
Subtotal (95% CI)	292/1885	439/1850	100.0		0.53 [0.44, 0.63]
Chi-square 16.53 (df = 17) Z = 7.18					

odds ratio for males is 0.43 (95% CI 0.29–0.64) and for females it is 0.36 (95% CI 0.23–0.57).

Postnatal surfactant

The reduction in RDS associated with antenatal corticosteroid therapy may seem less important in the post-surfactant era. This is not the case. Apart from the evident medical and economic advantages of preventing rather that treating RDS, there is evidence that antenatal exposure to corticosteroids potentiates the response to postnatally administered surfactant. Table 5.3 summarises a secondary analysis of data from the Survanta (surfactant) trials showing that adverse neonatal outcomes are lowest in the sub-group of babies exposed antenatally to corticosteroids and postnatally to corticosteroids (Jobe et al 1993)

Intraventricular haemorrhage

Corticosteroid therapy causes a highly significant reduction in the odds of periventricular haemorrhage. Because of the potential confounding effect of the differential in neonatal mortality on the diagnosis of intraventricular haemorrhage, this outcome is analysed by diagnosis at autopsy (typical odds ratio 0.29 (0.14–0.61)and by ultrasound (typical odds ratio 0.48 (0.32–0.72).

This benefit may, in part, reflect a domino effect of the reduced incidence of respiratory distress syndrome, but the profound effect on intraventricular haemorrhage was seen in the absence of a reduction in the risk of respiratory

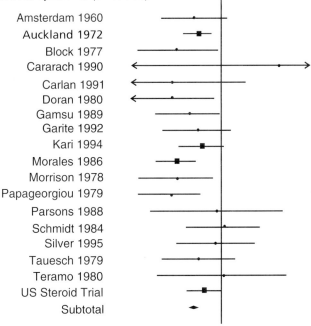

Fig. 5.2 Effect of antenatal corticosteroids on respiratory distress syndrome – graphical data representing odds ratios and 95% confidence intervals.

distress syndrome in the Garite et al (1992) trial and points to an independent benefit.

Necrotising enterocolitis

A marked effect (odds ratio 0.32, 95% CI 0.15–0.68) on the incidence of necrotising enterocolitis was reported in association with corticosteroid use in the US Collaborative Trial (Bauer et al 1984). Smaller trials (Kari et al 1994; Silver et al 1996) of poorer methodological quality do not show a benefit. The typical odds ratio is, therefore, 0.59 (95% CI 0.32–1.09). No effect on the incidence of patent ductus arteriosus or of bronchopulmonary dysplasia was seen. Only one trial reported on the incidence of neonatal jaundice and this result suggests a reduction in neonatal hyperbilirubinaemia in corticosteroid treated babies compared with controls.

Long-term effects on children

Lessons learned from medical history dictate caution in the use of hormonal preparations during pregnancy (Bibbo et al 1977) and underline the importance of long-term follow-up studies of children exposed to antenatal corticosteroids.

Children from three large trials have been followed in childhood (MacArthur 1982; Collaborative Group 1984; Smolders-de-Haas et al 1990).

Table 5.3 Effects of corticosteroids and surfactant: the Survanta prevention and rescue trials

	No Steroids No Surfactants	Steroids	Surfactant	Steroids + Surfactant
Number	566	46	555	57
Birthweight (g ± SD)	1021 ± 281	1013 ± 226	1013 ± 284	989 ± 201
Gestational age (weeks)	27.1 ± 2.6	27.5 ± 1.7	27.2 ± 2.6	27.4 ± 1.7
Air leaks (%)	23.3	13.3	11.3	1.7
Patent ductus (%)	44.2	21.7	47.0	27.6
Severe intraventricular haemorrhage (%)	22.6	10.9	24.6	6.9
Death from RDS (%)	19.6	6.5	7.2	0
28 Day death (%)	24.9	15.2	17.7	0

RDS = respiratory distress syndrome.

Follow-up data have been published on physical growth and development up to 3 years of age in children from the US trial (Collaborative Group 1984) up to 6 years of age in children from the Auckland trial (MacArthur 1982) and up to 12 years of age in children from the Amsterdam trial (Smolders-de-Haas et al 1990). None of these studies indicates that antenatal corticosteroid therapy has any effect on these parameters, nor is there any evidence that lung growth is affected. A variety of psychometric tests have been applied to survivors of these three trials at the ages already mentioned. No difference in the scores achieved by the two groups was found despite the fact that the preferential neonatal survival of children born after corticosteroid administration might be expected to have increased their risk of long-term neurological sequelae. The available evidence suggests that, if anything, antenatal corticosteroid administration may protect against neurological abnormality (hemiparesis, diplegia, quadriplegia, etc.).

Adverse maternal effects

Maternal infection

An increased risk of infection in mothers or an altered immunological response to an infectious process is one potential hazard of therapy. Eleven trials reported this outcome. The pooled odds ratio of 1.30 (95% CI 0.99–1.73) suggests a small increase in maternal infection which just stops short of statistical significance.

Maternal pulmonary oedema

Instances of pulmonary oedema have been reported in women being treated with corticosteroids in combination with intravenous fluids and other drugs, typically tocolytics (Stubblefield 1978). Case reports of such adverse events are important but lack denominators on which incidence rates can be based. Two cases of pulmonary oedema were reported by Morales et al (1986) in women who had both corticosteroids and magnesium sulphate – an incidence rate of 1.6%. Reports of cases of pulmonary oedema in women treated with corticosteroids and betamimetics are numerous. Katz et al (1981) reported an incidence rate of 5%.

Fluid overload, the presence of underlying heart disease and multiple pregnancy are significant risk factors (Finley et al 1984; King et al 1988). There appear to be no reports of the condition occurring in women treated with corticosteroids only.

Economic effects of antenatal corticosteroid therapy

Both the cost and duration of neonatal hospital stay are substantially reduced by antenatal corticosteroid therapy (Collaborative Group 1981; Garite 1992; Carlan 1991; Morales 1986). Using contemporary estimates of the cost of neonatal hospitalisation and of the number of babies at risk of respiratory distress syndrome, Avery (1984) estimated a potential annual savings to the US of $35 million. Present day estimates of the economic implications of antenatal corticosteroid therapy are altered by the availability of neonatal surfactant therapy, and by the possibility of using it either as prophylaxis or as treatment of respiratory distress syndrome. Only one trial (Kari et al 1994) reports on the effect of antenatal corticosteroid therapy on surfactant usage showing a reduced use of surfactant in treated babies (odds ratio 0.41 [0.19–0.90]). Mugford et al (1991) have attempted to estimate the cost implications of antenatal corticosteroid therapy in eligible patients based on a study of the cost of caring for neonates with and without respiratory distress syndrome at a variety of gestational ages. Using odds ratios for reduction in respiratory distress syndrome similar to those quoted in this chapter and, allowing for those deliveries that take place soon after admission to hospital, they estimate that a policy of intending to administer antenatal corticosteroids prior to delivery of all babies less than 35 weeks' gestation would result in a reduction in the average cost/baby of 10% with a 14% reduction in the average cost/survivor. Applied only to mothers of babies with gestational ages of less than 31 weeks, prenatal administration of corticosteroids would increase total costs by 7%, because of the greater cost of caring for babies of this gestation who would have survived, but this policy would have reduced the cost/survivor by 9%.

Preventing RDS in specific clinical situations

Preterm prelabour rupture of the membranes

Preterm prelabour rupture of the membranes (PROM) occurs in only 1% of all pregnancies, but precedes preterm delivery in 33% of babies born before 29 weeks (Hoekstra et al 1991). The proportion of preterm births associated with preterm prelabour rupture of the membranes is even higher if one excludes preterm births following elective preterm labour, twins and intrauterine fetal death. The effect of preterm prelabour rupture of the membranes on fetal lung maturation is controversial with some authors reporting an acceleration of fetal lung maturation and some disputing this (Wennergren et al 1986; Coustan 1987; Yoon et al 1973). The confusion here may relate to difficulties in choosing an appropriate control group with which to compare babies delivered preterm following PROM. Notwithstanding any effect that prelabour rupture of the membranes itself may have on fetal pulmonary maturity, the evidence derived from a meta-analysis of randomised trials of corticosteroid therapy following

PROM preterm indicates that the incidence of respiratory distress syndrome is substantially reduced by corticosteroid administration (typical odds ratio 0.44, 95% CI 0.32–0.60; Crowley 1992). There has been concern that the inherent susceptibility to infection of women with PROM might be increased or that the signs of infection might be masked, thereby, causing a delay in its diagnosis. Fifteen randomised controlled trials reported on the overall incidence of fetal or neonatal infection in corticosteroid cases compared with placebo-treated controls (Crowley 1997). No increase in perinatal infection was evident (typical odds ratio 0.82, 95% CI 0.57–1.19). However, the use of corticosteroids is associated with a small increase in the likelihood of perinatal infection when the membranes are already ruptured at trial entry (typical odds ratio 1.11, 95% CI O.50–2.43). The results of these meta-analyses support the use of corticosteroids to prevent RDS following preterm prelabour rupture of the membranes. A strategy of treating women with prelabour rupture of the membranes with corticosteroids followed by delivery 48 h later has been compared with expectant management in three randomized trials (Garite et al 1981; Iams et al 1985; Nelson et al 1985). This management is not associated with any advantage either in terms of either perinatal infection or respiratory distress syndrome.

The implications for clinical practice of this evidence are that women with preterm prelabour rupture of the membranes should be carefully evaluated for evidence of chorioamnionitis. In its absence, antenatal corticosteroids should be prescribed. The benefits for both mother and baby of perinatal antibiotic prophylaxis following PROM are currently being evaluated.

Maternal diabetes

Maternal diabetes predisposes the preterm infant to respiratory distress syndrome, especially when poorly controlled diabetes gives rise to fetal hyper-insulinism which blocks surfactant production by Type 2 pulmonary cells. Tight control of diabetes mellitus in pregnancy reduces the incidence of respiratory distress. The results of the randomized trials reviewed above do not permit an authoritative statement on the efficacy and safety of antenatal corticosteroids in women with insulin dependent diabetes as only 35 diabetic women were randomized across all available randomized controlled trials. Glucocorticoid therapy is likely to provoke insulin resistance and a deterioration in diabetic control which could potentially cause cortisol resistance in the fetal lung.

Maternal hypertensive disease

Hypertensive disease constitutes one of the main indications for elective preterm delivery. Respiratory distress syndrome is a major problem in the infants of hypertensive mothers and the evidence does not support the hypothesis that pre-eclampsia accelerates fetal lung maturation. Ninety women with hypertension were included in the first randomized trial of antenatal corticosteroid therapy (Howie & Liggins 1977). Twelve intrauterine fetal deaths occurred in 47 treated women compared with 3 among 43 controls (odds ratio 3.75; 95% CI 1.24–11.30). This understandably lead to a great reluctance to administer antenatal corticosteroid therapy to women with hypertension.

Subsequent analysis of these fetal deaths revealed that they occurred in women with proteinuria of greater than 2 g/day for more than 14 days. Women with hypertensive disease were included in 3 other trials (Collaborative Group 1981; Morrison et al 1978; Gamsu et al 1989) but only two of these (Collaborative Group 1981; Gamsu et al 1989) were able to provide a secondary analysis of intrauterine fetal deaths in this sub-group of women. No deaths occurred in either treatment or control arms of these trials. Observational data have not reproduced an excess risk of fetal death in association with corticosteroid therapy in women with pre-eclampsia (Lamont et al 1983).

Multiple pregnancy

Babies born preterm following multiple pregnancy are at increased risk of respiratory distress syndrome, with second twins being at particular risk. Two groups of investigators conducted a secondary analysis of the effect of corticosteroid therapy in reducing RDS in multiple pregnancies (Gamsu et al 1989; Burkett et al 1986). Burkett et al (1989) have quoted data from the Collaborative Group study to indicate that the effect of antenatal corticosteroid therapy is suboptimal in this situation. The odds ratio (0.79; 95% CI 0.33–1.91) quoted for the risk of respiratory distress syndrome in this group of babies is compatible with a treatment effect of equal magnitude to that seen in singleton babies. The apparently diminished treatment effect may represent a type 2 error, may be due to the subtherapeutic maternal plasma corticosteroid levels, (Burkitt et al 1986) or may indicate that the benefits of cortiocosteroid therapy are offset by the effects of perinatal hypoxia in second twins.

Single versus multiple doses of corticosteroid therapy

The course of threatened preterm labour is variable and unpredictable. All randomised trials of interventions, such as tocolysis and antenatal cortico-steroids, report significant numbers of both treatment and control subjects who remain undelivered 1 week or more following trial entry. Many women given antenatal corticosteroid therapy may even continue their pregnancies to term. The possibility arises of a late adverse effect of antenatal corticosteroid therapy on perinatal outcome. Such an effect was seen in association with antenatal thyrotropin releasing hormone (TRH). In a randomised trial of antenatal TRH plus corticosteroids versus corticosteroids alone, the worst outcomes were seen in the TRH-treated babies born more than 10 days after entering the study (Actobat Study Group 1995). There is no evidence from the randomised trials to suggest that a similar phenomenon occurs in association with antenatal corticosteroids. Animal studies are also reassuring (Jobe et al 1996).

In recent years, the practice has arisen of repeating treatment with antenatal corticosteroids in women who remain undelivered more than 1 week after treatment. The scientific basis to support this practice is weak. It is important to remember that all the evidence concerning the efficacy and safety of antenatal corticosteroids is based on trials of single courses of treatment. Babies delivered more that 7 days after trial entry showed a reduction in respiratory distress syndrome of a similar magnitude to those delivered earlier, however, the typical odds ratio is surrounded by wide confidence limits (0.41;

95% CI 0.18–0.98) due to the lower incidence of respiratory distress syndrome in both treated and control patients as pregnancy advances. Polk et al (1997) found no evidence that the benefits of betamethasone on lung compliance and lung volume in the neonatal lamb were enhanced by repeating treatment with betamethasone 1 week after initial treatment.

Repeated courses of antenatal corticosteroids could result in either immediate or long-term adverse effects not seen with single courses of treatment. Potential maternal risks include osteoporosis, immunosuppression and impaired glucose tolerance. There is a clear need for a multi-centre randomised trial to assess the risks and fetal benefits of single versus repeated doses of antenatal corticosteroids.

Key points for clinical practice

- Dexamethasone (24 mg) or betamethasone (24 mg) in 2–4 divided doses 24 h apart prior to preterm delivery accelerates the maturation of multiple organs and systems and reduces neonatal mortality, morbidity and the duration and cost of neonatal care.

- Antenatal corticosteroid therapy should be considered for all pregnant women from 24 to 37 weeks who are at increased risk of preterm delivery either because of preterm contractions or ruptured membranes or because of a fetal or maternal condition which makes delivery desirable.

- Antenatal corticosteroid therapy appears to be safe in the presence of maternal hypertension, however, the intrinsic fetal and maternal risks should be acknowledged. The need to complete the course of antenatal corticosteroid therapy should not take precedence over indications for urgent delivery in either the fetal or maternal interest.

- In cases of preterm prelabour rupture of the fetal membranes, the diagnosis of chorioamnionitis should be ruled out prior to the administration of corticosteroids.

- There is no scientific evidence to support the current practice of repeating antenatal corticosteroid therapy in women who remain undelivered 1 week following antenatal corticosteroid therapy. Research into the efficacy and safety of this approach is urgently indicated.

References

Avery ME 1984 The argument for prenatal administration of dexamethasone to prevent respiratory distress syndrome. J Pediatr 104: 240

Ballard R, Ballard P 1995 Scientific basis for antenatal steroid use. In: National Institutes of Health Report of the consensus development conference on the effect of corticosteroids for fetal maturation on perinatal outcomes. NIH Publication No 95-3784, Bethesda MD, pp 27–29

Bauer C R, Morrison J C, Poole W K et al 1984 Decreased incidence of necrotising enterocolitis after prenatal glucorticoid therapy. Pediatrics 73: 682–688

Bibbo M, Gill W B, Azizi F et al 1977 Follow-up study of male and female offspring of DES-exposed mothers. Obstet Gynecol 49: 1–8

Block M F, Kling O R, Crosby W M 1977 Antenatal glucocorticoid therapy for the prevention of respiratory distress syndrome in the premature infant. Obstet Gynecol 50: 186–190

Burkett G, Bauer C R, Morrison J C, Curet L B 1986 Effect of prenatal dexamethasone administration on prevention of respiratory distress syndrome in twin pregnancies. J Perinatol 6: 304–308

Cararach V, Sentis J, Botet F, De Los Rios 1990 A multi-centric prospective randomized study in premature rupture of membranes (PROM): respiratory and infectious complications in the newborn. In: Proceedings of the Twelfth European Congress of Perinatal Medicine, Lyon, France: European Congress of Perinatal Medicine

Carlan S J, Parsons M, O'Brien W F, Krammer J 1991 Pharmacological pulmonary maturation in preterm premature rupture of membranes. Am J Obstet Gynecol 164: 371

Chalmers I, Hetherington J, Elbourne D, Keirse M J N C, Enkin M 1989 Materials and methods used in synthesizing evidence to evaluate the effects of care during pregnancy and childbirth. In: Chalmers I, Enkin M, Keirse M J N C (eds) Effective care in pregnancy and childbirth. Oxford University Press, Oxford, pp 39–65

Collaborative Group on Antenatal Steroid Therapy 1981 Effect of antenatal steroid administration on prevention of respiratory distress syndrome. Am J Obstet Gynecol 141: 276–287

Collaborative Group on Antenatal Steroid Therapy 1984 Effect of antenatal steroid administration on the infant: long-term follow-up. J Pediatr 104: 259–267

Corbet A, Bucciarelli R, Goldman S et al US Exosurf Paediatric Group 1. 1991 Decreased mortality rate among small premature infants treated at birth with a single dose of synthetic surfactant: a multicentre controlled trial. J Pediatr 118: 277–284

Coustan D R 1987 Clinical aspects of antenatal enhancement of pulmonary maturity. Clin Perinatol 14: 697–711

Crowley P 1997 Corticosteroids prior to preterm delivery. In: Neilson J P, Crowther C A, Hodnett E D, Hofmeyr G J, Keirse M J N C (eds) Pregnancy and childbirth module of the Cochrane database of systematic reviews [updated 04 March]. Available in The Cochrane Library [database on disk and CDROM]. The Cochrane Collaboration; Issue 2. Oxford: Update Software; 1997. Updated quarterly

Crowley P 1992 Corticosteroids after preterm prelabour rupture of membranes. Obstet Gynecol Clin North Am 19: 317–326

Doran T A, Swyer P, MacMurray B et al 1980 Results of a double-blind controlled study on the use of betamethasone in the prevention of respiratory distress syndrome. Am J Obstet Gynecol 136: 313–320

Finley J, Katz M, Rojas-Perez M et al 1984 Cardiovascular consequences of beta-agonist tocolysis: an electro-cardiographic study. Obstet Gynaecol 64: 787–791

Gamsu H R, Mullinger B M, Donnai P, Dash C H 1989 Antenatal administration of betamethasone to prevent respiratory distress syndrome in preterm infants: report of a UK multicentre trial 1989. Br J Obstet Gynaecol 96: 401–410

Garite T J, Freeman R K, Linzey E M et al 1981 Prospective randomized study of corticosteroids in the management of premature rupture of the membranes and the premature gestation. Am J Obstet Gynecol 141: 508–515

Garite T J, Rumney P J, Briggs G G et al 1992 A randomized placebo-controlled trial of betamethasone for the prevention of respiratory distress syndrome at 24 to 28 weeks' gestation. Am J Obstet Gynecol 166: 646–651

Hoekstra R A, Jackson J C, Myers T F et al 1991 Improved neonatal survival following multiple doses of bovine surfactant in very premature neonates at risk for respiratory distress syndrome. Pediatrics 88: 10–18

Howie R N, Liggins G C 1977 Clinical trial of antepartum betamethasone therapy for prevention of respiratory distress in preterm infants. In: Anderson A B M, Beard R, Brudenell J et al (eds) Preterm labour: Proceedings of the Fifth Study Group of the Royal College of Obstetricians and Gynaecologists. RCOG, London, pp 281–289

Iams J D, Talbert M L, Barrows H, Sachs L 1985 Management of prematurely ruptured membranes: a prospective randomized comparison of observation versus steroids and timed delivery. Am J Obstet Gynecol 151: 32–38

Jobe A H, Mitchell B R, Gunkel J H 1993 Beneficial effects of the combined use of prenatal corticosteroids and postnatal surfactant on preterm infants. Am J Obstet Gynecol 168: 508–513

Jobe A H Polk D H Ervin M G et al 1996 Preterm betamethasone treatment of fetal sheep: outcome after term delivery. J Soc Gynecol Investig 3: 250–258

Kari A M, Hallman M, Eronen M 1994 Prenatal dexamethasone in conjunction with rescue therapy of human surfactant – a randomised placebo-controlled multicentre study. Paediatrics 93: 730–736

Katz M, Robertson P A, Creasy R K 1981 Cardiovascular complications associated with terbutaline treatment for preterm labor. Am J Obstet Gynecol 139: 605–608

Keirse M J N C 1984 Obstetrical attitudes to glucocorticoid treatment for lung maturation: time for a change? Eur J Obstet Gynaecol Reprod Biol 17: 247–255

King J F, Grant A, Keirse M J N C, Chalmers I 1988 Beta-mimetics in preterm labour: an overview of the randomized controlled trials. Br J Obstet Gynaecol 95: 211–222

Lamont R F, Dunlop P D M, Levene M I, Elder M I 1983 Use of glucocorticoids in pregnancies complicated by severe hypertension and proteinuria. Br J Obstet Gynaecol 90: 199–202

Lewis P J, de Swiet M, Boylan P, Bulpitt C J 1980 How obstetricians in the United Kingdom manage preterm labour. Br J Obstet Gynaecol 87: 574–577

Liggins G C 1969 Premature delivery of fetal lambs infused with glucocorticoids. J Endocrinol 45: 515–523

Liggins G C, Howie R N 1972 A controlled trial of antepartum glucocorticoid treatment for prevention of the respiratory distress syndrome in premature infants. Paediatrics 50: 515–525

MacArthur B A, Howie R N, Dezoete J A, Elkins J 1982 School progress and cognitive development of 6-year-old children whose mothers were treated antenatally with betamethasone. Paediatrics 70: 99–105

Morales W J, Diebel N D, Lazar A J et al 1986 The effect of antenatal dexamethasone on the prevention of respiratory distress syndrome in preterm gestation with premature rupture of membranes. Am J Obstet Gynecol 154: 591–595

Morrison J C, Whybrew W D, Bucovaz E T et al 1978 Injection of corticosteroids to the mother to prevent neonatal respiratory distress syndrome. Am J Obstet Gynecol 131: 358–366

Mugford M, Piercy J, Chalmers I 1991 Cost implications of different approaches to the prevention of respiratory distress syndrome. Arch Dis Child 66: 757–764

National Institutes of Health Consensus Development Conference Statement. 1995 Effect of corticosteroids for fetal maturation on perinatal outcomes. Am J Obstet Gynecol 173: 246–252

Nelson L H, Meis P J, Hatjis J M et al 1985 Premature rupture of membranes; a prospective, randomized evaluation of steroids, latent phase and expectant management. Obstet Gynecol 66: 55–58

Papageorgiou A N, Desgranges M F, Masson M et al 1979 The antenatal use of betamethasone in the prevention of respiratory distress syndrome. A controlled double-blind study. Paediatrics 63: 73–79

Parsons M T, Sobel D, Cummiskey K et al 1988 Steroid, antibiotic and tocolytic versus no steroid, antibiotic and tocolytic management in patients with preterm PROM at 25–32 weeks. In: Proceedings of the eighth annual scientific meeting of the Society of Perinatal Obstetricians. Society of Perinatal Obstetricians, Las Vegas, p 44

Polk D H Ikegami M Jobe A H et al 1997 Preterm lung function after retreatment with antenatal betamethasone in preterm lambs. Am J Obstet Gynecol 176: 308–315

Roberton N R C 1982 Advances in respiratory distress syndrome. BMJ 284: 917

Schmidt P L, Sims M E, Strassner H T et al 1984 Effect of antepartum glucorticoid administration upon neonatal respiratory distress syndrome and perinatal infection. Am J Obstet Gynecol 148: 178–186

Schutte M F, Treffers P E, Koppe J G et al 1980 The influence of betamethasone and orciprenaline on the incidence of respiratory distress syndrome in the newborn after premature labour. Br J Obstet Gynaecol 87: 127–131

Silver R K, Vyskocil C, Solomon S L et al 1996 Randomized trial of antenatal dexamethasone in surfactant-treated infants delivered before 30 weeks gestation. Obstet Gynecol 87: 683–691

Smolders-de Haas H, Neuvel J, Schmand B et al 1990 Physical development and medical history of children who were treated antenatally with corticosteroids to prevent respiratory distress syndrome: a 10 to 12 year follow-up. Paediatrics 86: 65–70

Stubblefield P G 1978 Pulmonary edema occurring after therapy with dexamethasone and terbutaline for premature labor: a case report. Am J Obstet Gynecol 155: 829–834

Tauesch H W, Frigoletto F, Kitzmiller J 1979 Risk of respiratory distress syndrome after prenatal dexamethasone treatment. Paediatrics 63: 64–72

Ten Centre Study Group 1987 Ten centre trial of artificial surfactant (artificial lung expanding compound) in very premature babies. BMJ 294: 991–996

Teramo K, Hallman M, Raivio K O 1980 Maternal glucocorticoid in unplanned premature labor. Pediatr Res 14: 326–329

Wennergren M, Krantz M, Hjalmarson O et al 1986 Interval from rupture of the membranes to delivery and neonatal respiratory adaptation. Br J Obstet Gynaecol 93: 799–803

Yoon J J, Harper R G 1973 Observations on the relationship between duration of membrane rupture and the development of idiopathic respiratory distress syndrome. Pediatrics 52: 161–168

Yusuf S, Peto R, Lewis T, Collins R, Sleight P 1985 Beta blockade during and after myocardial infarction: an overview of the randomised trials. Prog Cardiovasc Dis XXVII, 5: 336–371

Zoe J. Penn   Philip J. Steer

Preterm labour

Perinatal mortality in the UK has fallen by two-thirds over the last 30 years. Much of this fall has been due to the improved survival of preterm babies, largely brought about by advances in neonatal care. However, the incidence of preterm labour has not fallen significantly and neonatal intensive care is very expensive, placing an increasing (and increasingly questioned) burden on health service funding. In addition, survivors of extreme prematurity and their families may still face considerable long term morbidity in later life. Therefore, the accurate prediction, prophylaxis and management of preterm labour remains a challenge for all obstetricians.

AETIOLOGY AND PREDICTION OF PRETERM BIRTH

The aetiology of preterm birth is multifactorial, being associated with multiple pregnancy, ascending or systemic infections, pathology of the placenta, pathology of the uterus or pathology of the fetus. Each of these factors can operate singly or in combination. Some 30% of preterm births are preceded by prelabour preterm rupture of the membranes, 30% by idiopathic preterm labour and 30% by induction of labour or delivery for obstetric or medical reasons.

Sociodemographic variables

Sociodemographic variables are known to impact upon the incidence of preterm birth but the mechanism for this association is uncertain. Factors such as low

Zoe J. Penn MD MRCOG, Consultant Obstetrician, Chelsea and Westminster Hospital, 369 Fulham Road, London SW10 9NH, UK

Philip J. Steer BSc MD FRCOG, Professor and Head of Section, Academic Department of Obstetrics and Gynaecology, Imperial College School of Medicine, Chelsea and Westminster Hospital, 369 Fulham Road, London SW10 9NH, UK

socio-economic status, maternal age less than 16 years, being socially unsupported (single or separated), or cigarette smoking, are all independently correlated with preterm birth. However, the relative risk associated with each of these factors is only 1.5–2.0 and, therefore, the positive predictive value of each remains small. Other independent variables with even lower relative risks, which are nevertheless important from a public health point of view, include physical work during pregnancy (especially if it involves standing for more than 6 h per day), low body mass index (< 19), acute or chronic lung disease, poor social circumstances, stress in pregnancy and 'substance use' (especially heroin or cocaine). The relative risks associated with these factors are small. Ethnic origin is associated with considerable variation in the incidence of preterm birth defined as birth at less than 37 completed weeks of gestation, however, some of this variation is probably physiological rather than pathological. For example, babies of African ethnic origin are more mature than those of European origin at birth at any particular gestation and have, for example, about half the risk of respiratory distress syndrome (Richardson et al 1994). The incorporation of multiple factors into a composite risk scoring scheme has been attempted but has so far proved unsuccessful (e.g. Mercer et al 1996). Why this should be is not entirely clear. In addition, prevention strategies usually need to be targeted at specific aetiologies; for example antibiotics may be useful in preventing infection but seem unlikely to be of benefit in polyhydramnios – the reverse is true with indomethacin.

Cervical incompetence

Cervical incompetence is usually considered a rare cause of preterm labour, but some degree of cervical dysfunction may be involved in up to 17% of preterm labours. Recent work studying the biometry of the cervix suggests that cervical incompetence should not be considered a categorical variable (i.e. the cervix being either competent or incompetent) but rather as a continuum of competence from good to poor (Iams et al 1995). Guzman et al (1996) have reported static biometry of the cervix as well as active techniques of assessing the cervix and described both a transvaginal and transperineal approach to cervical visualisation that allows measurement of the upper and lower cervix and of any 'funnel' or 'wedge' above the internal os. Active assessment of the cervix involves the application of transfundal pressure down the axis of the uterus with the expectation that the pressure is transmitted transmurally, thereby increasing the intra amniotic pressure and stressing the upper cervix. Any degree of descent of the membranes or shortening of the endocervical canal as assessed by simultaneous transvaginal ultrasonography is judged to be a positive (adverse) response to transfundal pressure. It is not yet clear how well this positive response is correlated with the risk of preterm delivery. Iams et al (1995) showed that with cervical lengths less than the 10% percentile (2.5 cm) at 24 and 28 weeks, the relative risk of preterm birth was increased. The presence of funnelling, which was 5.9% and 8.6% at 24 and 28 weeks, respectively, was also a risk factor for preterm birth. The usefulness of this investigation as a screening test in a low risk population has not been prospectively evaluated and is likely to suffer from the same disadvantages as regular digital cervical assessment: that examinations at intervals of 4 weeks in the antenatal period are unlikely to be frequent enough to pick up early changes suggestive of an increased risk of preterm labour – more frequent assessments are impractical. Transvaginal ultrasound suffers from the additional disadvantage that it may prove even less acceptable to pregnant women than regular digital examinations.

Excessive uterine activity

Excessive uterine activity may play a part in a proportion of women with preterm labour. However, regular uterine activity monitoring has not been shown to be useful in reducing the preterm delivery rate in the general obstetric population (Iams et al 1987). A prospective evaluation of the signs and symptoms of preterm labour in the 7 days prior to the diagnosis of preterm labour showed that neither symptoms nor contraction monitoring strips indicated any significant changes more than 24 h before the diagnosis was made (Iams et al 1994). Roberts et al (1995) did find that the incidence of preterm labour was higher in women who experienced uterine irritability than in their general obstetric population (18.7% versus 11.0%), but the relative risk is lower than with many other high risk factors. This results in a high false positive rate which means that any prophylactic therapy, even if effective, is likely to have an unacceptable side-effect/benefit ratio.

Infection

Infection almost certainly has a role in many cases of preterm labour, but its mechanism of action is complex. Bacterial endotoxins and white blood cell cytokines have been implicated in changing the biochemistry of the cervix. Investigation of these biochemical changes has generated some promising diagnostic avenues. Fibronectin is a protein found in plasma and the extracellular matrix. It is thought to be involved in cell-to-cell adhesion. Fetal fibronectin is found in amniotic fluid and placental tissue and its presence in cervicovaginal secretions may be an indicator of loss of cervical and mucus plug integrity and may therefore signal impending preterm labour. These changes in the cervix may, in a proportion of cases, have been initiated by overt or subclinical urogenital infection. Preterm labour is associated with amnionitis in up to 70% of cases, but uncertainty remains as to whether this is cause or effect. Serial fibronectin assessment performed at 2 weekly intervals from 24 to 34 weeks gestation in asymptomatic women at high risk of preterm labour allows the identification of women at substantially increased risk of preterm delivery, both within 14 days of testing and prior to 37 weeks (Leeson et al 1996). The sensitivity and specificity of one positive swab for delivery prior to 37 weeks was 54% and 85%, respectively. Attempts to improve both sensitivity and specificity have led to its inclusion in risk scoring systems, combined with digital and ultrasonic evidence of cervical incompetence, suppression of fetal breathing, increased uterine activity, and the presence in the lower genital tract of tumour necrosis factor-alpha (TNFα), interleukin-6 (IL-6) and a variety of lower genital tract infections. If fetal fibronectin is assayed in the presence of signs and symptoms of preterm labour, but with intact membranes and a cervical dilatation of less than 2 cm, fetal fibronectin levels are more successful in predicting preterm birth before 37 weeks with a sensitivity of 63% and a specificity of 95.6% (Malak et al 1996). The exact role of fetal fibronectin in the prediction of preterm labour or delivery has yet to be defined but is likely to be within a combination of tests.

In the presence of ascending urogenital infection various pathogenic mechanisms are at work which may initiate premature labour. A variety of organisms, including *Bacteroides* spp. and Group B *Streptococcus* (GBS), produce proteases which may reduce the strength of the chorioamniotic membrane. In addition, *Escherichia coli* and GBS reduce the bursting pressure of the membranes in vitro. *Bacteroides* spp, anaerobic streptococci, and *Gardnerella vaginalis* all produce phospholipase A_2 in high concentrations. Phospoholipase A_2 is a precursor of prostaglandins which may play a part in the initiation of uterine activity. Phospholipase A_2 is stored in lysosomes in the fetal membrane cells and the destruction of lysosymes by bacterial toxins or inflammatory reactions may also liberate phospholipase A_2. Thus, bacteria in ascending infection all act by producing phospholipase A_2, endotoxins, proteinases and exotoxins which, in their turn, activate macrophages, leucocytes and monocytes which then synthesise cytokines. Bacterial endotoxins will stimulate the production of TNFα, IL-1 and prostaglandin E_2. These interleukins will, in turn, stimulate the arachidonic pathway and increase the production of prostaglandins. Cell mediated immune response is probably involved in the pathogenesis of a substantial proportion of preterm labours. The detection of many of these substances may be used in conjunction with fetal fibronectin to predict the occurrence of preterm labour, to increase the sensitivity of clinical markers of preterm labour and make therapy for preterm labour more targeted and logical (Inglis et al 1994).

The role of many pathogens in the aetiology of preterm labour has been investigated: the β-haemolytic *Streptococcus* (group B), *Ureaplasma urealyticum*, *Mycoplasma hominis*, *Chlamydia trachomatis*, *Trichomonas vaginalis* and *Neisseria gonorrhoeae* amongst others, but none has been definitively confirmed as having a causative role.

More recently, bacterial vaginosis has been suggested as the causative agent in up to 50% of cases of idiopathic preterm labour. Hay et al (1994) suggested that the odds ratio (OR) for preterm birth in the presence of bacterial vaginosis detected antenatally was 2.8. If bacterial vaginosis was detected before 16 weeks gestation, the risk of preterm birth and late miscarriage was increased with an odds ratio of 5.5. This effect was independent of other recognised risk factors such as previous preterm birth.

PREVENTION OF PRETERM BIRTH

Prevention of preterm birth implies either a recognised prevention strategy that can be applied to the whole population or that certain individuals at high risk of preterm birth can be identified and therapy targeted at this group.

Population strategies for the prevention of preterm birth have had limited success. The observation that preterm birth is more common in single and unsupported mothers led to the hypothesis that increased support in pregnancy might decrease the incidence of preterm birth. Boehm et al (1996) evaluated the role of daily telephone contact with mothers at risk of preterm labour in a randomised controlled trial and found that it did not affect the rate of preterm birth. There have been many such studies, some including nutritional support, health advice, assistance with fares and additional computerised risk assessment and ongoing and intensive education about the signs and symptoms of preterm labour. A meta-analysis of such studies confirmed that existing preterm birth prevention programmes have little benefit in reducing preterm birth and may only result in an increased rate of diagnosis of preterm labour (Hueston et al 1995).

In Continental Europe, regular cervical examination is carried out during the antenatal period to identify women with progressive changes in the cervix and thus identify those at increased risk of preterm labour. However, a recent randomised controlled trial of cervical examinations at every visit failed to show a significantly lower rate of preterm delivery in the 2803 women so examined (6.7%) compared with the 2799 women without such examination (6.4%) (Beukens et al 1994). Intermittent vaginal examinations at the usual intervals of antenatal visits are probably not sufficiently frequent to detect the short-term changes in the cervix that undoubtedly must herald preterm delivery. In support of this hypothesis, there was no evidence of increased interventions such as bedrest or tocolytics in the examination group; evidence that such strategies are effective is, in any case, lacking. An intervention study using transvaginal ultrasound of the cervical os and graded oral or subcutaneous tocolysis claimed that the rate of preterm birth was reduced in comparison to conventional care (Zalar 1996). In general, the usefulness of cervical assessment will be limited by the interval at which such assessments can be performed and the efficacy of any therapy that can be offered. Ultrasound of the cervix has been used most extensively to differentiate between threatened and actual preterm labour, to predict those who are more likely to deliver and as a guide as to those in whom more aggressive therapy might be warranted.

The use of home uterine activity monitoring continues to be a subject of controversy. The first reports by Katz et al (1985) were encouraging and suggested that the use of ambulatory tocodynamometry could result in the earlier detection of uterine contractions leading to preterm labour (Katz & Gill 1985, Katz et al 1986a,b). However, the first randomised controlled trial failed to find any significant benefits (Iams et al 1987, 1988). Some subsequent trials did find benefit (Hill et al 1990, Kosasa et al 1990, Watson et al 1990, Mou et al 1991) although others did not (Blondel et al 1992, Nagey et al 1993). The large CHUMS (Collaborative Home Uterine Monitoring Study) trial (Anonymous 1995), in which 1292 women were randomised showed no benefit. Meta-analyses have been equally divided. Grimes and Schultz (1992) came out against, whereas Colton et al (1995) came out generally in favour. Their meta-analysis was of six randomised controlled trials all performed in the US. The comparison made was between pregnancies with home monitoring of uterine activity and those given conventional care, controlled for the nursing contact factor. The outcomes studied were rates of preterm birth, preterm labour with cervical dilatation > 2 cm, infant referral to the neonatal intensive care unit and mean birth weight. Their analysis suggested that home uterine activity monitoring demonstrated significantly lower rates of preterm birth in singleton pregnancies, an increase in the mean birthweight in singleton pregnancies and a reduction in preterm labour combined with cervical dilatation of > 2 cm.

The most recently published randomised controlled trial in high risk pregnancies reported a 40% lower relative risk of preterm birth and a 50% lower risk of low birthweight and admission to the neonatal intensive care unit (Corwin et al 1996). These results seem promising but, in view of the lack of consistent evidence in the literature, the efficacy of ambulatory tocodynamometry needs further evaluation. The development of effective and safe techniques for suppressing uterine activity for more than 48 h might well transform the value of these 'early warning systems'.

Rather than waiting for the onset of premature contractions, and then trying to suppress them, a more fundamental therapy in appropriate cases would be to try and eradicate the urogenital infections which may invade the uterus from the genital tract. Trials of antibiotic therapy have been aimed at women with a high risk of preterm labour, with intact membranes and cervical dilatation less than 2 cm. In an unselected pregnant population, treatment of women with proven bacterial vaginosis with topical clindamycin cream successfully eradicated bacterial vaginosis but did not reduce perinatal mortality. However, in women with a preterm birth in the previous pregnancy who were found to have bacterial vaginosis in the index pregnancy and who were randomised to receive either metronidazole orally or a placebo, active treatment was shown to reduce admissions for episodes of preterm labour and reduce preterm birth, low birthweight and premature rupture of the membranes (Morales et al 1994). In a similar group of women at high risk of preterm birth with proven bacterial vaginosis, Hauth et al (1995) were able to demonstrate in a randomised trial that treatment with erythromycin and metronidazole decreased the rate of preterm birth. Clearly, as women at high risk of preterm labour become more specifically identified, the efficacy of any therapy in that group will appear to be greater.

If antibiotic therapy is applied to women in actual preterm labour, the results are more contradictory and the results of a randomised controlled trial are awaited. Norman et al (1994) showed that, in women with preterm labour and intact membranes, ampicillin and metronidazole significantly prolonged the pregnancy and decreased neonatal morbidity when used in conjunction with tocolytics and corticosteroids. On the other hand, Cox et al (1996) used antimicrobials (amoxycillin/clavulanic acid) in the treatment of preterm labour between 24 and 32 weeks gestation and found no reduction in the rate of preterm birth. They used neither corticosteroids nor tocolytics. The elucidation of markers for early ascending urogenital infection in conjunction with effective and well targeted antimicrobial treatment, in addition to tocolytics and specific anti prostaglandin agents is likely to make a real impact on the secondary prevention of preterm birth in the future.

A clearer picture may be emerging of the place of antibiotics in the presence of preterm prelabour rupture of the membranes (PPROM). Subclinical infection is a recognised cause of PPROM. In a systematic review of the trials (Mercer & Arheart 1995) of the use of antibiotics in PPROM, it was found that treatment was associated with a significant reduction in preterm delivery within one week of commencement of treatment together with a halving of the neonatal infection rate, although these benefits were not associated with a reduction in perinatal mortality. The optimal dose or duration of treatment is uncertain. The large UK multicentre trial (ORACLE) is comparing erythromycin, augmentin, or both against a placebo in the prevention of preterm birth. Since metronidazole, which is active against the organism(s) responsible for bacterial vaginosis, seems to be the most promising antibacterial so far, it will be interesting to see if the ORACLE trial shows any benefit to be gained from these antibiotics.

TOCOLYTIC THERAPY IN THE PREVENTION OF PRETERM DELIVERY

In many cases of preterm labour, tocolysis is inappropriate. Some are so near term that there would be little benefit in delaying birth. A high percentage have maternal or fetal indications for delivery and some are too advanced in labour or have vaginal bleeding, such that tocolysis would be contra-indicated. The remaining cases that are suitable amount to 6–20% of women in preterm labour. Tucker et al (1991) in a review of 13 119 singleton birth between 1982–6 in a US city reported 1445 preterm births (11%), but 630 (44%) of these were greater than 34 weeks gestation and treatment was therefore not indicated; 241 women had preterm premature rupture of the membranes and tocolysis was deemed inappropriate because of the risk of infection; in 238 women, birth was appropriate (26% had raised blood pressure, 22% had an intrauterine death, 16% had intrauterine growth retardation and 189 were 3 cm or more dilated); in only 147 was tocolysis possible, i.e. 5% of the of the 815 babies < 35 weeks, or just about 1% of the total births.

The best tocolysis would prolong pregnancy so that delivery would be expected at term. However, the results of meta-analyses indicate that β-sympathomimetics can be expected to prolong pregnancy by 24–48 h from the start of treatment and, therefore, have a limited effect on the total gestation (Lamont 1993). Kierse et al (1995) found the risk of delivery to be reduced from 27.9% to 10.6% and within 48 h, from 37% to 24%. The risk of perinatal death was reduced from 6.5% to 6%, which was not statistically significant. These hours may be crucial to the well-being of the neonate if they are used for transfer to a suitable tertiary neonatal unit and the administration of steroids.

The role of oral β-sympathomimetics as maintenance therapy after initial intravenous therapy for preterm labour has been evaluated in a meta-analysis of randomised controlled trials and has been shown to be of no benefit in reducing the incidence of preterm delivery, in increasing the interval to delivery or reducing the incidence of recurrent preterm labour (Macones et al 1995).

The use of intravenous β-sympathomimetics is a well established and proven intervention for the treatment of preterm labour. Important side effects include fluid overload and pulmonary oedema, myocardial ischaemia, hyperglycaemia, hypokalaemia and death. The search continues for newer and safer tocolytics with fewer side effects.

Indomethacin has been investigated as a tocolytic. It has important maternal fetal and neonatal side effects. Maternal side effects include peptic ulceration, gastrointestinal bleeding, thrombocytopaenia and allergic reactions. Fetal side effects include pulmonary hypertension due to premature closure of the ductus arteriosus, necrotising enterocolitis and intraventricular haemorrhage. Carlan et al (1995) performed a randomised double blind placebo controlled study of the use of oral sulindac after successful treatment of preterm labour with magnesium sulphate in 63 women and reported no reduction in the overall incidence of preterm delivery but an increase in the interval from the start of therapy until delivery or re-admission. The latter was achieved without observable adverse effects on the fetus. In comparison with intravenous ritodrine, indomethacin achieves similar results for delaying labour beyond 24 and 48 h but with the advantage of less maternal side effects (mainly headache, nausea and tinnitus; Morales et al 1989).

Calcium channel blockers, such as nifedipine, have been demonstrated to have a tocolytic effect in a few randomised trials (e.g. Glock et al 1993). Maternal side effects may be lower with nifedipine and its efficacy is promising, but important drug interactions have to be considered, particularly interaction with magnesium sulphate. The combination of the two drugs has been reported to cause neuromuscular blockade with respiratory failure (Snyder & Cardwell 1989, Ben-Ami & Giladi 1994), colonic pseudo-obstruction (Pecha & Danilewitz 1996), and severe vulval oedema (Trice et al 1996), particularly if the nifedipine is used in a non-sustained release form.

Oxytocin receptor blockers (such as atosiban) have shown recent promise (Goodwin et al 1994, 1996). Oxytocin levels in plasma, uterine oxytocin receptor concentrations and sensitivity to oxytocin have all been demonstrated to be higher in preterm labour. Studies comparing the efficacy of oxytocin receptor blockers in comparison with ritodrine are still ongoing and the results are awaited with interest. Atosiban's maternal side effects include nausea, headache, vomiting and chest pain, but failure of treatment due to maternal side effects is likely to be lower than ritodrine.

Preliminary reports suggest that glyceryl trinitrate transdermal patches may be useful as a tocolytic (Lees et al 1994) but randomised controlled trials are awaited.

CERVICAL CERCLAGE FOR PRIMARY AND SECONDARY PREVENTION OF PRETERM BIRTH

True cervical incompetence accounts for about 17% of preterm delivery. The role of cervical cerclage in the treatment of preterm labour was investigated in the MRC/MRCOG Trial published in 1993. This trial randomised 1,292 women with singleton and twin pregnancies to receive elective cerclage or not, the indication being clinicians' uncertainly about the value of cerclage in the management of their individual case. The overall preterm delivery rate in the 293 cases randomised was 28%; in the more important group delivering before 33 weeks, the rate was 13% in the group with cerclage compared to 17% in the group without ($P = 0.05$). The differences in the rate of miscarriage, stillbirth and neonatal death were not significant and the use of cerclage was associated with a doubling in the risk of postpartum pyrexia. The use of cervical cerclage will, therefore, prevent 1 preterm birth (before 33 weeks) for every 25 cerclages performed. The actual benefit of cervical cerclage in cases of cervical incompetence is probably greater than this trial would suggest, since the trial entry criteria were restricted to those women in whom the clinician was uncertain as to whether they would benefit or not. In those women where the diagnosis of cervical incompetence is more certain the magnitude of benefit is likely to be larger.

The place of emergency cervical cerclage is more difficult to define. A number of retrospective reviews of emergency cervical cerclage suggest some benefit in increasing the gestation. These have been largely uncontrolled and no randomised controlled trials are available.

The use of cervical cerclage, in cases where cervical incompetence has been suspected on the basis of examination or a history of surgery to the cervix in otherwise asymptomatic women with no pregnancy history suggestive of cervical incompetence, is unknown. The use of transvaginal ultrasound to define cervical changes that may indicate cervical weakness is attractive but has not been investigated. The prognostic significance of cervical shortening, funnelling and dilatation of the internal os and of the amniotic membranes, and efficacy of treatment with cervical cerclage, is uncertain.

ENHANCING LUNG MATURITY WITH CORTICOSTEROIDS

Crowley (1995) reviewed 15 trials including 3560 cases of preterm labour and the meta-analysis showed that the use of antenatal steroids reduces the chances of respiratory distress syndrome from 22.6% to 13.3% and the chance of neonatal death from 11.2% to 7.2%. However, many labours progress too quickly for a full course of steroids to be given or to take effect and probably only one half of the babies that could benefit theoretically are actually able to do so (see chapter 5 in this issue).

The available evidence shows that one course of steroids has a definite benefit on the maturity of the fetal lung. What is less certain is whether repeated doses of antenatal steroids are necessary. Animal models suggest that the repeated courses of steroids have the potential for impairing neurological development in the fetus. In addition the risks of osteoporosis and glucose intolerance occur in the mother. The published long term follow-up studies show no demonstrable developmental adverse outcomes in the child survivors of antenatal steroid administration. The current Royal College of Obstetricians and Gynaecologists Guidelines suggest that the use of antenatal steroids should be restricted to cases where the likelihood of preterm birth is high. The use of steroids in cases of PPROM will also reduce the incidence of respiratory distress syndrome without a significant increase in neonatal infection. The trials of antenatal steroid therapy were completed before the advent of neonatal lung surfactant. Whether lung surfactant and antenatal steroids have an additive value and whether lung surfactant will supplant or supersede antenatal steroid administration are uncertain.

The role of antenatal thyroid stimulating hormone (TRH) is under investigation and the trials so far have produced conflicting results. Thyroid hormones are known to influence lung development and TRH given to the mother readily crosses the placenta where the levels of thyroid hormone in the neonate will rapidly reach the levels achieved at term. There is some evidence that TRH given to the mother does not influence the incidence of respiratory distress syndrome (RDS) but may reduce the incidence of chronic lung disease (CLD), especially in babies weighing less than 1.5 kg (Morales et al 1989). It may be that combined therapy with TRH and corticosteroids will prove to be efficacious.

THE ROLE OF THE PLACE OF BIRTH

Tertiary care has been centralised in order to provide the highest quality of care for very preterm babies. Many of the interventions in the care of the mother in premature labour are designed primarily to allow '*in utero*' transfer, and permit delivery of the preterm baby in the tertiary centre. In the main, this has proved to be a successful policy, except that transfer prior to delivery may carry risks for the mother. In a study of '*in utero*' transfers in the Liverpool Region, UK, 66 of 190 women transferred in these circumstances had co-existing disease: 32 were receiving antihypertensives and/or anticonvulsants and 32 were receiving tocolytics. Postdelivery, 17 women needed prolonged intensive care (Ryan & Kidd 1989). Clearly, the condition of the mother should be taken into consideration as well as the optimum place of birth for the fetus.

OPTIMUM MODE OF DELIVERY

There is remarkably little evidence about the optimum mode of delivery of the preterm baby. The Cochrane review of this subject, by Grant (1995), reports that 'the data are not sufficient to justify a policy of caesarean delivery of the small baby'. The orthodox view is that the preterm vertex presentation may be allowed to deliver vaginally in the absence of any other indication for caesarean section but that the preterm breech will benefit from caesarean section. A series of small randomised controlled trials have been carried out in this area. Four were abandoned due to failure of recruitment, one was abandoned because of difficulties with eligibility criteria and one randomised reasonable numbers of women but then analysed the data by actual mode of delivery rather than the allocated mode of delivery. A systematic review of the data from these six randomised controlled trials, of babies presenting by the breech and by the vertex, found only 122 women to have been included (Grant et al 1996). The small numbers illustrate the difficulty of randomisation in this area of labour ward practice. The odds ratio of perinatal death was 0.32, in favour of caesarean section, although the confidence intervals overlapped zero. This is compatible with an important benefit to the very preterm baby from caesarean section. However, a policy of elective caesarean section was found to produce considerable morbidity for the mother (odds ratio 6.18, CI 1.27–30.14) and that this maternal morbidity was highly significant. In two cases, women had endotoxic shock, of whom one required an emergency hysterectomy. The other significant finding was that a policy of elective caesarean section will lead to a certain number of babies being delivered where the preterm labour was only threatened and would not have progressed. This in itself will have important implications for survival of the neonate. The results remain unconvincing and contradictory. In practice, clinicians will have to make individual decisions on the merits of each case and in close consultation with the parents and neonatal paediatrician.

In the delivery of the very preterm baby, the lower segment is often very poorly formed and adequate access to the baby will be difficult through a horizontal lower segment incision. Classical or De Lee caesarean section may be necessary to ensure the least traumatic delivery for the baby. Blood loss and post partum febrile morbidity are greater with classical caesarean section. The rupture rate in subsequent pregnancy is well known and has been reported to be as high as 6% (Halperin et al 1988). Moreover, the survival advantage for the fetus under 30 weeks seems to be negligible. Classical caesarean sections should be performed for the usual indications (poorly formed lower segment, transverse lie, etc.) and not as a universal panacea for the salvage of very preterm infants.

MONITORING LABOUR

The principles of fetal monitoring and fetal blood sampling remain the same in the care of the preterm baby in labour. Differences in the parameters between term and preterm babies include reduced short and long term fetal heart rate variability and slightly higher pH and pO_2 levels. Prolonged abnormalities in the fetal heart rate pattern will result in an increased incidence of respiratory distress syndrome and cerebral palsy in the survivors.

JUDGING THE APPROPRIATENESS OF CARE

The EPICURE study of all babies born in the UK between 22 and 26 weeks gestation in 1995 indicated that the handicap rates of surviving babies at these very early gestations can be as high as 50%. The improved survival of very preterm babies has lead to an increase in the rates of cerebral palsy; this may, in part, be due to multiple births secondary to the increase in rates of assisted conception. The conventional techniques of neonatal intensive care may have reached their limits and the survival rates, particularly the intact survival rates, have now plateaued. In the absence of new techniques in neonatal intensive care, or major advances in the primary or secondary prevention of premature delivery, the rates of preterm birth, perinatal mortality and cerebral palsy will remain the same. Interventions in relation to preterm delivery must be carefully evaluated and integrated into a psychosocial model in close collaboration with the general public to optimise the use of resources and increase satisfaction with maternity care.

Key points for clinical practice

- Prediction of preterm birth is imprecise and composite risk factor scoring has proved to be unreliable.

- Serial cervico-vaginal fibronectin measurements may prospectively identify women at risk of preterm birth.

- Tocolysis will only prolong gestation by a mean of 24-48 h.

- Cervical cerclage is an effective intervention for cervical imcompetence.

- Antenatal steroids reduce the incidence of respiratory distress syndrome and neonatal death.

- Vaginal delivery is conventionally preferred for the preterm vertex presentation.

- Caesarean section for the preterm breech may confer a small advantage on the neonate in terms of survival, but has considerable costs in terms of maternal morbidity.

References

Anonymous 1995 A multicenter randomized controlled trial of home uterine monitoring: active versus sham device. The Collaborative Home Uterine Monitoring Study (CHUMS) Group. Am J Obstet Gynecol 173: 1120–1127

Ben-Ami M, Giladi Y, Shalev E 1994 The combination of magnesium sulphate and nifedipine: a cause of neuromuscular blockade. Br J Obstet Gynaecol 101: 262–263

Blondel B, Breart G, Berthoux Y et al 1992 Home uterine activity monitoring in France: a randomized, controlled trial. Am J Obstet Gynecol 167: 424–429

Boehm F H, Glass C A, Reed G W 1996 Prevention of preterm birth. Role of daily telephone contact. J Reprod Med 41: 595–601

Buekens P, Alexander S, Boutsen M et al 1994 Randomised controlled trial of routine cervical examinations in pregnancy. Lancet 344: 841–844

Carlan S J, O'Brien W F, Jones M H, O'Leary T D, Roth L 1995 Outpatient oral sulindac to prevent recurrence of preterm labour. Obstet Gynecol 85: 769–774

Colton T, Kayne H L, Zhang Y, Heeren T 1995 A meta-analysis of home uterine activity monitoring. Am J Obstet Gynecol 173: 1499–1505.

Corwin M J, Mou S M, Sunderji S G et al 1996 Multicenter randomized clinical trial of home uterine activity monitoring: pregnancy outcomes for all women randomized. Am J Obstet Gynecol 175: 1281–1285

Cox S M, Bohman V R, Sherman M L, Levene K J 1996 A randomised investigation of antimicrobials for the prevention of preterm birth. Am J Obstet Gynecol 174: 206–210

Crowley P 1995 Corticosteroids prior to preterm delivery. In: Kierse M J N C, Renfrew M J, Neilson J P, Crowther C (eds) Pregnancy and Childbirth Module, In: The Cochrane Pregnancy and Childbirth Module, The Cochrane Collaboration (database on disk and CD-ROM) Oxford: Update Software

Glock J L, Morales W J 1993 Efficacy and safety of nifedipine versus magnesium sulfate in the management of preterm labor: a randomized study. Am J Obstet Gynecol 169: 960–964

Goodwin T M, Paul R, Silver H et al 1994 The effect of the oxytocin antagonist atosiban on preterm uterine activity in the human. Am J Obstet Gynecol 170: 474–478

Goodwin T M, Valenzuela G, Silver H, Hayashi R, Creasy G W, Lane R 1996 Treatment of preterm labor with the oxytocin antagonist atosiban. Am J Perinatol 13: 143–146

Grant A, Penn Z J, Steer P J 1996 Elective or selective caesarean delivery of the small baby? A systematic review of controlled trials. Br J Obstet Gynaecol 103: 1197–1200

Grimes D A, Schulz K F 1992 Randomized controlled trials of home uterine activity monitoring: a review and critique. Obstet Gynecol 79: 137–142

Guzman E R, Benito C, Hanley M 1996 Sonography in the evaluation of the cervix during pregnancy. Curr Opin Obstet Gynecol 8: 99–105

Halperin M E, Moore D C, Hannah W J 1988 Classical versus low-segment transverse incision for preterm caesarean section: maternal complications and outcome of subsequent pregnancies. Br J Obstet Gynaecol 95: 990–996

Hay P E, Lamont R F, Taylor Robinson D 1994 Abnormal bacterial colonisation of the genital tract and subsequent preterm delivery and late miscarriage. BMJ 308: 295–298

Hauth J C, Goldenberg R L, Andrews W W, DuBard M B, Copper R L 1995 Reduced incidence of preterm delivery with metronidazole and erythromycin in women with bacterial vaginosis. N Engl J Med 333: 1732–1736

Hill W C, Fleming A D, Martin R W et al 1990 Home uterine activity monitoring is associated with a reduction in preterm birth. Obstet Gynecol 76: 13S–18S

Hueston W J, Knox M A, Eilers G, Pauwels J, Lonsdorf D 1995 The effectiveness of preterm birth prevention educational programmes for high risk women: a meta-analysis. Obstet Gynecol 86: 705–712

Iams J D, Johnson F F, O'Shaunessy R W, West L 1987 A prospective randomised controlled trial of home uterine activity monitoring in pregnancies at high risk of preterm labor. Am J Obstet Gynecol 157: 638–643

Iams J D, Johnson F F, O'Shaughnessy R W 1988 A prospective random trial of home uterine activity monitoring in pregnancies at increased risk of preterm labor. Part II. Am J Obstet Gynecol 159: 595–603

Iams J D, Johnson F F, Sonek J, Sachs L, Gebauer C, Samuels P 1995 Cervical incompetence as a continuum: a study of ultrasonographic cervical length and obstetric performance. Am J Obstet Gynecol 172: 1097–1106

Inglis S R, Jeremias J, Kuno K et al 1994 Detection of tumour necrosis factor-α, interleukin-6 and fetal fibronectin in the lower genital tract in pregnancy: relation to outcome. Am J Obstet Gynecol 171: 5–10

Katz M, Gill P J 1985 Initial evaluation of an ambulatory system for home monitoring and transmission of uterine activity data. Obstet Gynecol 66: 273–277

Katz M, Gill P J, Newman R B 1986 Detection of preterm labor by ambulatory monitoring of uterine activity: a preliminary report. Obstet Gynecol 68: 773–778.

Katz M, Gill P J, Newman R B 1986 Detection of preterm labor by ambulatory monitoring of uterine activity for the management of oral tocolysis. Am J Obstet Gynecol 154: 1253–1256

Kierse M 1995 Beta-mimetics in preterm labour. In: Kierse M, Renfrew M, Neilson J, Crowther C (eds) The Cochrane Pregnancy and Childbirth Database. Oxford: Update Software

Kosasa T S, Abou-Sayf F K, Li-Ma G, Hale R W 1990 Evaluation of the cost-effectiveness of home monitoring of uterine contractions. Obstet Gynecol 76: 71S–75S

Lamont R 1993 The contemporary use of beta-agonists. Br J Obstet Gynaecol 100: 890–892

Lees C, Campbell S, Jauniaux E et al 1994 Arrest of preterm labour and prolongation of gestation with glyceryl trinitrate, a nitric oxide donor. Lancet 343: 1325–1326

Leeson S C, Maresh M J, Martindale E A et al 1996 Detection of fetal fibronectin as a predictor of preterm delivery in high risk asymptomatic pregnancy. Br J Obstet Gynaecol 103: 48–53

Mercer B M, Arheart K L 1995 Antimicrobial therapy in expectant management of preterm premature rupture of the membranes. Lancet 346: 1271–1279

Macones G A, Berlin M, Berlin J A 1995 Efficacy of oral beta-agonists maintenance therapy in preterm labour: a meta-analysis. Obstet Gynecol 85: 313–317

Malak T M, Sizmur F, Bell S C, Taylor D J 1996 Fetal fibronectin in cervicovaginal secretions as a predictor of preterm birth. Br J Obstet Gynaecol 103: 648–653

Mercer B M, Goldenberg R L, Das A et al 1996 The preterm prediction study: a clinical risk assessment system. Am J Obstet Gynecol 174: 1885–1895

Morales W J, Angel J L, O'Brien W F, Knuppel R A 1989 Use of ampicillin and steroids in premature rupture of the membranes: a randomised study. Obstet Gynecol 73: 721–726

Morales W J, Schorr S, Albritton J 1994 Effect of metronidazole in patients with preterm birth in preceding pregnancy and bacterial vaginosis: a placebo controlled double blind trial. Am J Obstet Gynecol 171: 345–347

Mou S M, Sunderji S G, Gall S et al. 1991 Multicenter randomized clinical trial of home uterine activity monitoring for detection of preterm labor. Am J Obstet Gynecol 165: 858–866

MRC/RCOG Working Party on Cervical Cerclage 1993 Final report of the MRC/RCOG multicentre randomised trial of cervical cerclage. Br J Obstet Gynaecol 100: 516–523

Nagey D A, Bailey-Jones C, Herman A A 1993 Randomized comparison of home uterine activity monitoring and routine care in patients discharged after treatment for preterm labor [see comments]. Obstet Gynecol 82: 319–323

Norman K, Pattinson R C, de Souza J, de Jong P, Moller G, Kirsten G 1994 Ampicillin and metronidazole treatment in preterm labour: a multicentre randomised controlled trial. Br J Obstet Gynaecol 101: 404–408

Pecha R E, Danilewitz M D 1996 Acute pseudo-obstruction of the colon (Ogilvie's syndrome) resulting from combination tocolytic therapy. Am J Gastroenterol 91: 1265–1266

Richardson D K, Torday J S 1994 Racial differences in predictive value of the lecithin/sphingomyelin ratio. Am J Obstet Gynecol 170: 1273–1278

Roberts W E, Perry Jr K G, Naef 3rd R W, Washburne J F, Morrison J C 1995 The irritable uterus: a risk factor for preterm birth. Am J Obstet Gynecol 172: 138–142

Ryan T, Kidd G 1989 Maternal morbidity associated with in-utero transfer. BMJ 229: 1383–1385

Snyder S W, Cardwell M S 1989 Neuromuscular blockade with magnesium sulfate and nifedipine. Am J Obstet Gynecol 161: 35–36

Trice L, Bennert H, Stubblefield P G 1996 Massive vulvar edema complicating tocolysis in a patient with twins. A case report. J Reprod Med 41: 121–124

Tucker J, Goldenberg R, Davis R, Copper R, Winkler C, Hauth J 1991 Etiologies of preterm birth in an indigent population: is prevention a logical expectation. Obstet Gynecol 77: 343–347

Watson D L, Welch R A, Mariona F G et al 1990 Management of preterm labor patients at home: does daily uterine activity monitoring and nursing support make a difference? Obstet Gynecol 76: 32S–35S

Zalar Jr R W 1996 Transvaginal ultrasound and preterm labour: a non-randomised intervention study. Obstet Gynecol 88: 20–23

James J. Walker

Advances in the management of severe pre-eclampsia and antihypertensive therapy

Since 1950, in the UK, a dramatic fall has occurred in the maternal mortality and morbidity from pre-eclampsia/eclampsia (Fig 7.1; Department of Health 1996). Compared to many other parts of the world, complications of pre-eclampsia are now relatively rare with the incidence of eclampsia in the UK of 4.9/10 000 deliveries (Douglas & Redman 1994). These changes coincided with introduction of the National Health Service and free, generalised antenatal care for all. The reduction of maternal morbidity does not result from the management of the acute disease, but mainly the screening and intervention that comes with organised antenatal care and the improved health of the community. This is the mainstay of obstetric practice and any change in the pattern of care must take this into account. Because of this service, most hypertensive women are diagnosed early in the disease process when intervention can reduce the incidence of severe disease and eclampsia. If antenatal care reduces the incidence of the condition, the experience obtained in its management by the majority of obstetricians is similarly reduced. Despite the reduction in the incidence of severe disease, pre-eclampsia/eclampsia remains one of the main causes of maternal mortality and morbidity in the UK (Department of Health 1996). The continuing importance of this disease and its relative rarity increases the need for protocols and guidelines for the acute management. Since the risk from hypertension and eclampsia are not the only problems encountered (Table 7.1; Duley et al 1995), these protocols need to address all aspects of the disease particularly pulmonary oedema which has now become the main cause of maternal death and morbidity (Table 7.2; Department of Health 1996).

As far as the baby is concerned, perinatal mortality and morbidity is related to placental insufficiency and to the complications of premature delivery (Friedman & Neff 1976). The level of maternal blood pressure is not a significant factor.

James J Walker MD FRCP(E) FRCP(G) FRCOG, Head, Department of Obstetrics and Gynaecology, St James University Hospital, Beckett Street, Leeds LS9 7TF, UK

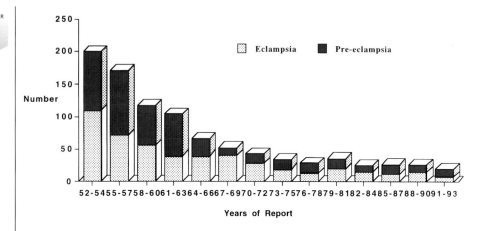

Fig. 7.1 The change in the number of maternal mortalities associated with pre-eclampsia/eclampsia since 1950.

Because of these multifaceted problems, the management of pre-eclampsia/eclampsia requires multiple, separately targeted, strategies.

SCREENING FOR HYPERTENSION IN PREGNANCY

It is important that effort is put to developing antenatal care systems that allow close vigilance and easy referral for all the pregnant women at risk. Greater attention should be made to those with specific risk factors such as family history, past history and pre-existing hypertension. Not only must the women be seen regularly, but action must be taken if an abnormality is found. This is the basis of the stepwise system of management of pregnancy hypertension (Table 7.3). The development of proteinuria, increasing oedema or the addition of clinical symptoms such as headache, visual disturbance or abdominal pain

Table 7.1 The maternal sequelae of severe hypertension in pregnancy

Major

    Cerebral vascular accident
    Haemolysis elevated liver enzymes and low platelets (HELLP)
    Convulsions
    Occipital lobe blindness
    Pulmonary oedema
    Aspiration syndrome
    Post partum haemorrhage
    Renal failure
    Liver failure and liver rupture
    Deep venous thrombosis

Complications of treatment

    Sedation and aspiration
    Fluid overload
    Caesarean section

Table 7.2 The causes of maternal death documented in the Confidential Enquiries over the last 23 years

Year	Cerebral	Pulmonary	Hepatic	Renal	Other
1970–72	25	8	5	3	6
1973–75	23	7	14	1	4
1976–78	21	4	5	0	3
1979–81	17	8	8	0	3
1982–84	21	3	0	0	1
1985–87	11	12	1	1	2
1988–90	14	10	1	0	2
1991–93	5	11	0	1	3
Total	137	63	34	6	24

increases the concern. Similarly, any pregnant woman with a presenting symptom of headache, abdominal pain, nausea or just feeling unwell should have her blood pressure checked and her urine tested for proteinuria as pre-eclampsia can present under many guises. Closer assessment can be carried out by open referral to an Antenatal Day Assessment Unit (ADAU; Walker 1993). The purpose of an ADAU is to investigate the significance of the hypertension and look for the presence of systemic disease. The majority of hypertensive women will have benign disease and can be managed totally as outpatients with no intervention apart from the monitoring of the mother and fetus. However, around 25% of the hypertensive patients require admission to hospital for further acute management (Walker 1987).

THE USE OF ANTIHYPERTENSIVE AGENTS

On first presentation, the hypertension is the primary risk to the mother and needs to be controlled. During the 1980s, there was an increase in the use of antihypertensive drugs amongst obstetricians (Hutton et al 1992) and this has been associated with a reduction in maternal and neonatal death from pre-eclampsia, particularly in maternal deaths related to cerebral pathology (Table 7.2; Department of Health 1996). The most recent meta-analysis of antihypertensive therapy in pregnancy has shown that early treatment reduces not only hypertensive crisis but also neonatal complications, such as respiratory distress syndrome (Collins & Duley 1994). Therefore, there is good evidence that early aggressive use of antihypertensive therapy is beneficial to both mother and baby. The meta-analysis does not compare different drugs. It probably does not matter which drugs are used as long as attendant staff are experienced in their use and they are safe. The most common drugs used in the UK are methyldopa, labetalol and nifedipine (Hutton et al 1992). No one therapy can control all patients and increasing doses of drug and combination therapies are often required (Walker 1996). Care should be taken not to reduce the blood pressure too quickly. The use of intravenous hydrallazine is associated with abnormalities of fetal heart rate (Visser & Wallenburg 1995a). Studies have suggested that this may be due to a combination of acute vasodilatation and a reduced plasma volume. Hydrallazine has been used successfully combined with plasma expansion but

Table 7.3 The stepwise management of pregnancy hypertension

Screening
> Screen women for the risk or signs of hypertension in pregnancy
> Monitor those at risk in a Antenatal Day Unit

Prior to delivery
> Regularly updated management protocols
> Early involvement of senior medical staff
> Stabilisation with antihypertensive drugs if required
> Prophylactic steroid administration if the pregnancy is under 34 weeks
> Consider the need for magnesium sulphate
> Continuing monitoring for signs of disease progression
> Delivery of the baby on the best day, the best way and in the best place

---

the results are no better than with antihypertensive therapy alone (Visser et al 1994). Oral labetalol and nifedipine appear to be at least as good as hydrallazine (Walker et al 1983, Visser & Wallenburg 1995a) without the need of plasma expansion and invasive monitoring.

In St James's University Hospital, Leeds (SJUH), the antihypertensive regimen used is oral labetalol with a starting dose of 200 mg tid (Table 7.4). This can be increased steadily to a maximum of 300 mg qid. If control is not achieved, 10 mg oral nifedipine retard is given twice a day and this is increased to a maximum of 60 mg a day. These drugs have been shown in animal experiments not to reduce placental or maternal peripheral blood flow in human pregnancy (Walker 1991).

Oral therapy can be used in acute hypertension management. Labetalol compares favourably with hydrallazine and is more predictable (Walker et al 1983). Nifedipine can also be used, but care should be taken, especially with sublingual usage, as sudden falls in blood pressure may occur (Impey 1993). The oral route is safer and as effective. The combination of nifedipine and magnesium sulphate was thought to be potentially dangerous due to synergism but many centres have extensive experience without problem with this combination.

Table 7.4 A suggested antihypertensive regime

Acute management
> Labetalol 200 mg orally repeat hourly until control is achieved

or
> Nifedipine 10 mg orally (not sublingual)

or
> Labetalol 50 mg by slow i.v. bolus

followed by
> Labetalol infusion starting at a rate of 60 mg/h doubling every 15 min
> until control is achieved or a maximum of 480 mg is reached

Starting daily dose for chronic therapy
> Labetalol 200 mg three times daily

increasing to
> Labetalol 300 mg four times daily

with the addition of
> Nifedipine retard 10 mg twice a day

increasing to
> Nifedipine retard 60 mg a day in divided doses

If oral therapy is not successful, intravenous labetalol 50 mg given by slow bolus followed by labetalol infusion will lower blood pressure in the majority of patients (Mabie et al 1987). Blood pressure control should be achieved prior to delivery, if at all possible, and especially before intubation for general anaesthetic before caesarean section as an acute blood pressure rise can occur (Ramanathan et al 1988).

The aim of therapy is to stop the rise of blood pressure and achieve a moderate fall but not to normalise the level. Therapy should be increased until a fall of around 10 mmHg is achieved and, once control is adequate, an increase in dosage may subsequently be required to maintain control. Severely pre-eclamptic/eclamptic patients often present acutely, often out of hours and all staff should be familiar with the management protocols and the aims of therapy.

USE OF ANTICONVULSANT AGENTS

Eclampsia is a common presentation in many parts of the world, but now a rare occurrence in the UK, occurring in 1/2,000 of all pregnant women (Douglas & Redman 1994). The majority of patients convulse once and do not convulse again (Duley et al 1995). The risks to the mother and baby from eclampsia appear to be more related to the degree of pre-eclampsia pre-existing the convulsion rather than the eclampsia itself. Evidence of prodromal signs, particularly headache and abdominal pain, are present in most patients who have a convulsion; however, about 20% of patients will convulse unexpectedly, often with normal blood pressure, and no sign is specific for the development of eclampsia (Duley et al 1995). The clinical assessment of hyperreflexia has never been demonstrated as an accurate predictor although widely used as such. However, it is of great value as a clinical measure of magnesium toxicity. If the reflexes are absent, magnesium toxicity should be suspected and the medication stopped.

If convulsions have occurred, anticonvulsants are required. A large multicentre study has shown that magnesium sulphate is superior to both phenytoin and diazepam (Duley et al 1995). Both the reconvulsion rates and maternal deaths were found to be significantly reduced by magnesium sulphate as compared to either diazepam or phenytoin. Although there is now no doubt what preparation to use (Table 7.5), it is important to note that no treatment will completely prevent seizures and reconvulsion rates vary between 5% and 20% (Duley et al 1995). Both the i.v. and i.m. regimens of magnesium sulphate, used in the study, were similar to those previously published. No evidence suggests that one route is superior to any other. Both regimens use a slow i.v. loading dose of 4–5 g magnesium sulphate that can be used to treat the convulsion. This should be given over 20 min as a faster bolus may produce cardiac arrest. There is no need to use diazepam initially to stop the seizure. Whether the i.m. or the i.v. maintenance dosage is used depends on the preference and facilities of the centre. The i.m. route has the advantage of ease of use, although i.v. therapy may provide better blood levels. One of the concerns many obstetricians have is the fear of magnesium toxicity. This study used clinical evaluation alone and showed that the toxicity did not occur; the side effects from magnesium were no worse than from diazepam and significantly less than those found with

Table 7.5 Anticonvulsant therapy to be used in the eclamptic patient

Either the i.v. or i.m. regimen of magnesium sulphate can be used
i.v. regimen
Loading dose of 4–5 g intravenously (i.v.) over 20 min Infusion of 1 g/h for 24 h
i.m. regimen
A loading dose of 4–5 g intravenously (i.v.) over 20 min 5 g into each buttock intramuscularly (i.m.) Further 5 g i.m. every 4 h (provided the respiratory rate was > 16/min, urine output > 25 ml/h, and knee jerks were present)
For recurring convulsion
A further 2–4 g given i.v. over 10 min
If magnesium toxicity is suspected: suggested by the absence of reflexes and repiratory depression
Stop magnesium infusion 1 g of calcium gluconate should be given

phenytoin. Therefore, using these dose regimens, there is no need to check magnesium levels or to have this facility available at all times. Magnesium levels are useful in the management of treatment failures.

The role of prophylactic magnesium sulphate in women with pre-eclampsia is less clear. If in doubt, it is probably safer to give magnesium sulphate than not, but it is not without risk and, in some series, the only deaths have come from magnesium toxicity. The risk of eclampsia in women with pre-eclamspia is probably around 1/200 and there is no evidence that magnesium will reduce this (Moodley & Moodley 1994). However, if a prophylactic anticonvulsant is to be used, magnesium sulphate is the drug of choice (Lucas et al 1995).

CONTINUATION OF THE PREGNANCY

Once the patient has been stabilised, a plan of action should be made by a senior doctor. After convulsion has occurred, continuation of pregnancy cannot be justified in the UK setting, but there is no urgency to deliver the baby. The mother requires to be assessed and stabilised and the fetus may be acutely affected but will quickly recover. A carefully planned delivery over the next few hours should be carried out, so that all the relevant carers are in place and ready to look after the mother and baby.

In the absence of convulsions, prolongation of the pregnancy is possible, in most cases, for an average of 15 days (Walker 1991). This has been shown to improve the outcome for the baby without detriment to the mother. Rushing the delivery in the maternal interest is not of benefit to the mother and can lead to increased morbidity for the baby, as the gestation at delivery influences the outcome of the baby more than any other parameter (Friedman & Neff 1976). However, the mother's condition must be stable so that prolongation of pregnancy does not jeopardise her life. The situation should be constantly reassessed and the management plan regularly reviewed by a senior doctor

Table 7.6 The management plan for the continuing care of the women with severe pre-eclampsia

Maternal management

> Keep blood pressure controlled with antihypertensive drugs
> Use the average of four blood pressure readings for monitoring
> At least twice weekly serum uric acid, platelet count and
>   liver function tests
> Test for the presence of proteinuria ± quantification

Fetal management

> Prophylactic steroids given if the gestation is below 34 weeks
> An initial ultrasound assessment of fetal weight
> Doppler ultrasound assessment of umbilical blood flow velocity
>   twice a week
> Daily cardiotocographs
> At least twice weekly ultrasound for liquor volume

Care after delivery

> Continuing close monitoring of the mother within a closely
>   monitored environment
> Careful fluid balance and use of diuretics if required
> Reduction of antihypertensive agents as indicated
> Stopping anticonvulsants after 48 h if stable

Follow-up

> Long term follow-up to make sure that the blood pressure resolves
> Discussion concerning what has gone on and the significance
>   for the future

(Table 7.6). A woman who is stable may not remain so. The plan of management is more along the lines of 'not needing delivery now' rather than 'lets deliver her tomorrow'.

If delivery within the next few days is thought to be a possibility and the gestation is less than 34 weeks, prophylactic steroids should be given to encourage fetal lung maturity. Dexamethasone 12 mg given i.m., twice, 12 h apart is the regimen used in SJUH. The aim is to prolong the pregnancy for at least 48 h to achieve maximum effect although, if the delivery is earlier, some benefit will be gained.

Delivery should be carried out if there is strong maternal or fetal reasons prior to 48 h being completed. After 48 h, if a further prolongation for more than a week is not thought to be achievable, delivery should be carried out when the mother is stable and the baby has received maximum benefit from the prophylactic steroids. Transfer of the mother prior to delivery may be necessary for the optimum care for mother or her newly born, possibly premature baby.

ASSESSMENT OF THE HYPERTENSIVE DISORDER

Antihypertensive therapy lowers blood pressure and should not be expected to do anything else. It is important to emphasise that, if pregnancy is going to be continued, close monitoring of the mother is required using blood pressure monitoring, proteinuria, maternal urates (Redman et al 1976) and platelet

Recent Advances in Obstetrics and Gynaecology 20

count (Redman et al 1978) to monitor disease progression. Fetal well-being should be followed using cardiotocography and ultrasound for fetal growth, umbilical artery Doppler velocity wave forms and liquor volume estimations.

Blood pressure measurement

Abnormality of blood pressure is the primary diagnostic criteria in pregnancy hypertension. However, blood pressure is variable and can fluctuate on a minute-to-minute basis (Halligan et al 1995). Therefore, a single elevated blood pressure reading needs to be confirmed, preferably by the average of 4–5 readings before it is used in management decisions (Walker 1996), Automatic blood pressure recorders often measure diastolic blood pressure several mmHg lower than the normal sphygmomanometer and this should be taken into account when patients are on these machines in the acute situation.

The presence of hypertension can, in itself, put the mother at increased risk of cerebral vascular accident but the systemic involvement is the hallmark of pre-eclampsia and the hypertension is part of the progressive disorder. The major morbidity factors like renal failure, liver failure and pulmonary oedema are associated with these systemic changes.

Proteinuria

The testing of the urine for proteinuria is the simplest and most readily available test. The association of proteinuria with eclamspia has been known for over 100 years. Urine stick testing will overestimate the presence of proteinuria and this should always be confirmed by a 24 h collection for quantification. The importance of proteinuria is that it helps to confirm the diagnosis of pre-eclampsia with the concomitant increased risks (Friedman & Neff 1976). Once protein is present, changes in the amount does not reflect increasing severity of disease and, on its own, should not influence the decision to deliver. Lowering blood pressure is associated with a reduction of the proteinuria and similarly this does not imply the risks have diminished.

Uric acid measurement

Uric acid rises in pre-eclampsia and is a better predictor of fetal death than blood pressure itself (Redman et al 1976). The reason for the rise in uric acid is not totally clear, but is partly due to impairment of renal tubular function reducing excretion. This renal involvement is probably due to ischaemia of the renal medulla and is not a sign of renal failure. Some of the rise in uric acid is due to increased production secondary to tissue damage from ischaemia. Therefore, uric acid is a surrogate marker of tissue involvement in pre-eclampsia and a useful adjunct to other monitoring tests. Serial testing is of particular benefit as a rising level is indicative of disease progression and increased risk.

Platelet count

Platelet counts fall in pre-eclampsia and are associated with progressive disease and worsening outcome (Redman et al 1978). In recent years, the combination of haemolysis, elevated liver enzymes and low platelets has been described as the HELLP syndrome (Weinstein 1982). Although this is undoubtedly associated with increased maternal and fetal morbidity, it is not a new phenomenon but more a new description of previously described pathological findings. Serial samples should be taken to watch for the developing trends. Falling counts are of concern and can give some guidance about the timing of the delivery. If a platelet count of below 100 is found, a full coagulation screen, blood film and LFTs should be carried out as this can give further information about the progression of the disease and the future maternal risk (Roberts et al 1994). The presence of HELLP syndrome is of concern, particularly with severe thrombocytopenia, and usually implies the need for delivery, although cases of conservative management have been reported (Visser & Wallenburg 1995b).

If the platelet count is higher than 100, then it is unlikely that the coagulation screen will be abnormal. In these cases, there is no need to carry out a coagulation screen and no risk from epidural analgesia.

Liver function tests

These are not true liver function tests but are measurements of enzymes contained largely in liver cells. Disruption of these cells leads to release of the enzymes into the circulation and, hence, a rise in levels. The most sensitive change is seen in Ast but there is also a rise in Alt which is easier to measure in an emergency laboratory. A rise in liver enzymes is always significant and needs to be followed carefully. Severe liver impairment is associated with liver rupture which is rare but can be fatal.

In pre-eclampsia, DIC is a rare complication in the absence of abruption. The coagulation defects seen are usually related to HELLP syndrome with liver function impairment leading to an intrinsic coagulation defect.

FETAL ASSESSMENT

The assessment of the maternal disease does not give accurate information about the well-being of the baby. Once the mother is stabilised, specific fetal assessment tests should be carried out. The main risks to the fetus are placental insufficiency and prematurity. Investigations are directed at the assessment of fetal health, fetal growth and placental blood flow.

Cardiotocography

Cardiotocography is the mainstay of fetal monitoring in most units. It gives information concerning the fetal well-being at that time but has little predictive value. It can be repeated regularly and easily without need of expensive equipment or highly skilled personnel and can be particularly reassuring to the mother herself. Although tracings from below 30 weeks can be misleading, it is the change in the trace that is most informative.

As long as the tracing is reactive with good variability, all would appear to be well with the fetus. If accelerations or variability are lost, then this would imply deterioration in the fetal state and the presence of decelerations must be seen as sinister at any time.

Cardiotocography should be repeated as often as thought necessary depending on the severity of the situation; daily tracings in women hospitalised on antihypertensive therapy would seem sensible.

Fetal ultrasound assessment

Ultrasound assessment of fetal size is valuable as a one-off measurement to assess the fetal growth at the time of the initial admission and provides useful information about the expected fetal weight to the paediatricians if the baby is to be delivered. Expected fetal weight allows estimates of the chances of survival of the baby that can be used in discussion with the parents about management decisions. Serial growth studies are of less value as they should not be done more often than every 2 weeks and the average length of prolongation of pregnancy in severe disease is only 15 days (Sibai et al 1994).

Liquor volume estimation is of less value in the earlier gestations where close fetal assessment is usually being carried out (Schucker et al 1996). Reduced liquor volume is associated with fetal growth restriction and serial estimations are of value as reducing liquor volume can be indicative of increasing fetal compromise.

Placental blood flow

Reduced uterine artery Doppler is associated with an increased incidence of placental insufficiency and pre-eclampsia (Bower et al 1993). It can be used as a screening test in normal pregnancy. In established disease, it is of less value (Hanretty et al 1988) but it still can give an indication whether fetal growth restriction is likely to be present.

Umbilical Doppler artery assessment is of greater value (Fairlie 1991) where serial investigations can be used to follow pregnancies under treatment. If end diastolic flow is present, therapy can be continued in an attempt to prolong the pregnancy, as the baby will normally be able to tolerate prolongation of pregnancy and antihypertensive therapy (Fairlie 1991).

Monitoring protocol

Although single tests can give information about the maternal and fetal well-being, serial sampling adds to this by demonstrating the rate of progression. Proteinuria should be quantified and serial uric acid levels and platelet counts taken, at least on a twice weekly basis. A cardiotocograph should be carried out daily and at least twice weekly ultrasound estimation of liquor volume and umbilical artery Doppler velocity wave forms should been done. A particular area of concern is that of liver impairment and the development of HELLP syndrome. Liver function tests or a minimum of at least the Alt or Ast should be carried out on a twice weekly basis. This, along with the platelet count, will screen for early signs. If the liver function tests and the platelet counts remain normal, HELLP syndrome and coagulation abnormalities are not present. If HELLP syndrome is thought to be developing, a full coagulation screen and a blood film, looking for fragmented red cells and evidence of haemolysis, should be carried out.

PLANNING THE DELIVERY

Delivery is the ultimate cure of pre-eclampsia. The timing of delivery effects the outcome for both mother and baby. However, most maternal deaths occur postpartum. A rushed delivery in an unstable patient probably adds to her risk rather than reduces it. A delay in delivery in a sick patient may be treacherous. Any transfer of the women should be at an early stage, while she is stable and communication should be between senior doctors in each hospital.

If delivery has been decided upon before 32 weeks, it should be carried out by elective caesarean section, unless this is more dangerous for the mother. A long induced labour can add to the problems of fluid overload and the difficulties of blood pressure control. After 34 weeks, a vaginal delivery is aimed at and the chances of this being successful have been greatly increased by the use of vaginal prostaglandins. Antihypertensive therapy is continued throughout labour to help control blood pressure.

The choice of anaesthetic in caesarean section is important. General anaesthetic can add to the risk to the mother since intubation and extubation can cause a rise in both systolic and diastolic blood pressure as well as heart rate (Ramanathan et al 1988). An epidural or spinal block would seem far safer allowing delivery to take place with the patient awake and speeds recovery. Care should be taken that the fluid load is kept to a minimum and a colloid solution may be preferable to crystalline which passes quickly across the capillaries into the interstitial space.

During labour, an epidural is also beneficial but not to control blood pressure as this is a pathological effect rather than a physiological one. By allowing adequate pain relief, it can stop the rise in blood pressure often associated with labour. It also allows a planned delivery and easy transition to caesarean section if this is thought necessary. There is no reason to shorten routinely the second stage of labour by instrumental delivery as long as the mother is pushing well and remains stable.

After delivery, drugs containing ergometrine should not be used in the third stage of labour, i.v. syntocinon is the preferred option.

CARE AFTER DELIVERY

Continued close monitoring is required in a suitable environment. An initial improvement may be seen, but most will worsen again to some degree within 48 h. Women with severe disease should be kept in the high dependency areas and not be transferred to the postnatal wards until parameters begin to return to normal.

The main cause of maternal mortality in this condition is now pulmonary oedema (Table 7.2; Department of Health 1996) and is probably due to various underlying mechanisms within the pre-eclamptic woman, including a low albumin and an increased capillary leak. Post-delivery, a relative oliguria is not uncommon, occurring in about 30% of patients with severe disease. This does not require therapy as urine output will recover in its own time. Renal impairment is a rare complication (Table 7.2) and can usually be managed easily. If there is any doubt about renal function, urinary osmolality should be checked. If the urine is concentrated, then renal function is satisfactory and the reduced output is related to a reduced renal perfusion which will improve gradually. If it is not, then renal failure is present and a renal failure regimen should be put in place. There is no evidence, however, that oliguria, especially in the presence of concentrated urine, leads to renal failure. Fluid challenges are potentially dangerous in pre-eclampsia as much of the fluid will be lost from the vessels into the interstitial fluid aggravating the existing tissue oedema. If fluid is to be given, colloid should be used up to a maximum of 500 ml and not repeated unless an adequate urinary response has been achieved.

Invasive monitoring is usually not necessary and central venous pressure (CVP) lines can be misleading (Cotton et al 1985). In pre-eclampsia, pulmonary oedema, because of increased interstitial fluid, can occur in the presence of a low CVP. If a central line is used, it is important that the CVP level is not higher than 5 mmHg or 7 cm H_2O. If the CVP is higher than this, diuretics should be used to reduce it. One of the best methods of assessing pulmonary oedema is continuous measurement of oxygen saturation using a pulse-oximeter. It is far safer and sensible to run a patient 'dry' and restrict intravenous fluids than to run the risk of pulmonary overload. Total fluid replacement should not exceed an hourly rate of 80 ml. Most of the problems of fluid overload begin around 16 h after delivery with severe problems occurring at 24–48 h. This is associated with a failure of the normal postpartum diuresis. If the patient is in positive balance or has evidence of pulmonary oedema, 40 mg of frusemide should be given which usually produces a positive response. This can be followed by 20 g of mannitol to reduce tissue fluid and the probability of pulmonary and cerebral oedema, increase oxygen saturation, and improve blood pressure control.

Therefore, after delivery, management should be aimed at maintaining blood pressure control and carefully monitoring the fluid balance. If convulsions occur, anticonvulsant therapy can be added. The majority of postnatal convulsions occur within the first 24 h so anticonvulsant therapy is usually continued for 48 h post-delivery. If the patient is well, especially if prophylactic anticonvulsant is being used in the absence of any convulsions, this therapy can be stopped within 24 h.

Antihypertensive therapy should be reduced after delivery depending on the blood pressure. There may be a significant drop within the first 24 h with a rise again after 48 h. Antihypertensive drugs may be necessary for some weeks after delivery.

FOLLOW-UP

The patient should be followed up until normal blood pressure has returned. The diagnosis of the underlying cause of the hypertension in pregnancy may not be apparent until after the pregnancy is over. If blood pressure has not returned to normal by 6 postpartum weeks, the patient should be referred for further investigation as the cause is unlikely to have been pre-eclampsia.

A postnatal visit should be carried out to assess the recovery of the woman and to discuss the significance of what happened and what might happen in the future.

Key points for clinical practice

- Be aware of the signs of developing pre-eclamspia and refer to Antenatal Day Units for assessment.

- Develop protocols agreed by the obstetricians, anaesthetists and midwives and regularly discuss and update them.

- Use antihypertensive drugs to lower the blood pressure and stabilise the mother prior to transfer or delivery.

- Continue to monitor the mother and fetus for signs of disease progression.

- Use antenatal steroids to mature fetal lungs if required and deliver in the best way on the best day.

- Continue vigilance after delivery, taking particular care with fluid balance.

- Follow-up after delivery to make sure the mother returns to normal.

References

Bower S, Bewley S, Campbell S 1993 Improved prediction of pre-eclampsia by 2-stage screening of uterine arteries using the early diastolic notch and color Doppler imaging. Obstet Gynecol 82: 78–83

Collins R, Duley L 1994 Any antihypertensive therapy for pregnancy hypertension. In: Enkin M W, Keirse M J N C, Renfrew M J, Neilson J P (eds) Pregnancy and childbirth module, Cochrane Database of Systematic Reviews: Review No. 04426, Disk Issue 1. Cochrane Updates on Disk, Oxford

Cotton D B, Gonik B, Dorman K, Harrist R 1985 Cardiovascular alterations in severe pregnancy-induced hypertension: relationship of central venous pressure to pulmonary capillary wedge pressure. Am J Obstet Gynecol 151: 762–764

Department of Health, Welsh Office, Scottish Home and Health Department, Department of Health and Social Security, Northern Ireland 1996 Report on confidential inquiries into maternal deaths in the United Kingdom 1991–93. HMSO, London

Douglas K A, Redman C W G 1994 Eclampsia in the United Kingdom. BMJ 309: 1395–1400

Duley L, Carroli G, Belizan J et al 1995 Which anticonvulsant for women with eclampsia – evidence from the collaborative eclampsia trial. Lancet 345: 1455–1463

Fairlie F M 1991 Doppler flow velocimetry in hypertension in pregnancy. Clin Perinatol 18: 749–778

Friedman E A, Neff R K 1976 Pregnancy, outcome as related to hypertension, edema, and proteinuria. Perspect Nephrol Hypertens 5: 13–22

Halligan A, Shennan A, Thurston H, deSwiet M, Taylor D 1995 Ambulatory blood-pressure measurement in pregnancy – the current state-of-the-art. Hypertens Pregnancy 14: 1–16

Hanretty K P, Whittle M J, Rubin P C 1988 Doppler uteroplacental waveforms in pregnancy-induced hypertension: a re-appraisal. Lancet i: 850–852

Hutton J D, James D K, Stirrat G M, Douglas K A, Redman C W G 1992 Management of severe pre-eclampsia and eclampsia by UK consultants. Br J Obstet Gynaecol 99: 554–556

Impey L 1993 Severe hypotension and fetal distress following sublingual administration of nifedipine to a patient with severe pregnancy-induced hypertension at 33 weeks. Br J Obstet Gynaecol 100: 959–961

Lucas M J, Leveno K J, Cunningham F G 1995 A comparison of magnesium-sulfate with phenytoin for the prevention of eclampsia. N Engl J Med 333: 201–205

Mabie W C, Gonzalez A R, Sibai B M, Amon E 1987 A comparative trial of labetalol and hydralazine in the acute management of severe hypertension complicating pregnancy. Obstet Gynecol 70: 328–333

Moodley J, Moodley V V 1994 Prophylactic anticonvulsant therapy in hypertensive crises of pregnancy – the need for a large, randomized trial. Hypertens Pregnancy 13: 245–252

Ramanathan J, Sibai B M, Mabie W C, Chauhan D, Ruiz A G 1988 The use of labetalol for attenuation of the hypertensive response to endotracheal intubation in preeclampsia. Am J Obstet Gynecol 159: 650–654

Redman C W, Beilin L J B, Wilkinson B H 1976 Plasma urate measurements in predicting fetal death in hypertensive pregnancy. Lancet i: 1370–1374

Redman C W, Bonnar J, Beilin L 1978 Early platelet consumption in pre-eclampsia. BMJ 1: 467–469

Roberts W E, Perry K G, Woods J B, Files J C, Blake P G, Martin J N 1994 The intrapartum platelet count in patients with HELLP (hemolysis, elevated liver-enzymes, and low platelets) syndrome – is it predictive of later hemorrhagic complications? Am J Obstet Gynecol 171: 799–804

Schucker J L, Mercer B M, Audibert F, Lewis R L, Friedman S A, Sibai B M 1996 Serial amniotic-fluid index in severe pre-eclampsia – a poor predictor of adverse outcome. Am J Obstet Gynecol 175: 1018–1023

Sibai B M, Mercer B M, Schiff E, Friedman S A 1994 Aggressive versus expectant management of severe preeclampsia at 28 to 32 weeks gestation – a randomized controlled trial. Am J Obstet Gynecol 171: 818–822

Visser W, Vanpampus M G, Treffers P E, Wallenburg H C S 1994 Perinatal results of hemodynamic and conservative temporizing treatment in severe pre-eclampsia. Eur J Obstet Gynecol Reprod Biol 53: 175–181

Visser W, Wallenburg H C S 1995a A comparison between the hemodynamic effects of oral nifedipine and intravenous dihydralazine in patients with severe preeclampsia. J Hypertens 13: 791–795

Visser W, Wallenburg H C S 1995b Temporising management of severe preeclampsia with and without the HELLP-syndrome. Br J Obstet Gynaecol 102: 111–117

Walker J J, Greer I, Calder A A 1983 Treatment of acute pregnancy-related hypertension: labetalol and hydralazine compared. Postgrad Med J 59: 168–170

Walker J J 1987 The case for early recognition and intervention in pregnancy induced hypertension. In: Sharp F, Symonds E M (eds) Hypertension in pregnancy. Proceedings Sixteenth Study Group of the Royal College of Obstetricians and Gynaecologists. Perinatology Press, New York, pp 289–299

Walker J J 1991 Hypertensive drugs in pregnancy. Antihypertension therapy in pregnancy, pre-eclampsia, and eclampsia. Clin Perinatol 18: 845–873

Walker J J 1993 Day-care obstetrics. Br J Hosp Med 50: 225–226

Walker J J 1996 Care of the patient with severe pregnancy induced hypertension. Eur J Obstet Gynecol Reprod Biol 65: 127–135

Weinstein L 1982 Syndrome of hemolysis, elevated liver enzymes, and low platelet count: a severe consequence of hypertension in pregnancy. Am J Obstet Gynecol 142: 159–167

Richard Johanson

Advances in assisted vaginal delivery with vacuum extractor

Assisted vaginal delivery using the vacuum extractor is a procedure which has become integral to the practice of obstetrics worldwide. However, the choice of the vacuum extractor in preference to the forceps remains a source of debate in some countries (Drife 1996). Although the vacuum extractor has traditionally been used in the non-English speaking countries of Northern Europe, Asia and Africa (Hillier & Johanson 1994), recent surveys from the USA and the UK (Meniru 1996, Bofill et al 1996) suggest that there is a relative increase in the use of vacuum extraction. This confirms a trend away from the forceps and towards the vacuum established in the previous decade (Stephenson 1992).

In this review, I intend to examine differing practices of assisted delivery, ways of avoiding assisted delivery, the evidence for and against using the vacuum extractor, developments in equipment and technique, medicolegal implications and developments in training.

VARYING INTERVENTION RATES

The rates at which obstetricians intervene vary enormously. Assisted vaginal delivery may occur as infrequently as 1.5% of deliveries, for example in the Czech Republic, or as frequently as 15%, for example in Australia and Canada (Stephenson 1992). Whilst intervention rates have been steadily falling in the USA, they have remained relatively constant in other parts of the world, for example in Scotland and Norway (Notzon 1990). Even within countries, there are marked differences in rates of intervention which are important. Elferink-Stinkens and co-workers (1996) found that even after adjusting for many clinical risk factors, interdepartmental differences in The Netherlands of

Richard Johanson BSc MA MD MRCOG, Senior Lecturer in Perinatology, Academic Department of Obstetrics and Gynaecology, Maternity Department, North Staffordshire Hospital Trust, City General, Newcastle Road, Stoke-on-Trent ST4 6QG, UK

intervention rates were both clinically relevant and statistically significant. In the UK, differing rates of intervention, including assisted delivery (ranging from 4–26%!) have been found (Middle & Macfarlane 1996) and have been noted as a cause for concern (Audit Commission 1997).

The overall rate of assisted delivery required to provide an optimal neonatal and maternal outcome is by no means clear. At a recent RCOG consultant conference, a questionnaire was administered by the author to discussion group participants, an average operative vaginal delivery rate of 10.5% was found (range 4–20%). In answer to a further question about optimal intervention rates, the consensus was that they should be lower (an average of 8.5% [range 5–15%]).

Traditional interventionist practices are slowly giving way to a more flexible approach in most labour wards. Careful consideration of the indication for assisted delivery should allow some operative interventions to be avoided; a number of practices have been shown to be associated with lower instrumental vaginal delivery rates.

AVOIDING ASSISTED DELIVERY

Various approaches and techniques may help to achieve low assisted delivery rates. Avoiding unnecessary inductions of labour and correct diagnosis of spontaneous labour will reduce the numbers of women who suffer 'dysfunctional labour'. A number of techniques have been shown in controlled studies to reduce the need for assisted delivery (Enkin et al 1995); these include companionship in labour, active management of the second stage with Syntocinon and upright posture in the second stage (De Jong et al 1997). Intelligent decision making will reduce intervention rates. An example might be, undertaking fetal scalp sampling rather than a delivery in selected cases where fetal heart rate decelerations occur in the second stage. Epidural anaesthesia is associated with higher instrumental delivery rates; siting the epidural later in labour, letting the epidural wear off and the modern use of lower motor block regimens will all reduce the risk of instrumental delivery. It has now been widely recognised that there is no need to limit arbitrarily the length of the second stage of labour; this is particularly important when an epidural is being used. Being more liberal about 'delay', given that the fetal condition is good, is reasonable practice.

Avoiding instrumental vaginal delivery by elective caesarean section or by optimising the chances of a normal birth?

Although there is currently a vogue for choosing caesarean section rather than vaginal delivery, long-term follow-up of large cohorts of women has clearly demonstrated that the optimal mode of delivery is a normal vaginal birth, with both caesarean section and instrumental delivery more likely to be associated with residual morbidity at 1 year (Glazener et al 1995). Every effort should be made to facilitate a normal vaginal delivery. There will, nevertheless, remain an important group of women where assistance is required for maternal, fetal or combined indications. The debate continues (principally in English speaking countries) about the relative merits of the vacuum extractor and forceps.

Table 8.1 Meta-analysis of controlled trials comparing vacuum extraction and forceps delivery (Johanson & Menon 1997)

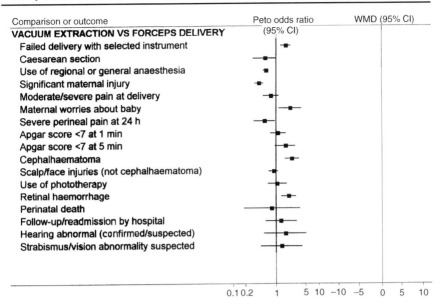

Why vacuum extraction rather than forceps?

Evidence from randomised controlled trials with respect to maternal outcome

The controlled trials comparing vacuum extraction and forceps delivery have recently been reviewed (Johanson & Menon 1997). The overall meta-analysis of the review is summarised in Table 8.1. The vacuum extractor is more likely to fail than the forceps, principally because it is not possible to pull as hard with this instrument. Interestingly, however, the overall caesarean section rate was found to be significantly lower with the vacuum extractor, suggesting that it might be more effective than forceps in some situations, for example deflexed occipito-posterior positions. An overall reduction in regional and general anaesthesia was found with the use of the vacuum extractor rather than forceps and the studies which reported the maternal perception of pain showed less discomfort in the vacuum extractor group. Overall, with the vacuum extractor there was a significant reduction in severe maternal injuries, which mirrors decades of observational data.

Observational studies on maternal morbidity

Maternal morbidity following assisted vaginal delivery, and particularly following forceps delivery, has been the focus of a considerable amount of research in recent years. Faecal incontinence, to a large extent previously unrecognised, has been widely documented. The commonest cause in healthy women is unrecognised damage to the anal sphincter during childbirth. Of women having their first vaginal delivery, 13% develop incontinence or urgency and 30% have structural changes shown by anal endosonography

(Kamm 1994) and the commonest predisposing cause of damage was the use of forceps. Sultan and co-workers (1993), in an observational study, identified anal sphincter defects in 81% of women delivered by forceps compared to 21% amongst vacuum extractor patients and 36% in control patients. In a second study by Sultan et al (1994), matched controls were compared to a group of 34 women who had sustained rectal sphincter injury at delivery and once again forceps delivery was significantly implicated. Bladder function may also be affected by instrumental vaginal delivery; e.g. Chien and co-workers (1994) found that women delivered with Kielland's forceps were more likely to have higher residual bladder volume than controls.

What are the relative effects of the vacuum and forceps on the fetus/neonate; evidence from the randomised controlled trials?

The appearances of the neonatal scalp following vacuum delivery are a frequent source of concern for parents, even though the vast majority of the changes seen are both superficial and temporary. The chignon, which is more dramatic with metal cups than the pliable silicone rubber cups, is in reality no more than a marked caput, but can be disconcerting. The vacuum extractor is significantly more likely to cause a cephalhaematoma than forceps (Johanson & Menon 1997), with the largest study suggesting an incidence of around 10%. A cephal-haematoma is subperiosteal and is limited usually to a single cranial bone, most often one of the parietals. Fahmy (1971) found that factors significantly related to cephalhaematoma formation included high station of the fetal head, suction for more than 10 min, more than one cup detachment and fetal weight greater than 3.6 kg. Other scalp and facial injuries are relatively more common with forceps, in particular facial nerve palsy.

In the literature, there has been a suggestion that vacuum extraction is more likely to result in jaundice than delivery with forceps. This is not supported by evidence from controlled trials where similar proportions of babies (approximately 4%) in each group have required phototherapy (Johanson & Menon 1997). Although the vacuum extractor is associated with a higher incidence of retinal haemorrhage than forceps (50% compared to 30%), there is no evidence that this is linked with any adverse long-term outcome.

The combined evidence obtained from all controlled trials only allows conclusions to be drawn about relatively common outcomes (1175 babies in the vacuum extractor group and 1155 babies in the forceps group). Rarely, more serious injuries do occur with both vacuum extractor and forceps instrumental delivery; from the data that exists, it is not possible to judge which instrument is more dangerous with inappropriate use.

Observational data on serious neonatal injuries

Rare adverse outcomes with the vacuum extractor include subgaleal haematomas and intracranial haemorrhage. Intracranial haemorrhage also occurs with forceps delivery. Careful practice will minimise these risks.

Subgaleal haematomata

A subgaleal haematoma, otherwise known as a subaponeurotic haematoma, is caused by the rupture of the diploic vessels in the loose subaponeurotic tissues of the scalp. The subaponeurotic space stretches from the orbital ridges to the nape of the neck and, if filled, would exsanguinate the newborn. With increasing use of the vacuum extractor, the neonatal paediatrician should be prepared to encounter greater numbers of infants with this complication (Vacca 1996). Benaron (1993) highlights the importance of being aware of this complication when hypovolemic shock occurs after birth, in the presence of ballottable cranial fluid. Subgaleal haemorrhage and the use of the metal cup vacuum extractor has clearly been documented. The association with silicone rubber cups has only rarely been reported; two cases have been described (Florentino-Pineda et al 1994) and the authors suggest that the diagnosis of subgaleal haemorrhage should be considered in any infant with a scalp swelling and a falling haematocrit. This type of bleed can be significant yet easily missed as it tends to manifest late in the postnatal course, some days after delivery (Ahuja et al 1969).

The overall incidence of subgaleal haemorrhage has been described in Malaysia as 1.6/1000 live births (Boo 1990). Benaron (1993) found the incidence of this complication in the general population to be 5/10 000 compared to 50/10 000 silastic vacuum extractor deliveries and 160/10 000 Malmstrom vacuum deliveries. As no cases were described in the controlled trials (over 1000 vacuum extractor delivered babies), this estimate (16/1000) may reflect local practices or a lower threshold for diagnosis.

Intracranial haemorrhage

Intracranial haemorrhage is a more serious threat to the newborn than scalp haemorrhage. Plauche (1979) found a 0.35% incidence of intracranial haemorrhage in a review of over 14 000 vacuum extractions. Teng and Sayre (1997) had one infant with a subdural and subarachnoid haemorrhage in a series of 123 deliveries. In their review of the literature, they demonstrated the difficulties of interpreting uncontrolled data as adverse outcomes are likely to be published and true denominator data are difficult to obtain. Sims and co-workers (1986) found all intracranial ultrasounds to be normal in 23 clinically asymptomatic term infants with cephalhaematoma. However, one vacuum delivered infant with a cephalhaematoma, skull fracture and abnormal neurologic examination was found to have intracranial haemorrhage. Jeannin and colleagues (1984) found all intracranial ultrasounds to be normal, even following 28 mid-pelvic vacuum extractor procedures with a mean duration of 11 min. On the other hand, other authors have reported a high incidence of intracranial bleeding, and Avrahami and co-workers (1993), using CT scanning, found bleeding around the tentorium in all 10 (selected) babies examined.

Neurological injuries

Other rare adverse events include neurological injuries. Transient neonatal lateral rectus paralysis has been found to be more common in vacuum extracted deliveries (3.2%) than in forceps deliveries (2.4%) when compared to babies born spontaneously (0.1%) or by caesarean section (0%) (Galbraith 1994); this is thought to be related to a transient sixth nerve palsy. Possibly the abducens nerve is injured due to cranial distortion, which compresses the nerve during its transit through the petrous segment of the temporal bone (deGrauw et al 1983).

Rare adverse neonatal events with forceps

Similar injuries are described with the use of forceps. O'Driscoll and co-workers (1981), found traumatic intracranial haemorrhage in first born infants to be highly related to delivery with obstetric forceps. A recent report demonstrated the close association between high cervical spinal cord injury in neonates and delivery with forceps (Menticoglou et al 1995).

Reducing the risks of serious adverse neonatal events

Overall, the risks of perinatal trauma using the vacuum extractor correlate with the length of the application and time to delivery, the station of the fetal head at the commencement of the delivery and the difficulty of the delivery. Risks increase significantly with attempts at combined vacuum/forceps delivery where the forceps is used after the failed vacuum.

Long-term effects of instrumental vaginal delivery

Follow-up at 9 months of a randomised controlled comparison cohorts (Carmody et al 1986) found no difference in developmental delay in the two groups, with one child in each group showing problems. In a case controlled study of 295 children delivered by vacuum, there was no difference in the incidence of neurological abnormalities when compared to 302 controls (Ngan et al 1990). Seidman and co-workers (1991) documented the results of draft intelligence testing results in medical examinations at the age of 17 years in Israel. The data did not suggest any adverse associations with either form of instrument at delivery compared to normal deliveries, indeed, the instru-mental deliveries had slightly higher IQs! Wesley and co-workers (1993) looked at the long-term development of children born by forceps compared to normal delivery and found no significant cognitive development differences.

Indications and contra-indications for delivery with the vacuum extractor

Traditional indications for instrumental delivery include 'delay' and 'distress'. In addition, conditions requiring a shortening of the second stage are usually included. The vacuum extractor is contra-indicated with a face presentation. Previously, acute fetal distress has been given as a reason for preferring forceps, as has prematurity, and forceps have been suggested for patients who have had fetal scalp sampling.

Vintzileos and co-workers (1996) found no adverse effect of the vacuum extractor on cord blood acid base changes, when used in cases of fetal distress. In two controlled trials (Johanson et al 1993, Vacca et al 1983), delivery with the vacuum extractor was quicker in cases of fetal distress than delivery with forceps. Morales and co-workers (1995) reviewed neonatal morbidity following the vacuum extraction of preterm infants with birth weights of

1500–2499 g and found no significant effects, suggesting that the vacuum extractor could be used, if indicated, in this group of preterm infants. Fetal haemorrhage in association with vacuum extraction following fetal blood sampling has been reported (Roberts & Stone 1978). However, this case report was not supported by evidence from a larger series. Lee (1970) found no cases of this complication in a prospective study of 63 vacuum deliveries following fetal scalp sampling and no cases were reported in the controlled trial carried out in the North West Midlands (Johanson et al 1993).

Which cup?

The resurgence of interest in the vacuum extractor over the last 10 years has largely been related to the introduction of silicone rubber cups. These, and the more traditional metal cups, are described in full for the interested reader by Vacca (1992) who also goes into great depth about technique and outcome after assisted delivery.

Both clinical and laboratory studies suggest that the silicone rubber cups are more likely to fail in the presence of excessive caput (Muise et al 1993, Chenoy & Johanson 1992). Soft cups, although they are more likely to fail, are associated with less scalp disfiguration and frequently the only evidence of the application is redness of the skin. This justifies their use in the majority of situations, but selective use of the metal cups is advised where the baby is large, the delivery is anticipated to be more difficult and in the presence of a large amount of caput. Since the earlier work by Bird (1976), a scientific approach to successful vacuum delivery has been developed (Vacca 1990). Essentially, this entails the application of the metal cup in the midline over the occiput to ensure good flexion. Where there is significant deflexion prior to application (i.e. only the anterior fontanelle is palpable), the occipito-posterior (OP) cup should be used. This unique instrument allows the head to flex and, invariably, this is followed by spontaneous rotation to the occipito-anterior position as the presenting part encounters the pelvic floor. In our experience (Johanson et al 1993) the silicone cup is used in 50% of cases, the anterior silicone cup (usually the 5–6 cm diameter) in approximately 35% of cases and the OP cup in the remainder (Fig. 8.1). Other developments, such as the O'Neil cup or the 'new generation' series of Bird cups, have not been widely adopted (Hillier & Johanson 1994).

Which vacuum source?

The initial hand pumps have given way to electrical and foot pumps (Fig. 8.2). A recent controlled study comparing electrical and foot pumps demonstrated no advantage in the use of the electric pump, which is more expensive (Gabrawi et al 1997). Wiper and co-workers (1996) concluded that wall suction is an unreliable source of vacuum.

Manner of application of the vacuum

Application of the vacuum has traditionally been in a stepwise manner, over the course of 8–10 min. Lim and co-workers (1997) carried out a controlled trial

A

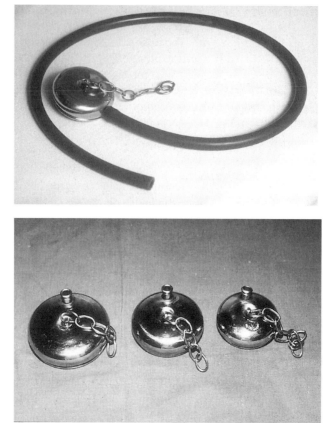

B

C

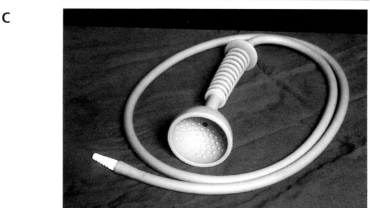

Fig. 8.1 Vacuum caps. (**A**) OP (Bird); (**B**) OA (Bird) 4, 5, 6 cm metal; (**C**) silicone rubber.

of stepwise compared to rapid application of the vacuum. In the rapid method, the negative pressure was taken to 0.8 kg/cm^2 in one step. The total duration of ventouse vacuum extractor application in the rapid method was 8 min compared to 14 min in the stepwise method and no significant differences were found in terms of cup detachment or scalp injury.

Special indications for delivery with the vacuum extractor

Meniru and colleagues (1996) found that over 60% of obstetricians who responded to their survey would consider using the vacuum extractor prior to full dilatation. It is important to recognise that use prior to full dilatation raises the risk of cervical injury, not to mention difficulty in delivering the baby. In

A

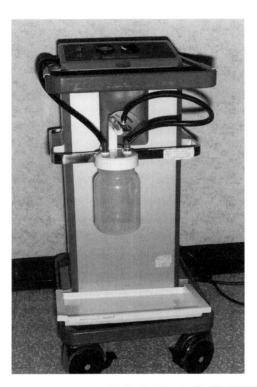

B

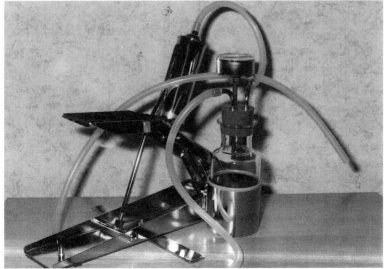

Fig. 8.2 Vacuum pumps. (**A**) Electrical (Egnell-Ameda); (**B**) foot (Menox).

the 1988–1990 Confidential Enquiries into Maternal Deaths (Department of Health 1994), two women died when the cervix had been torn during the use of the vacuum extractor and this injury had not been recognised despite heavy bleeding. This special usage has not been evaluated in controlled trials but common sense would dictate that it should be reserved for those cases with fetal distress where delivery is imminent and where labour is progressing well (and not situations with late 1st stage delay). Clearly, this is a situation for expert and not novice use. A second special indication for the use of the vacuum extractor is delivery of the second twin, presenting by vertex and where fetal distress is present or another indication for delivery. In this situation, the 4 cm metal cup or the small silicone rubber cup may be used.

In a small number of cases, a trial of vacuum extractor may be indicated in theatre. Where this was carried out by an experienced obstetrician in theatre with facilities for immediate caesarean section, there was no associated increased morbidity of either the mother or the baby (Revah et al 1997). However, this study was not a controlled trial and the results have to be interpreted with caution.

Technique

Technique of delivery is extensively discussed in currently available reviews and textbooks (O'Grady et al 1995, Vacca 1992). In the *Road to Success* with the Ventouse video (Johanson 1992), the following points are made with respect to why failures in assisted delivery occur.

1. Failure to use the correct instrument. The silicone rubber cup will often fail if it is used with deflexion of the head, excess caput, a big baby or a prolonged second stage of labour.

2. Inadequate initial assessment of the case:
   (a) The head being too high. A classic mistake is to assume that because caput can be felt below the ischial spines, the head must be engaged.
   (b) Mis-diagnosis of the position and attitude of the head.

3. Anterior or lateral placement increases the failure rate. The correct placement is mid-line over the occiput.

4. Traction in the wrong direction.

5. Rarely adequate traction is not possible even with a metal cup because of excessive caput. Such cases should be delivered by caesarean section unless the head is well down when forceps can be used.

6. Poor maternal effort. Maternal pushing contributes substantially to the success of the delivery. Adequate encouragement and instruction should be given and the forceps may be preferred if the patient is under general anaesthesia.

7. True failure due to cephalopelvic disproportion is rare.

Minimising medico-legal risk

Legal issues related to vacuum extraction as well the assessment of risk have both been well covered in a recent textbook on vacuum extraction by O'Grady and co-workers (1995), who have reviewed court files, insurance company reports, medical case reviews and the commentary of seasoned litigators and medical experts. They conclude that these sources indicate that the bulk of malpractice litigation involving instrumental delivery derives from four broad obstetric categories:

1. Failure to exercise adequate and informed medical judgment when assessing what cases are appropriate for an instrumental operation and when that intervention should take place.

2. Failure to understand or accept the limitations of the procedure itself and plan in advance for possible failure.

3. Failure to abandon timely a trial of instrumental delivery. Particularly the failure to eschew improperly prolonged, repeated or excessive traction efforts in the presence of poor (or no) progress.

4. Failure to assess properly the position of the fetal head in relationship to the pelvic outlet and attempting to advance the fetal head by traction against the resistance of an unfavourable pelvic diameter or fetal position (i.e. unrecognised cephalopelvic disproportion).

These demonstrate a failure to fulfil the basic requirements:

1. Clear medical indications for the procedure.

2. Absence of cephalopelvic disproportion.

3. Concomitant preparation for caesarean delivery with immediate availability of all requisite personnel in the case of a trial of instrumental delivery.

4. Undertaking all cases of instrumentation as if they were truly a trial, with the requirements that the obstetrician remain willing to abandon an attempted instrumental delivery in favour of a caesarean operation when no descent occurs following reasonable traction effort(s).

5. An operator/surgeon with demonstrable knowledge and skill in performing deliveries with the chosen instrument (either vacuum extractor or forceps).

Every assisted delivery with a vacuum extractor or forceps should be clearly documented. Any cases that are not documented become indefensible and documentation should be complete. The record of the delivery should include, at least, the indication for the procedure, anaesthesia, personnel present, instruments used, station, position and deflexion of the fetal head at commencement of the operation and any complications, as well as a detailed description of how they were managed.

O'Grady et al (1995) conclude their chapter on legal issues by reminding the obstetrician that the process of consent should include active participation by the patient in decision making and an acceptance by her of a responsibility for making an informed choice.

Training in the use of the vacuum extractor

It is essential that whoever undertakes a vacuum delivery should have been adequately trained and supervised. Since training has traditionally been in forceps deliveries, doctors who are expected to carry out vacuum extractor delivery may be inexperienced in the technique.

Observational studies suggest a wide range of ability amongst registrars working on labour ward. Iffland and co-workers (1996) reviewed all cases of emergency caesarean section carried out by five registrars, all of whom had been in the grade for at least one year. Marked differences were found between the registrars and the proportion of caesarean sections carried out at full dilatation and failed vaginal operative deliveries. With a view to ensuring that registrars have adequate experience, we are currently developing models for teaching vacuum extractor delivery in the classroom situation.

Who should do vacuum deliveries?

A number of authors are of the opinion that the use of the vacuum extractor should not be confined to medical staff (Rajkhowa et al 1995). A hospital survey found that the majority of respondents agreed with the statement that 'midwives should conduct ventouse deliveries' (Rajkhowa et al 1995). Hayes (1997) has described the results of a series of 144 midwife ventouse deliveries. The success rate was over 90% with 50% of the women not requiring an episiotomy. Hayes concludes that the midwives in this series 'could truly be called practitioners within their own right with the needs of women rather than the needs of any traditional role as the fundamental guide to their conduct!'

CONCLUSIONS

Over the past decade there has been an increased awareness of the wide discrepancies in obstetric practice both around the world and within countries. Overall, we should be aiming to reduce intervention rates. Where instrumental delivery is required, on the basis of risk of maternal injury, the vacuum extractor remains the instrument of first choice. Both the vacuum extractor and forceps have the potential to seriously injure babies and strict rules for their use should be adhered to and documented. The future will see more classroom teaching with simulators and scenarios. It is possible that assisted vaginal delivery may be undertaken by midwives.

Acknowledgements

I would like to thank Mrs Paula Aucock and Miss Nicola Leighton for their assistance in preparing this chapter.

References

Ahuja G L, Willoughby M L N, Kerr M M, Hutchinson J H 1969 Massive subaponeurotic haemorrhage in infants born by vacuum extraction. BMJ iii: 743–745

Key points for clinical practice

- Every effort should be made to avoid an instrumental vaginal delivery.

- Where indicated, current evidence continues to support the RCOG audit standard that the 'ventouse is the instrument of first choice for vaginal delivery'.

- Rare adverse fetal/neonatal events do occur with the vacuum extractor; it is particularly important to be aware of and to recognize a subgaleal (subaponeurotic) haematoma.

- The soft cups are suitable for over 50% of deliveries but there is an important place for the metal anterior cups and a vitally important place for the occipitoposterior (OP) cup.

- Whichever instrument is used indications should be clear, informed consent obtained, and the operator should be suitably trained or supervised.

- Failures are most commonly due to unrecognised occipito-posterior positions or a non-engaged head. Use of the soft cups when there is a large amount of caput will often result in failure.

- By the 21st century ,training with models in classroom situations will be standard practice.

Audit Commission 1997 First class delivery: improving maternity services in England and Wales. Abingdon: Audit Commission Publications

Avrahami E, Frishman E, Minz M 1993 CT demonstration of intracranial haemorrhage in term newborn following vacuum extractor delivery. Neuroradiology 35: 107–108

Benaron D A 1993 Subgaleal hematoma causing hypovolemic shock during delivery after failed vacuum extraction: a case report. J Perinatol 13: 228–231

Bird G C 1976 The importance of flexion in vacuum extractor delivery. Br J Obstet Gynaecol 83: 194–200

Bofill J A, Perry K G, Roberts W E, Morrison J C 1996 Forceps and vacuum delivery: a survey of North American residency programs. Obstet Gynecol 88: 622–625

Boo N 1990 Subaponeurotic hemorrhage in Malaysian neonates. Singapore Med J 31: 207

Carmody F, Grant A, Mutch M, Vacca A, Chalmers I 1986 Follow-up of babies delivered in randomized comparison of vacuum extraction and forceps delivery. Acta Obstet Gynecol Scand 65: 763–766

Chenoy R, Johanson R B 1992 A randomised prospective study comparing delivery with metal and silicone rubber vacuum extractor cups. Br J Obstet Gynaecol 99: 360–363

Chien P F W, Agustsson P, Patel N B et al 1994 The effect of obstetric forceps delivery on postpartum bladder function. J Obstet Gynecol 14: 410–415

De Jong P R, Johanson R B, Baxen P, Adrians V D, Van der Westhuisen S, Jones P W 1997 Randomised trial comparing the upright and supine positions for the second stage of labour. Br J Obstet Gynaecol 104: 567–571

deGrauw A J, Rottenveel J, Cruysberg J R 1983 Transient sixth nerve paralysis in the newborn infant. Neuropaediatrics 14: 164–165

Department of Health 1994 Report on Confidential Enquiries into Maternal Deaths in the United Kingdom 1988–1990. London: HMSO

Drife J O 1996 Choice and instrumental delivery. Br J Obstet Gynaecol 103: 608–611

Elferink-Stinkens P M, Brand R, le Cessie S, Van Hemel O J S 1996 Large differences in obstetrical intervention rates among Dutch hospitals, even after adjustment for population differences. Eur J Obstet Gynecol Reprod Biol 68: 97–103

Enkin M, Keirse M J N C, Renfrew M J, Neilson J P 1995 Guide to Effective Care in Pregnancy and Childbirth, 2nd edn. Oxford: Oxford University Press.

Fahmy K 1971 Cephalhematoma following vacuum extraction. J Obstet Gynaecol Br Commonw 78: 369

Florentino-Pineda I, Ezhuthacan S G, Sineni L G et al 1994 Subgaleal hemorrhage in the newborn infant associated with silicone elastomer vacuum extractor. J Perinatol 14: 95–100

Gabrawi E, Johanson R B, Jones P 1997 A random controlled trial of two different vacuum extractor pumps: new foot pump and electric pump. J Obstet Gynecol In press

Galbraith R S 1994 Incidence of neonatal sixth nerve palsy in relation to mode of delivery. Am J Obstet Gynecol 170: 1158–1159

Glazener C M A, Abdalla M, Stroud P, Naji S, Templeton A, Russell I T 1995 Postnatal maternal morbidity: extent, causes, prevention and treatment. Br J Obstet Gynaecol 102: 286–287

Hayes S 1997 Ventouse deliveries by midwives; our role or encroachment on the role of the obstetrician. MIDIRS Midwifery Digest 7: 197–200

Hillier C, Johanson R B 1994 Worldwide survey of instrumental delivery. Int J Obstet Gynecol 47: 109–114

Iffland C A, Gordon H 1996 Failed forceps and ventouse: an audit of registrars in training. J Obstet Gynecol 16: 83–85

Jeannin P, Afschrift M, Voet D et al 1984 Cranial ultrasound after forceful midpelvis vacuum extraction at term. J Perinatol Med 12: 319–323

Johanson R B 1992 The Road to Success using the Ventouse Video. North Staffs Hospital, Department of Obstetrics and Gynaecology

Johanson R B, Rice C, Doyle M et al 1993 A randomised prospective study comparing the new vacuum extractor policy with forceps delivery. Br J Obstet Gynaecol 100: 524–530

Johanson R B, Menon V 1997 Vacuum extraction vs forceps delivery. In: Neilson J P, Crowther C A, Hodnett E D, Hofmeyr G J, Keirse M J N C (eds) Pregnancy and Childbirth Module of the Cochrane Database of Systematic Reviews (updated 03 June 1997). Available in The Cochrane Library (database on disk and CDROM). The Cochrane Collaboration; Issue 3. Oxford: Update Software

Kamm M A 1994 Obstetric damage and faecal incontinence. Lancet 344: 730–733

Lee K H 1970 Vacuum extraction after fetal blood sampling. Aust NZ J Obstet Gynecol 10: 205

Lim F T H, Holm J P, Schuitemaker N W E, Jansen F H M, Hermans J 1997 Stepwise compared with rapid application of vacuum in ventouse extraction procedures. Br J Obstet Gynaecol 104: 33–36

Meniru G I 1996 An analysis of recent trends in vacuum extraction and forceps delivery in the United Kingdom. Br J Obstet Gynaecol 103: 168–170

Menticoglou S M, Perlman M, Manning F A 1995 High cervical spinal cord injury in neonates delivered with forceps: report of 15 cases. Obstet Gynecol 86: 589–594

Middle C, Macfarlane A 1996 Labour and delivery of 'normal' primiparous women: analysis of routinely collected data. Br J Obstet Gynaecol 102: 970–977

Morales R, Adair C D, Sanchez-Ramos L et al 1995 Vacuum extraction of preterm infants with birth weights of 1,500–2,499 grams. J Reprod Med 40: 127–130

Muise K L, Duchon M A, Brown R H 1993 The effect of artificial caput on performance of vacuum extractors. Obstet Gynecol 81: 170–173

Ngan H Y S, Miu P, Ko L et al 1990 Long-term neurological sequelae following vacuum extractor delivery. Aust NZ J Obstet Gynecol 30: 111–114

Notzon F C 1990 International differences in the use of obstetric intervention. JAMA 263: 3286–3291

O'Driscoll K, Meagher D, MacDonald D, Geoghegan F 1981 Traumatic intracranial haemorrhage in firstborn infants and delivery with obstetric forceps. Br J Obstet Gynaecol 88: 577–581

O'Grady J P, Gimovsky M L, McIlhargie C J 1995 Vacuum Extraction in Modern Obstetric Practice. The Parthenon Publishing Group

Plauche W C 1979 Fetal cranial injuries related to the delivery with the Malmstrom vacuum extractor. Obstet Gynecol 53: 750–757

Rajkhowa M, Abukhalil I, Chapman G et al 1995 Should midwives conduct ventouse deliveries? Br J Midwifery 3: 88–91

Revah A, Ezra Y, Farine D, Ritchie K 1997 Failed trial of vacuum or forceps – maternal and fetal outcome. Am J Obstet Gynecol 176: 200–204

Roberts I F, Stone M 1978 Fetal haemorrhage, complication of vacuum extractor after fetal blood sampling. Am J Obstet Gynecol 132: 109

Seidman D S, Laor A, Gale R et al 1991 Long-term effects of vacuum and forceps delivery. Lancet 337: 1583–1585

Sims M E, Halterman G, Jasani N, Vachon L, Wu P Y K 1986 Indicators for routine canial ultrasound scanning in the nursery. J Clin Ultrasound 14: 443–447

Stephenson P A 1992 International differences in the use of obstetrical interventions. Copehagen: WHO.EUR/ICP/MCH 112, Conference proceedings

Sultan A H, Kamm M A, Bartram C I, Hudson C N. 1993 Anal sphincter trauma during instrumental delivery. Int J Obstet Gynecol 43: 263–270

Sultan A H, Kamm M A, Hudson C N, Bartram C I 1994 Third degree obstetric anal sphincter tears: risk factors and outcome of primary repair. BMJ 308: 887–891

Teng F Y, Sayre J W 1997 Vacuum extraction: does duration predict scalp injury? Obstet Gynecol 89: 281–285

Vacca A, Grant A, Wyatt A, Chalmers I 1983 Portsmouth operative delivery trial: a comparison of vacuum extraction and forceps delivery. Br J Obstet Gynaecol 64: 431–443

Vacca A 1990 The place of the vacuum extractor in modern obstetric practice. Fetal Med Rev 2: 103–122

Vacca A 1992 Handbook of Vacuum Extraction in Obstetric Practice. London: Edward Arnold

Vacca A 1996 Birth by vacuum extraction: neonatal outcome. J Paediatr Child Health 32: 204–206

Vintzileos A M, Nochimson D J, Antsaklis A, Varvarigos I, Guzman E R, Knuppel R A 1996 Effect of vacuum extraction on umbilical cord blood acid-base measurements. J Matern Fetal Med 5: 11–17

Wesley B D, van den Berg B J, Reece E A 1993 The effect of forceps delivery on cognitive development. Am J Obstet Gynecol 169: 1091–1095

Wiper D W, Duchon M A, Muise K L 1996 Vacuum sources in obstetrics. J Reprod Med 41: 444–446

Advances in assisted vaginal delivery with vacuum extractor

Karl W. Murphy

Reducing the complications of caesarean section

Today, the caesarean operation is one of the most commonly performed surgical procedures. This in itself attests to its safety and acceptability to women, but is not the whole story. Unfortunately, caesarean sections are associated with a great deal of maternal morbidity, and in this chapter we will examine the nature of this morbidity and the evidence which supports the use of various prophylactic measures. Obviously, a lower caesarean rate will mean a reduction in the overall incidence of complications, but this is a separate issue and will not be addressed here. In addition, caesarean related anaesthetic complications will not be covered in this chapter, being a subject which is best dealt with by our anaesthetic colleagues.

GENERAL PRINCIPLES

Nielson and Hokegard (1984) identified the following risk factors for complications at caesarean: excessive speed, lack of experience, gestational age below 32 weeks, low station of the vertex and ruptured membranes pre-operatively. Proper planning is essential to avoid or minimise problems at caesarean. Full knowledge of obstetric, medical and surgical history of both mother and fetus (for example – previous incisions, details of previous surgery, anatomical aberrations) is vital, though not infrequently overlooked. Issues such as previous anaesthetic problems, or allergies to antibiotics should be ascertained. The operator should anticipate blood loss and technical difficulties: size and position of the fetus and placental site. Proper planning will reduce the incidence of intra-operative complications.

Mr Karl W. Murphy MD MRCOG MRCPI DCH, Consultant Obstetrician and Gynaecologist, Subspecialist in Fetomaternal Medicine, St Mary's Hospital, Praed Street, London W2 1NY, UK

Maternal mortality

There are data to show that delivery by caesarean is associated with a 5-fold increase in maternal mortality compared with vaginal delivery after the exclusion of severe antenatal complications and medical disorders (Lilford et al 1990). Hypertensive disorders, pulmonary embolism, haemorrhage, sepsis and anaesthesia are the main causes of obstetric death amongst women delivered by caesarean section as reported in the Confidential Enquiry into Maternal Deaths in the UK 1991–1993. In this chapter, however, we are particularly interested in the use of techniques and prophylactic measures which might prevent mortality and morbidity resulting from the surgery itself.

The 1991–1993 report of the Confidential Enquiry into Maternal Deaths in the UK raised the complex issue of increased mortality related to unplanned caesarean operations. Compared with the previous triennium, there was a fall in the number of maternal deaths related to elective caesarean, but a significant rise in mortality related to unplanned emergency operations. Lilford's data on maternal mortality suggest that, after excluding medical disorders and severe antenatal complications, the relative risk for emergency intrapartum compared with elective caesarean is approximately 1.7:1.0. These data reduce the temptation to justify repeat caesarean solely on the basis that the likelihood of a successful vaginal birth is low and, in the absence of other problems, the use of elective caesarean to obviate the risks of emergency surgery cannot be justified.

The authors of the 1991–1993 Confidential Enquiry alluded to the lack of senior obstetric input into many of the unplanned caesareans which resulted in fatalities. Those involved in the provision of obstetric services need to take this on board, although the current restructuring of training and planned consultant expansion should help to alleviate this problem in the future.

THROMBOEMBOLISM

Thromboembolism remains an important cause of maternal mortality and morbidity after caesarean. Those women affected tend to be young relative to the population they come from, so there is great potential for long-term morbidity. Clinical diagnosis of thromboembolism is unreliable and up to 70% of those who suffer a fatal pulmonary embolism may exhibit no warning signs. Therefore, all women undergoing caesarean section should have a risk-assessment performed and the type of thromboprophylaxis employed should be based on the result of this assessment, in accordance with recent RCOG Working Party Guidelines (1995). In the absence of risk factors, women undergoing elective caesarean require only early mobilisation and adequate hydration as thromboprophylaxis. Women are considered to be at moderate risk of thromboembolism if one of the risk factors listed in Table 9.1 is present.

For women at moderate risk of thromboembolism, heparin prophylaxis should be considered, as it is more effective than protective stockings. Women at high risk include those with hereditary hypercoagulable conditions, such protein C and S deficiency, activated protein C resistance, antithrombin III deficiency, those with a positive antiphospholipid antibody screen or sickle cell

Table 9.1 Women are considered to be at moderate risk of thromboembolism if one of the risk factors is present

Age above 35 years	Pre-eclampsia
Weight above 80 kg	Immobility > 4 days
Para 4 or more	Major illness
Significant varicose veins	Emergency C. Section in labour
Current infection	Postpartum haemorrhage

anaemia, those undergoing major pelvic surgery, and those with three or more moderate risk factors (Table 9.1). For high-risk women who have not already been on heparin treatment during their pregnancy, prophylactic heparin combined with stockings are advisable . Unfractionated heparin may be given as 5000 i.u. BD subcutaneously, or alternatively, enoxaparin 20 mg can be given subcutaneously once daily. A 5 day course should be completed, even when early mobilisation occurs, when the risk is low or moderate. For high-risk cases, the heparin should be continued for a period of 6 weeks postpartum. Breastfeeding is not contra-indicated on heparin or warfarin.

HAEMORRHAGE

Haemorrhage with the need for blood transfusion is one of the more common intra-operative complications at caesarean. It is also potentially one of the most serious complications. The average blood loss at caesarean is about 0.7–1.0 l (Pritchard et al 1962). Much of this loss comes from the placenta, and, therefore, blood transfusion is not required. Anticipation is the clinician's most effective strategy for coping with haemorrhage. Factors associated with haemorrhage (blood loss > 1.5 litres) at caesarean section include: placenta praevia, previous postpartum haemorrhage, obesity, prolonged second stage of labour, pre-eclampsia, general anaesthesia, amnionitis, preterm caesarean, and classical uterine incision. Combinations of these factors increase the risk synergistically. Previous caesarean increases the risk of placenta praevia (Taylor et al 1994) and, therefore, it is wise to check the placental site by ultrasound in women undergoing repeat caesarean. Appropriate precautions would then include the presence of an experienced operator at the caesarean and cross matching of an adequate amount of blood. As there is evidence that the need for blood transfusion is greater when trainees perform the operation without supervision (Dickason & Dinsmoor 1992), the former precaution might avoid the need for blood transfusion altogether. The combination of an anterior placenta praevia and a uterine scar is particularly worrying, and the possibility of accreta and the need for hysterectomy should be anticipated and discussed fully with the mother prior to elective surgery. Appropriate anticipation would also allow the mother to consider autologous blood transfusion in particular situations if supported by the local Blood Transfusion Service. There is some evidence that autologous blood transfusion can be employed safely in pregnancy, thereby reducing the risk of transmitting infectious agents at transfusion (McVay et al 1989).

Minimising blood loss at operation

Having anticipated the risk of haemorrhage and taken the appropriate precautions, the next strategy is to minimise blood loss at operation. Wide lateral dissection of the bladder should be avoided, as this may provoke bleeding from the broad ligament engorged venous plexuses. Using bandage scissors to cut the uterine incision concave upwards may be preferable to tearing the uterus digitally, which results in a concave downward incision and may make less use of the room available on both sides. One randomised controlled trial, however, failed to demonstrate any difference in blood loss at caesarean between these two methods of opening the uterus (Rodriguez et al 1994), so the decision can be left to operator preference.

Probably the commonest reason for haemorrhage at caesarean is extension of the uterine incision during delivery of the fetal head. This typically occurs in advanced labour when the lower segment is thin and the fetal head is deeply engaged. A posterior position of the occiput aggravates the situation. Again, anticipation is the key: the mechanisms of normal vaginal delivery should be remembered so that the operator never tries to deliver the fetal head through the incision in the posterior position. The unfavourable diameters presenting and thin lower segment make an extension of the incision inevitable. The operator should allow sufficient time for the head to disimpact from the pelvis, applying gentle horizontal traction with cupped fingers, and once disimpacted the head should be manually rotated and the occiput delivered anteriorly through the incision. With care, this manoeuvre allows a surprisingly easy delivery of the moulded occipitoposterior head, and minimises the risk of extending the incision. The use of disimpaction from below by a third assistant may be helpful, but sometimes this manoeuvre causes the occipitoposterior head to deflex and the fetal chin presents at the incision. The operator should replace the chin, flex and rotate the head and deliver it in the occipitoanterior position.

Spontaneous expulsion of the placenta at caesarean significantly reduces blood loss, by about 300 ml in one study (Mc Curdy et al 1992). In addition, it probably also reduces the incidence of fetomaternal haemorrhage at placental separation and, thereby, the risk of maternal isoimmunisation. Therefore, the clinician should avoid the temptation to shear manually the placenta from the uterine wall in the interest of making haste. Oxytocic drugs reduce blood loss at caesarean section, and oxytocin 10 I.U. intravenously is usually preferred to syntometrine, because the latter has a tendency to cause vomiting.

After delivery of the baby, bleeding from the uterine incision edges may be profuse and it is wise to stem this rapidly. Four Green-Armytage clamps, two for the angles and two for the most vascular areas anteriorly and posteriorly can be helpful in controlling blood loss prior to suturing. Rapid closure of the uterus minimises blood loss, and great care should be taken to incorporate fully both angles in the suture. Where angle bleeding is particularly profuse, it may be wise to suture them separately.

Strategies to control haemorrhage

It is beyond the scope of this chapter to discuss, in detail, the management of haemorrhage at caesarean section, but there are a number of strategies to avoid hysterectomy in this situation, and hysterectomy should invariably be seen as a last resort. Remember that profuse haemorrhage can itself lead to disseminated intravascular coagulation (DIC) and that checking the coagulation screen and replacing clotting factors or platelets may reduce the need for further surgical intervention.

When the underlying cause of haemorrhage at caesarean is uterine atony, therapeutic manoeuvres include vigorous massage of the exteriorised uterus, intramyometrial injection of prostaglandin 2 alpha (Carboprost), and an intravenous oxytocin infusion. For troublesome bleeding from a low-lying placental site, options include: the above drugs, the application of direct pressure over the bleeding surface using hot packs, and the use of figure-of-eight sutures in the placental bed. For persistent bleeding there are a number of further measures. Unilateral or bilateral ligation of the uterine arteries has been used very successfully by some workers (O'Leary 1995). The author describes a mass suture technique which involves ligating the uterine arteries and veins bilaterally incorporating almost the full thickness of the myometrium in each suture. The authors had only 10 failures, where hysterectomy was required, in a series of 265, and follow up revealed subsequent normal menstruation in all cases. Another interesting technique, which has been used to avoid hysterectomy, has been described by Lynch et al (1997): the B-Lynch Brace Suturing Technique, in which a single suture enveloping the body of the uterus reduces total uterine blood flow. Although this technique remains to be evaluated, it has the advantage that the operator can ascertain its success at the time of insertion. When bleeding from the lower segment is particularly troublesome, it may be necessary to use some figure-of-eight sutures in addition to the brace suture. Another variation is a circular suture for placenta accreta (Cho et al 1991) using interrupted chromic catgut sutures 2 cm long and placed at 1 cm intervals around the bleeding area deep into the muscle on the serosal surface of the uterus. Ligation of the internal iliac arteries is a more widely recognised procedure for the control of haemorrhage, but it is technically more difficult to accomplish safely, and there is a substantial failure rate (Evans & McShane 1985).

INFECTION

As many as one in four women in the untreated groups of randomised, controlled trials of antibiotics at caesarean developed a wound infection, fever or endometritis. Serious infections were uncommon in any of the trials, but even for elective caesarean up to one in ten women may develop a wound infection (Beattie et al 1994). Because so many variables can alter the risk the reported rates of infection vary widely: for endometritis 0–86%, for wound infection 0–24%, for urinary tract infection 1–34%, and for febrile morbidity 0–66%. Therefore, there is a substantial risk of infectious morbidity for women undergoing both emergency and elective caesareans. Wound infection in particular can be emotionally devastating for the woman who is generally unprepared for it. They also have major cost implications not least by delaying hospital discharge.

Clinical predictors of postpartum endometritis are still poor with an overall positive predictive value of about 50%. Recognised risk factors for infectious morbidity after caesarean include: maternal obesity – for wound infection in particular; prolonged ruptured membranes; emergency intrapartum surgery preceded by multiple vaginal assessments and the use of fetal scalp electrodes; and bacterial vaginosis – for endometritis in particular. Urinary tract infections are also a problem post-caesarean with reported rates of bacteriuria of 20% post-catheterisation (Leigh et al 1990).

The mother's endogenous vaginal flora is thought to be responsible for most cases of postpartum endometritis. With ruptured membranes and prolonged labour, genital tract flora may reach the uterine cavity. Isolation of the group B beta haemolytic *Streptococcus*, *Enterococcus faecalis* and bacterial vaginosis from the upper vaginal tract is significantly associated with postpartum endometritis (Heather-Watts et al 1991). Wound infections may be caused by amniotic fluid contaminated with vaginal bacteria from labour, and also by direct contamination with skin flora. Organisms such as *Staphylococcus epidermis*, *Enterococcus faecalis*, *Staphylococcus aureus*, *Escherichia coli* and *Proteus mirabilis*, in that order, account for the majority of wound infections. *Staph. aureus* accounts for up to 25% of wound infections and most are nosocomial in nature. The genital mycoplasmas are also commonly isolated from the genital tract of women after caesarean and warrant further consideration as primary pathogens.

Infection prophylaxis

Good surgical techniques must underpin any attempts to reduce the rate of infectious morbidity at caesarean. These principles will be examined below. Antibiotic prophylaxis has had a major beneficial impact on infectious morbidity post-caesarean, so that it is no longer considered ethical to conduct trials which compare antibiotics with placebo in women undergoing either elective or emergency surgery (Enkin et al 1989). Cochrane overviews of 69 randomised controlled trials of antibiotics given at the time of caesarean operation have demonstrated unequivocally that there is a statistically significant and clinically important reduction in postpartum febrile morbidity/endometritis (OR = 0.30, 95% CI = 0.27–0.34), in wound infection (OR = 0.38, 95% CI = 0.31–0.45), and in serious infection (OR = 0.24, 95% CI = 0.19–0.30).

The higher infection rates following emergency surgery are well known, and it is, therefore, widespread practice to administer antibiotics to women undergoing caesarean in labour. However, the evidence from 17 randomised controlled trials evaluating the use of prophylactic antibiotics at elective caesarean is also unequivocal: their use is associated with a statistically significant and clinically important reduction in the incidence of postpartum febrile morbidity or endometritis (OR = 0.30, 95% CI = 0.21–0.42), and wound infection (OR = 0.45, 95% CI = 0.23–0.88). The magnitude of risk reduction is similar to that recorded for emergency caesarean, although the absolute risk reduction is smaller. Serious infection after elective caesarean is rare and although the reduction here is also of the same order, it does not reach statistical significance (Enkin et al 1989).

No particular antibiotic has been shown to be superior to all others, and most authors use a second or third generation cephalosporin (for example:

Cefoxitin or cefotaxime). The optimal time of administration is at the time of bacterial contamination, as demonstrated by Burke (1961) in the animal model. A single dose given intravenously, after the umbilical cord has been clamped, is effective and avoids any placental transfer. The slight delay from the mother's perspective is balanced by the reduced risk to the baby of culture failure in suspected infection. Peritoneal irrigation with antibiotics, although effective, is probably less efficacious than systemic administration and, therefore, offers no particular advantage.

Detailed histological studies of the uterine decidua and myometrium have helped to explain why antibiotic prophylaxis sometimes fails. Again, wide variations in failure rates have been reported. Incipient or subclinical infection may already be present, with myometrial inflammation and polymorph cell invasion, such that antibiotic treatment rather than prophylaxis may be indicated (Gonik et al 1992). These authors speculate that it may be possible to identify this subgroup in the future by means endometrial biopsy at caesarean and the application of rapid DNA probe technology.

There are a number of concerns with universal antibiotic administration. Anaphylaxis with beta-lactams is rare, reported to occur in 1/10 000 cases. At least two maternal deaths have been reported from anaphylaxis after cephalosporin prophylaxis in the US. Another concern is that of bacteriological shifts in colonising flora and resistance patterns. Some workers have demonstrated a reduction in benign vaginal flora with a concomitant increase in Gram-negative facultative anaerobes following antibiotic prophylaxis (Gibbs et al 1981). These concerns have led some to argue that the risk of routine antibiotic prophylaxis outweigh the benefits. The counter arguments are that anaphylaxis is rare, the operating theatre is one of the safer places to be when it occurs, and that any institution employing routine antibiotic prophylaxis needs an on-going bacteriological programme to monitor shifts in vaginal flora. In addition, shortening the duration over which antibiotics are given may help to discourage the development of resistance. Concerns about widespread resistance following use of routine antibiotic prophylaxis must be balanced against the clear benefits for the individual. Current problems with methicillin-resistant *Staph. aureus* (MRSA) control in many UK hospitals emphasise the need to remain vigilant, and to be prepared to alter unit policies if necessary.

Other measures which may also reduce the risk of infection post-caesarean include the following: pre-operative skin preparation, chlorhexidine gluconate 0.5% in 70% isopropyl alcohol offers similar protection to two-stage iodophor preparation (iodine plus polyvinyl pyrolidone); there are some data now to suggest that the newer iodophar impregnated adhesive film is protective, provided that it is not dislodged at surgery; avoiding shaving of the skin (use clippers); minimising tissue trauma; avoiding manual removal of the placenta where the surgeon's 'vaginally-contaminated' hand shears it from the uterine wall (Yancy et al 1994); closure of Camper fascia; improved aseptic technique, which has been shown to reduce infection rates at caesarean, in particular limiting the number of people in theatre (Frost et al 1989); and wound infection surveillance with reporting back to individual surgeons. The high rates of urinary tract infections at caesarean could also be reduced by careful attention to aseptic technique, and by removing the catheter immediately after the bladder is emptied pre-operatively (Leigh et al 1990).

SURGICAL TECHNIQUES FOR CAESAREAN

Skin incision and entry

The skin incision is usually made in the line delineating the pelvic groove, about 2 cm above the pubic symphysis. A skin incision length of less than 15 cm is associated with increased difficulty delivering the fetus for both the Pfannenstiel and the Maylard incisions. The Allis Forceps measures approximately 15 cm in length and can be useful as a guide, particularly for the less experienced operator (Finan et al 1991). The Maylard incision involves incising the rectus muscles transversely about 2 cm above the symphysis, without separating them from the sheath, so as to provide more room for the delivery in an emergency. Blunt finger dissection of the fascial tissue may be appropriate for the first caesarean but is less so for repeat operations. It is particularly important to open the parietal peritoneum high anteriorly to avoid excising an unexpectedly high bladder, a finding which may be present in advanced labour in the primiparous woman as well as in those who have adhesions from previous surgery.

Uterine incision

Before making the uterine incision, it is important to assess the degree of uterine rotation which can lead to injury of the lateral uterine vessels by blind incision to the anteriorly rotated side. A good bladder flap must then be fashioned allowing plenty of room for the uterine incision, 2–3 cm above the bladder base, but avoiding excessively wide dissection laterally with its attendant risk of bleeding. In obstructed second stage labour, the low transverse uterine incision must be made high to avoid opening into the vagina. To avoid injury to the fetus, the uterus should be incised carefully over a 2–3 cm length and the membranes should be left intact while inserting a finger between the fetus and the uterine wall until after the uterine lower segment has been cut (or torn). If more room is needed, then a J shaped incision should be made into the upper segment on the most accessible side, but an inverted T incision should be avoided if at all possible because of its poor long-term healing potential. If the placenta covers the lower segment anteriorly, it is nearly always possible to lift the placental edge to deliver the fetus rather than incising directly into placental tissue.

The vertical uterine incision in the lower segment is popular in some countries and does have the advantage that the incision completely avoids the large uterine vessels bilaterally, but extensive bladder dissection is needed, and it is virtually impossible to keep the vertical incision in the 10–12 cm of the lower segment. Furthermore, unwanted extension of the incision is usually down towards the bladder. That said, numerous studies attest to its safety as an alternative to the transverse uterine incision, particularly with respect to subsequent risks of scar dehiscence (Naef et al 1995). The Classical incision is reserved for situations when safe delivery via the transverse incision is impossible: extreme prematurity before the formation of the lower segment (before 26 weeks gestation); preterm breech presentation with prolonged ruptured membranes; transverse lie with the back down especially if the membranes are ruptured (if they are not external cephalic version may allow a transverse incision); and dense adhesions to the bladder or large fibroids obstructing the lower segment. Placenta praevia in general is no longer regarded as an indication for classical uterine incision. Neither is speed of operation! Triplets can be delivered safely through a transverse uterine incision (Mordel et al 1993).

Delivery of the fetus

The delivery of the deeply engaged head has already been discussed. A high mobile head at a repeat elective caesarean can also pose considerable difficulty and the operator needs to employ fundal pressure or Wrigley's forceps to assist the delivery. It is wise to be practised with the forceps in this situation, so as to minimise trauma in a particularly difficult case. It should be reiterated that the same manoeuvres used to deliver a fetus vaginally should be employed in delivering the fetus transabdominally. The fetal head should always be rotated to and delivered in the occipitoanterior position. The use of intravenous nitroglycerine to relax the uterus at difficult caesareans has been described but needs to be evaluated rigorously before its use can be recommended.

Urinary tract and bowel injury

Urinary tract injury is uncommon at caesarean section: bladder damage 0.3% and ureteral damage < 0.1% are commonly quoted figures.

Bladder damage

The bladder can be damaged at repeat caesarean when it may be particularly adherent to the lower segment, and this can occur even with blunt dissection when tissues are heavily fibrosed. The lower the bladder injury the greater the risk of subsequent fistula. If there is doubt, methylene blue dye via the urethral catheter may help. The tear can be repaired in two layers with 3.0 polyglycolic acid (dexon) suture. The integrity of the repair does not need to be tested. A urinary catheter is left in situ until microscopic haematuria clears and prophylactic antibiotics are administered.

Ureteral damage

The commonest cause of ureteric injury is an attempt to control parametrial bleeding following lateral extension of the uterine incision. Ligation or partial ligation of the ureter for a short time usually causes few problems, but clamping may cause crush injury and devitalisation of the tissue. If a clamp is placed on the ureter it should be removed immediately and a urological expert should be consulted. The important thing is to recognise any damage at the time of the operation so as to minimise subsequent morbidity. Opening the peritoneum high-up, dissecting the fibrosed bladder off the lower segment carefully, and taking the steps outlined previously to avoid extension of the uterine incision laterally should help the operator to avoid these problems altogether.

Bowel injury

Bowel injury is extremely rare at caesarean and almost all cases have adhesions secondary to previous surgery or infection. Small injuries may be repaired, suturing at right angles to the bowel axis in two layers, using 4.0 polyglycolic acid for the first layer and 4.0 silk for the second.

Surgical closure

After delivery, the uterus should not normally be exteriorised as traction on the pelvic viscera may be painful for the woman with regional anaesthesia. The uterine incision can be closed safely with a continuous locking, single layer suture (commonly Polyglactin (vicryl) No.1 suture). The traditional second imbricating layer was borrowed directly from the technique used to repair the vertical incision early in the 20th century and may increase tissue ischaemia and delay healing. Histological studies, hysterographic studies, and animal investigations have demonstrated that a single layer of suture in the uterine incision provides the best anatomical result and the strongest scar (Jelsema et al 1993). In addition, other studies have shown that compared with double layer closure of the uterus single layer closure reduces the risk of endometritis, decreases the operating time and is not associated with an increased rate of dehiscence in a subsequent trial of labour (Tischendorf 1987, Winkler et al 1986). Additional sutures will be required in up to 50% of cases to achieve haemostasis but, overall, there is still a significant reduction in the amount of suture material used. The use of uterine stapling devices have produced conflicting results and may offer little advantage over traditional closure methods. Classical incisions should be closed in three layers with a 'baseball' suture for the final line using a fine needle. When closing the rectus sheath, it is important to take large bites, at least 1 cm, with thick suture material to minimise the risk of tearing through.

Complete surface repair of large defects in the peritoneum is usually completed within 5–8 days (Di Zerega & Rodgers 1992). Ischaemia profoundly adversely affects the normal healing process and numerous animal studies show that suturing the peritoneum actually increases the incidence of adhesions. Moreover, both animal and human studies (Hull & Varner 1991, Pietrantoni et al 1991) demonstrate clearly that non-approximation of these layers does not increase infection rates, ileus, incisional hernia or dehiscence at 1 year follow-up. Recent reviews have concluded that it is both safe and prudent to omit peritoneal closure in the majority of pelvic operations.

The routine use of a suction drain placed beneath the rectus sheath after caesarean has been helpful in some randomised, controlled trials, but not in others (Saunders & Barclay 1988), and probably should be reserved for persistent oozing. However, closure of the Camper fascia, usually using a 3.0 plain catgut or vicryl running suture, has been shown to reduce the risk of haematoma formation in randomised, controlled trials (Del Valle et al 1992). The protective effect is even more marked in the obese woman. Alternatively en-bloc closure requires less suture material and shortens closure time, which in turn may reduce the risk of postoperative infection. For patients at high risk of postoperative dehiscence mass closure using the Smeade-Jones technique is recommended. Polydioxanone suture (PDS) retains its strength for up to 6 weeks and is ideal for such cases.

Three methods of skin closure were compared in a recent, prospective (though not randomised) Danish trial (Lindholt et al 1994). Predictably, the best cosmetic outcome both from the mother's and obstetrician's perspective was obtained using a subcutaneous rather than a percutaneous skin suture. Subcuticular prolene has the advantage over dexon that it can be removed completely early in the postoperative period.

Postoperative measures

Many well conducted studies have demonstrated the safety of early feeding after caesarean (within 6 h) (Kramer et al 1996). Early feeding is associated with earlier return of bowel sounds and no increase in gastrointestinal morbidity.

Early discharge (day 2) has also been shown to be safe (Brooten et al 1994), with up to 80% of mothers meeting the criteria required for early discharge. Outcome measures were no different from normal and there was no increase in re-admissions. This is an area which could be looked at more closely in the UK where typically mothers are not discharged until the fourth or fifth postoperative day.

Key points for clinical practice

- Caesarean sections are associated with higher rates of maternal morbidity and mortality than vaginal delivery.

- The increased maternal risks associated with unplanned caesarean operations do not in general justify elective caesarean to avoid the risks of emergency surgery.

- All women undergoing caesarean section should have a thrombo-embolism risk assessment performed to determine their postoperative thromboprophylaxis requirements.

- Anticipation is the key to safe caesarean sections and an experienced operator should be present at all operations where complications are predicted.

- Delivery of the fetal vertex in the occipitoanterior position at caesarean helps to prevent extension of the uterine incision angles and thereby lessens the risk of haemorrhage and iatrogenic trauma.

- Hysterectomy for haemorrhage at caesarean should be seen as a last resort and clinicians should be familiar with the variety of techniques available to avoid it.

- Antibiotic prophylaxis should be offered to all women undergoing caesarean section in labour. Routine antibiotic prophylaxis should also be seriously considered for elective caesarean sections.

- A continuous, locking single-layer suture is optimal for uterine closure. It is both safe and prudent to omit suturing the peritoneum after caesarean delivery, although the Camper fascia should be sutured routinely.

- Early feeding within 6 h of caesarean is safe, and women who have had uncomplicated operations may be considered for early discharge after 2 days.

References

Beattie P G, Rings T R, Hunter M F, Lake Y 1994 Risk factors for wound infection following caesarean section. Aust NZ Obstet Gynecol 34: 398–402

Brooten D, Roncoli M, Finkler S et al 1994 A randomised trial of early hospital discharge and home follow-up of women having caesarean birth. Obstet Gynecol 84: 832–838

Burke J F 1961 The effective period of preventive antibiotic action in experimental incisions and dermal lesions. Surgery 50: 161

Cho J Y, Kim S J, Cha K Y et al 1991 Interrupted circular suture: bleeding control during caesarean delivery in placenta praevia accreta. Obstet Gynecol 78: 876–879

Del Valle G O, Combs P, Qualls C, Curet L B 1992 Does closure of Camper fascia reduce the incidence of post-caesarean superficial wound disruption? Obstet Gynecol 80: 1013–1016

Dickason L A, Dinsmoor M J 1992 Red blood cell transfusion and caesarean section. Am J Obstet Gynecol 167: 327–332

Di Zerega G S, Rodgers K E 1992 The Peritoneum. New York: Springer, 11–23

Enkin M W, Enkin E, Chalmers I, Hemminki E 1989 Prophylactic antibiotics in association with caesarean section. In: Chalmers I, Enkin M W, Keirse M J (eds), Effective Care in Pregnancy and Childbirth. Oxford: Oxford University Press, 1246–1269

Evans S, McShane P 1985 SGO 160: 250

Finan M A, Mastrogiannis D S, Spellacy W N 1991 The Allis test for easy caesarean delivery. Am J Obstet Gynecol 164: 772–774

Frost L, Pedersen M, Seiersen E 1989 Changes in hygienic procedures reduces infection following caesarean section. J Hosp Infect 13: 143–148

Gibbs R S, St Clair P J, Castillo M S, Castoneda Y S 1981 Bacteriologic effects of antibiotic prophylaxis in high-risk caesarean section. Obstet Gynecol 57: 277–282

Gonik B, Shannon R L, Shawar R, Costner M, Seibel M 1992 Why patients fail antibiotic prophylaxis at caesarean delivery: histological evidence for incipient infection. Obstet Gynecol 79: 179–184

Heather Watts D, Hillier S L, Eschenbach D A 1991 Upper genital tract isolates at delivery as predictors of post-caesarean infections among women receiving antibiotic prophylaxis. Obstet Gynecol 77: 287–290

Hull D B, Varner M W 1991 A randomised study of closure of the peritoneum at caesarean delivery. Obstet Gynecol 77: 818–821

Jelsema R D, Wittingen J A, Vander Kolk K J 1993 Continuous non-locking, single-layer repair of the low transverse uterine incision. J Reprod Med 38: 393–396

Kramer R L, Van Someren J K, Qualls C R, Curet L B 1996 Post-operative management of caesarean patients: the effect of immediate feeding on the incidence of ileus. Obstet Gynecol 88: 29–32

Leigh D A, Emmanuel F X, Sedgwick J, Dean R 1990 Post-operative urinary tract infection and wound infection in women undergoing caesarean section: a comparison of two study periods in 1985 and 1987. J Hosp Infect 15: 107–116

Lilford R J, Van Coeverden De Groot H A, Moore P J, Bingham P 1990 The relative risks of caesarean section (intrapartum and elective) and vaginal delivery: a detailed analysis to exclude the effects of medical disorders and other acute pre-existing physiological disturbances. Br J Obstet Gynaecol 97: 883–892

Lindholt J S, Moller-Christensen T, Steele R E 1994 The cosmetic outcome of the scar formation after caesarean section: percutaneous or intracutaneous suture? Acta Obstet Gynecol Scand 73: 832–835

Lynch C B, Coker A, Lawal A H, Abu J, Cowen M 1997 The B-Lynch surgical technique for the control of massive postpartum haemorrhage: an alternative to hysterectomy? Five cases reported. Br J Obstet Gynaecol 104: 372–375

McCurdy C M, Magann E F, McCurdy C J, Saltzman A K 1992 The effect of placental management at caesarean delivery on operative blood loss. Am J Obstet Gynecol 167: 1363–1367

McVay P A, Hoag R W, Hoag M S, Toy P T 1989 Safety and use of autologous blood transfusion during the third trimester of pregnancy. Am J Obstet Gynecol 160: 1479–1488

Mordel N, Ezra Y, Benshushan A et al 1993 Transverse versus longitudinal uterine incision in caesarean delivery of triplets. J Reprod Med 38: 695–696

Naef R W, Ray M A, Chauhan S P et al 1995 Trial of labour after caesarean delivery with a lower segment, vertical uterine incision: is it safe? Am J Obstet Gynecol 172: 1666–1674

Nielsen T F, Hokegaard K 1984 Caesarean section and intraoperative surgical complications. Acta Obstet Gynecol Scand 63: 103–108

O'Leary J A 1995 Uterine artery ligation in the control of post-caesarean haemorrhage. J Reprod Med 40: 189–193

Pietrantoni M, Parsons M T, O'Brien W F et al 1991 Peritoneal closure or non-closure at caesarean. Obstet Gynecol 77: 293–296

Pritchard J A, Baldwin R M, Dickey J C, Wiggins K M 1962 Blood volume changes in pregnancy and the puerperium. II. Red cell loss and changes in apparent blood volume during and following vaginal delivery, caesarean section, and caesarean section plus total hysterectomy. Am J Obstet Gynecol 84: 1271–1282

Rodriguez A I, Porter K B, O'Brien W F 1994 Blunt versus sharp expansion of the uterine incision in low-segment transverse caesarean section. Am J Obstet Gynecol 171: 1022–1025

Saunders N J, Barclay C 1988 Closed suction wound drainage and lower-segment caesarean section. Br J Obstet Gynaecol 95: 1060–1062

Taylor V M, Kramer M D, Vaughan T L, Peacock S 1994 Placenta praevia and prior caesarean delivery: how strong is the association? Obstet Gynaecol 84: 55–57

Tischendorf D 1987 The single layer uterine suture in caesarean section: a comparative study. Geburtshilfe Frauenheilkd 47: 117–121

Winkler V M, Ruckhaberle K E, Saul S et al 1986 Clinical experiences with a single layer uterine suture in caesarean section. Zentralbl Gynakol 108: 1039–1042

Yancy M K, Clark P, Duff P 1994 The frequency of glove contamination during caesarean delivery. Obstet Gynecol 83: 538–542

Ann Johnson

Cerebral palsy and its relationship with pregnancy and delivery

In the last 15 years it has become increasingly clear that brain damage and maldevelopment may originate at any time from conception onwards. The clinical effects of such damage may be diverse, but there are recognisable clusters of neurological signs and symptoms which are included under the umbrella term of 'cerebral palsy'. These include difficulty with controlling movement, altered muscle tone, additional unwanted movements and varying degrees of associated sensory and intellectual impairment. The condition is non-progressive, but the disability arising may have profound implications for the child, the family and health and educational services.

For many years, attention has focused on birth as the most likely time at which brain injury resulting in this type of clinical picture occurs. Although it is possible for hypoxic–ischaemic damage to occur at this time, there is now considerable evidence that in many children with cerebral palsy, brain injury has occurred well before the time of birth.

In this chapter we will consider the response of the developing brain to hypoxic–ischaemic insults at different stages of gestation, the ways of visualising and studying the resulting lesions and clinical risk factors for cerebral palsy with particular attention to the times at which these may exert their effect.

EARLY BRAIN DEVELOPMENT

Brain development continues from a few days after conception until well into the second decade. By 30 days, the central nervous system begins to roll to form a tube and failure of this results in a neural tube defect (NTD). Between 7 and 16 weeks, nerve cells migrate from the germinal layer lining the

Ann Johnson MD ERCP, Developmental Paediatrician, National Perinatal Epidemiology Unit, Radcliffe Infirmary, Oxford OX2 6HE, UK

ventricles out to the cortex and central nuclei. Failure of this to happen results in a neuronal migration disorder (NMD). NMDs include various types of cortical dysplasia, such as lissencephaly in which the brain surface appears smooth, and polymicrogyria in which the brain surface is irregular with multiple small gyri. In general, therefore, insults to the brain which occur in the first few months of intra-uterine life will result in brain malformation.

From 28 weeks of gestation onwards, glial cells migrate into white matter and wrap a myelin sheath around nerve fibres. This process of myelination continues into adult life. It is between 28 and 36 weeks of gestation that areas of white matter, with their high metabolic rate, are so vulnerable to hypoxic–ischaemic damage. Acute, single or repeated episodes of hypoxia or more prolonged periods of chronic hypoxia at this time can result in white matter damage with cellular necrosis particularly in areas close to the ventricles (periventricular leucomalacia). If there are larger areas of necrosis, there may be large cystic areas, either unilateral or bilateral.

In contrast, as gestation progresses, asphyxial damage is found particularly in grey matter, that is the cortex and basal nuclei. Some areas are particularly vulnerable, such as the so-called 'watershed zones' which are distal areas where the blood supply from the terminal vessels of the main cerebral arteries is most precarious. The middle cerebral artery area is commonly involved, sometimes the thalamus and basal ganglia and, if the asphyxia is very severe, the brain stem also.

These interruptions in normal development can be associated with a clinical picture which is included under the umbrella term of 'cerebral palsy'. The severity and extent of the motor signs, and any additional intellectual and sensory signs will depend on the extent and site of the brain injury.

TIMING OF BRAIN INJURY

It is clear, therefore, that the gestational age of the fetus at the time when an insult occurs will determine the type of response in brain tissue. There has, therefore, been a good deal of interest in ways of visualising brain lesions, assessing the likely gestational age at which they occurred and then, in the light of that information, drawing inferences about whether the events which precipitated the injury, occurred before, during or after birth.

NEUROPATHOLOGICAL STUDY

Examination of the brains of babies who die either before birth or within a few days of birth show evidence of ischaemic white matter injury in approximately one-fifth (Squier & Keeling 1991). This white matter injury may be diffuse, or the lesions may be focal, cystic and multiple. Among stillbirths, these lesions must have arisen in pregnancy, as have the well established cystic lesions seen in babies who die within a few days of birth. It is plausible that had these babies survived, they might have had cerebral palsy. The lesions are located in the areas of the descending motor tracts and are similar to those described in autopsy studies of children with cerebral palsy. It may be difficult, however, to determine the exact timing of brain injury from these autopsy studies;

subsequent postnatal brain growth and development, secondary hydro-cephalus or atrophy can alter brain appearance considerably. There is scope for further work on the correlation of clinical and pathological findings in children with cerebral palsy who die in early childhood.

Fetal and neonatal neuro-imaging

Ultrasonography

Although recent advances in sonographic examination of the fetal brain have meant that fetal brain lesions may now be visualised during pregnancy, we remain limited in our ability to monitor brain development *in utero*. Apart from neural tube defects and evidence of ventriculomegaly, occasionally large haemorrhagic or cystic lesions may be detected, but this is uncommon (Achiron et al 1993).

Neonatal cranial ultrasound in preterm babies is now used routinely in many nurseries and it has been possible to search systematically for well-established lesions present at birth or the appearance of cystic lesions within a few days of birth. It is generally accepted that cysts will not be apparent until at least 10 days after an injury. However, these early onset lesions are not common (Murphy et al 1996, de Vries et al 1996) and a far more usual scenario is an apparently normal image immediately after birth and the subsequent development of echodense then echolucent lesions reflecting a postnatal haemorrhagic–ischaemic injury (Levene 1990). It is possible that not all lesions are detected on an early neonatal cranial ultrasound. Hope et al (1988) showed that 28% of non-haemorrhagic hypoxic–ischaemic lesions detected at autopsy are not identified on ultrasound and it remains to be seen if in the future more refined techniques will allow the more precise timing of lesions.

Other methods of neuro-imaging

Other neuro-imaging techniques may also be helpful in establishing the time of onset of lesions. Computerized tomography has been used particularly in the study of changes in the brain appearance in babies who appear asphyxiated at birth (Roland & Hill 1992). The radiation dose is not inconsiderable and the technical difficulties of moving sick babies to the equipment are daunting. As a result, magnetic resonance imaging (MRI) in the neonatal period has been more widely adopted as a way of detecting white matter changes and myelination defects, and studying the characteristics of the brain changes in term babies who appear to have had a hypoxic–ischaemic event around the time of birth and monitoring the changes over time. A characteristic pattern of injury is seen with damage to basal ganglia, thalamus and internal capsule, as well as the subcortical white matter and the cortex, that is, the typical response of the term brain to a hypoxic insult (Rutherford et al 1996). The later outcome of the baby correlates well with the severity of the MRI changes.

Methods of studying cerebral haemodynamics and function

The introduction of non-invasive methods of studying brain function rather than structure has perhaps been the most exciting advances in this area.

Doppler ultrasound has been used to measure cerebral blood flow velocity waveforms in cerebral vessels in the fetus and newborn (Mari & Deter 1992). Magnetic resonance spectroscopy (MRS) can be used to measure concentrations in brain tissue of phosphorus metabolites reflecting energy metabolism (Roth et al 1992); near infrared spectroscopy (NIRS) can be used at the bedside to measure brain oxygenation at cellular level, from which information on cerebral blood volume can be derived (Edwards et al 1988). These techniques have provided valuable information on brain function and haemodynamics during labour, during the neonatal period and following hypoxic–ischaemic injury. From these studies, it appears that following such injury and resuscitation, there is a biphasic type of injury, with initial loss of high energy phosphates, a recovery phase and then a secondary energy failure with cell death (Wyatt et al 1989). These techniques, which are currently available for research purposes only, may in future become available to identify which babies have had a severe hypoxic insult, to monitor brain function in the period following this, and act as a guide to the possible value of cerebroprotective therapies aimed at preventing or reducing the effects of secondary energy failure.

Neuro-imaging in later childhood

With increasing experience in the use and interpretation of MRI in children, there has been considerable interest in scanning children with cerebral palsy. Although there is yet to be a study of a total geographically defined population of children with cerebral palsy, observations on selected series suggest that up to one-third of CP children born at term have evidence of brain maldevelopment on MRI (Truwit et al 1992). This is a less common finding in CP children born preterm, in whom it is more likely to find evidence of PVL (periventricular leucomalacia) compatible with an ischaemic insult in the vulnerable period of 28–36 weeks gestation (Krageloh-Mann et al 1995). Preterm delivery occurs during this period and it is often not possible to determine the time of onset of the lesion in relation to birth. A further 12–16% of term CP children scanned have evidence of a late third trimester lesion, the timing and appearance of the lesion being compatible with hypoxia–ischaemia around the time of birth (Krageloh-Mann et al 1995).

As neuro-imaging techniques are made more available to CP children, it is likely that more lesions arising in early pregnancy will be detected. Relating the clinical signs during pregnancy and around birth and later scan findings may shed light on the significance and interpretation of clinical observations of fetal and neonatal state. For example, CP children with a brain maldevelopment may show signs of fetal distress and severe depression at birth leading to a diagnosis of birth asphyxia. Here, however, the signs of distress are the result of the pre-existing brain injury and not the cause of the brain injury.

Having considered the types of brain injury, the influence of gestational age on the type of response, and ways of directly visualising brain lesions, we now need to examine the clinical correlates of such lesions (Table 10.1). In other words, what are the risk factors for cerebral palsy and what do these tell us about the time of origin of a lesion?

Table 10.1 Known causes of cerebral palsy

Conception	Chromosomal abnormalities	Autosomal, X-linked, translocations/deletions
Pregnancy	Infection	Rubella, toxoplasmosis, cytomegalovirus, herpes, listeriosis, others
	Developmental	Malformations, neuronal migration disorders
	Vascular	Fetal hypoxic–ischaemic damage
	Toxins	Alcohol, lead, mercury, others
	Metabolic	Iodine deficiency
Labour and delivery	Intrapartum hypoxia –ischaemia	major obstetric event (unavoidable/avoidable)
Neonatal	Neonatal hypoxia – ischaemia	neonatal complications especially in preterm babies
Post-natal	Trauma or infection	

RISK FACTORS FOR CEREBRAL PALSY

Genetic factors

Families with multiple family members or siblings with cerebral palsy are not common. Karyotyping of affected children in such families and indeed more detailed investigation of CP children without a family history has revealed a number of different chromosome anomalies, particularly small translocations and deletions (Hughes & Newton 1992). Other genetically determined conditions which give rise to a CP-like clinical picture include neuro-cutaneous disorders, storage diseases and other metabolic disorders. Whether or not these children should be included under the umbrella term of cerebral palsy is a source of debate. Many are so labelled, at least initially, and this highlights the need for a full and careful assessment of all children with CP to exclude an underlying genetically determined disorder.

Presence of congenital anomalies

It has been recognised for a number of years that children with CP are more likely to have congenital anomalies, both major and minor, than children without CP (Coorsen et al 1991). Ectodermal defects arising early in fetal life will give rise to abnormalities of CNS, skin, and teeth. It has been of interest, therefore, that tooth enamel defects and abnormal palmar creases and finger print patterns have all been described in CP children (Bhat et al 1992). These markers of aberrant embryonic development support an early prenatal origin to CP in such children and need to be sought in all CP children.

Pre-existing maternal conditions and known early pregnancy risk factors

Extremes of maternal age (Cummins et al 1993), long menstrual cycle (Torfs et al 1990), and excessively long or short interpregnancy gap (Nelson & Ellenberg 1986) have all been identified as risk factors. It is not known how these factors operate, but it likely that they reflect a risk of abnormal early embryonic development. Intra-uterine infection with rubella, toxoplasmosis and cytomegalovirus can all cause brain injury, as can intra-uterine exposure to methyl alcohol, lead, mercury and probably other, as yet unrecognised, toxins. These are all probably rare causes of cerebral palsy.

Maternal thyroid dysfunction

Maternal thyroid dysfunction in pregnancy, both hyperthyroidism and the need for thyroid supplementation has been associated with an increased risk of CP in the baby (Nelson & Ellenberg 1986). Although not a commonly found risk factor, two recent observations have highlighted the importance of normal thyroid hormone homeostasis in early brain development. Blood thyroxine levels are related to gestational age and in one-third of babies born before 27 weeks of pregnancy, severe hypothyroxinaemia is found. On follow-up, the group with severe hypothyroxinaemia was at increased risk of cerebral palsy and intellectual delay compared with those with normal thyroxine levels (Reuss et al al 1996, den Ouden et al 1996). There is interest in evaluating thyroid replacement therapy in such babies (van Wassener et al 1996) and randomised

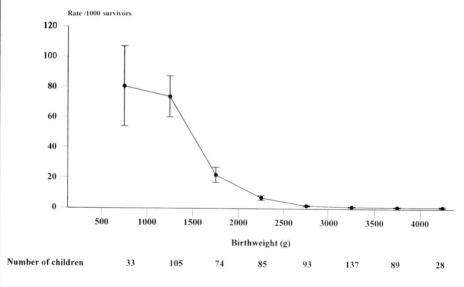

Fig. 10.1 Cerebral palsy rate/1000 survivors, with 95% confidence limits, by birthweight group among children born 1984–1991 (excluding postnatal cases) From Oxford Register of Early Childhood Impairments (1997).

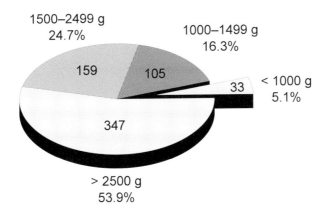

1500–2499 g
24.7%

1000–1499 g
16.3%

159   105

33   < 1000 g
5.1%

347

> 2500 g
53.9%

Fig. 10.2 Children with cerebral palsy born between 1984–1991 (total = 644; excluding postnatal cases) From Oxford Register of Early Childhood Impairments (1997).

trials are ongoing. A second observation was in a report of the one year follow-up of a randomised controlled trial of thyrotrophic releasing hormone (TRH) to mothers at risk of preterm labour (Crowther et al 1997). The babies of mothers who received TRH showed less advanced development compared to the control babies at the age of one year. Further follow-up will be needed for the clinical significance to be evaluated. However, these observations, together with the emerging evidence that maternal TRH does not appear to confer short-term benefit in the neonatal period, have led to the recommendation that TRH is not used in the management of threatened preterm labour.

Preterm birth

Preterm birth and low birthweight have a strong association with cerebral palsy. The rate of cerebral palsy per 1000 survivors for babies weighing less than 1 kg at birth is 80 times the rate for babies weighing more than 2.5 kg at birth (Fig. 10.1). Although only 1% of liveborn babies weigh less than 1.5 kg at birth, 20% of all children with CP are in this birthweight group (Fig. 10.2). During the 1980s, the rate of CP per 1000 livebirths among these very low birthweight babies increased (Pharoah et al 1990) and this was attributed to an increased rate of survival. There is some evidence that the rate of cerebral palsy has levelled off in the early 1990s, although 1 in 12 surviving babies weighing less than 1 kg will have cerebral palsy.

There is considerable interest in the possible explanations for this increased risk of cerebral palsy in babies born early (Fig. 10.3). One explanation is that an *in utero* ischaemic insult will result in both preterm birth and white matter damage resulting in later CP. Alternatively, preterm birth results in the delivery of a baby who is particularly vulnerable in the intrapartum and neonatal period to circulatory instability and subsequent brain hypoxia and ischaemia. A third possibility is that cerebral palsy represents the endpoint of a continuum of adverse effects that occur throughout the period of white matter vulnerability; these effects may occur before, during or after birth. A better understanding of the sequence of events which culminate in cerebral palsy in preterm babies could determine timing of preventive measures.

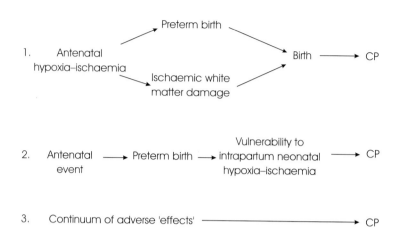

Fig. 10.3 Sequence of events in preterm birth and cerebral palsy.

Multiple births

Babies born of multiple pregnancies have 6 times the risk of cerebral palsy compared with singletons, and babies of higher order births have a 20-fold increase in risk (Pettersen et al 1993, Pharoah & Cooke 1996). This is partly accounted for by the increased risk of preterm delivery among multiples but, even within gestational age groups, multiples have a higher risk than singletons. Other complications of multiple pregnancy may contribute. The concordance rate for CP is higher among monozygotic than dizygotic twins suggesting that placental vascular anastomoses and instability of the fetal circulation may be factors. Antenatal loss of a co-twin is associated with a high risk of CP in the surviving twin and it has recently been suggested that unrecognised early loss of a twin could account for a proportion of unexplained CP children (Pharoah & Cooke 1996). This hypothesis will be difficult to test but, if sustained, there would be implications for assisted conception techniques and selective fetocide.

Pre-eclampsia

Babies of mothers with pre-eclampsia who are born before 33 weeks gestation are at a lower risk of cerebral palsy than babies of mothers without pre-eclampsia (Murphy et al 1995). A previous report showed that there is a reduction in the rate of germinal layer and intraventricular haemorrhage in preterm babies of pre-eclamptic mothers (Kuban et al 1992). A number of reasons for this reduced risk of neurological damage have been suggested. In some centres where magnesium sulphate is used in the management of pre-eclampsia, a neuro-protective effect on the fetus is postulated (Nelson & Grether 1995). This is supported by a similar risk reduction for CP when magnesium sulphate is used as a tocolytic in the absence of pre-eclampsia. These are observational studies, however, and whether there is a causal link between magnesium sulphate and a reduction in preterm cerebral palsy, or whether it is the underlying conditions which carry a reduced risk of cerebral palsy is uncertain. This can be best resolved with a randomized controlled trial and a multicentre trial in Australia is underway. An alternative explanation for the reduced risk of CP in very preterm babies of mothers with pre-eclampsia, is that these babies may die *in utero* or in the neonatal period. Although fetal death is clearly a danger in these high risk women, observational studies suggest that with a carefully timed elective delivery the risk of death or cerebral palsy in these babies is low.

In the term baby, maternal pre-eclampsia is a risk factor for CP, and placental insufficiency, with cerebral ischaemia may contribute (Gaffney et al 1994). This is supported by the observation that intra-uterine growth retardation, with or without pre-eclampsia, in term babies is also a risk factor for cerebral palsy.

Intra-uterine growth retardation (IUGR)

IUGR a risk factor for CP in term babies (Blair & Stanley 1990, Gaffney et al 1994) and also associated with ischaemic white matter lesions in babies who die *in utero* or early in the neonatal period (Gaffney et al 1994). Chronic hypoxia resulting in growth retardation may also be associated with cerebral ischaemia. Under both experimental conditions of intra-uterine hypoxia (Ashwal et al 1980), and growth retardation and in the human growth retarded fetus (Wladimoroff 1989), cerebral perfusion initially increases without alteration of regional distribution of blood flow within the brain. With severe and prolonged hypoxia, however, cerebral blood flow decreases and high metabolic areas such as areas where myelination is proceeding are vulnerable. This decreased blood flow has also been detected by Doppler techniques (Vyas et al 1990) and current work on the follow-up of growth retarded babies with abnormal blood flow velocity waveforms will provide further clarification.

One further group of CP babies among whom intra-uterine growth retardation appears to be an important risk factor are those who weigh between 1.5 and 2.5 kg at birth. Babies in this birthweight group have a 12-fold increase in rate of CP compared to babies weighing over 2.5 kg. Most of these babies do not have complications of prematurity in the neonatal period and, indeed, most of them are not admitted to a special care nursery. Their high risk of cerebral palsy is more likely related to antenatal cerebral injury or maldevelopment rather than intrapartum or neonatal events. Further work is needed in this area.

Maternal infection

Prolonged rupture of the membranes, maternal infection and chorioamnionitis are all associated with an increased risk of cerebral palsy particularly in preterm babies (Grether et al 1996, Murphy et al 1995). There are a number of possible mechanisms for this. Leviton (1993) suggested that some pregnant women mount an excessive response to infection, producing tumour necrosis factor (TNF) which results in altered cerebral circulation and a risk of brain ischaemia. TNF stimulates prostaglandin production (Romero & Mitchell 1989), and high prostaglandin E_2 concentration has been found in association with very early preterm labour when chorionitis is present (Hillier & Krohn 1988).

These types of observations have led to an interest in evaluating the use of antibiotics in delaying delivery in women with threatened preterm labour (Mercer & Arheart 1995). The ongoing MRC preterm antibiotic uncertainty study (ORACLE) may provide an opportunity to also test the effect of antibiotics in reducing the risk of later cerebral palsy in the babies.

Birth asphyxia

A huge literature debates whether or not intrapartum hypoxia–ischaemia is a cause of cerebral palsy and, if so, how it can be recognised. The term 'birth asphyxia' is not easily defined as no routine direct method is available to measure fetal oxygenation at the cellular level in pregnancy and during labour and delivery (Blair 1993). Indirect markers of fetal state are widely used, such as changes in fetal heart rate, pattern of fetal movement, and presence of meconium; more recent approaches have been use of Doppler ultrasound to estimate umbilical artery and cerebral artery velocity waveforms. Fetal acidosis can be measured in capillary scalp blood or umbilical cord blood and are assumed to reflect cellular acidosis. Signs of neonatal depression and neurological abnormality are used to infer that a preceding hypoxic event has occurred. Although useful in guiding clinical management, all these markers have a low sensitivity and specificity for later cerebral palsy.

The current position may be summarised as follows:

1. Experimental animal evidence indicates that damage to the fetal and neonatal brain occurs after prolonged and severe hypoxia. The response to an acute hypoxic event can be modified by previous metabolic and hypoxic stress.

2. Babies who have had a recent hypoxic event are ill in the neonatal period – they are profoundly depressed at birth and show signs of neurological dysfunction, usually seizures and often respiratory depression.

3. Such babies will have evidence of hypoxic damage to other organs such as myocardium, kidney and gastro-intestinal tract.

4. Intrapartum hypoxia–ischaemia is an unlikely cause of CP in the absence of a major clinically identifiable hypoxic event during labour or delivery, such as a major antepartum haemorrhage, ruptured uterus or cord prolapse.

Using these stringent criteria, no more than 10% of all children with cerebral palsy have had an intrapartum hypoxia–ischaemia and many of these will be unavoidable. Some observers estimate that an even lower proportion of CP is birth related (The Australian and New Zealand Perinatal Society 1995).

While the debate continues, there are a number of important therapeutic challenges. Firstly, there is considerable interest in targeting new therapies at preventing the secondary energy failure following hypoxia. A number of different agents have been identified which can potentially do this, including magnesium, allopurinol, insulin growth factors and others. Although there has been extensive animal work in this area, it is not easy to mount clinical trials in human subjects. The agents used are potentially toxic and the selection of recruits for the trials is a problem. As we have seen, the markers of birth asphyxia have a high false positive rate for cerebral palsy, that is, most babies with these markers will have a good outcome without a new experimental treatment. However, the effects of birth related hypoxic injury may be ameliorated if the therapeutic window between the initial injury and secondary energy failure can be successfully exploited. Further trials will be needed in due course.

Secondly, until newer and more precise techniques of evaluating fetal state and compromise become available, we will need to remain cautious when considering the origins of cerebral palsy in a child. Clinical markers thought to reflect birth asphyxia may reflect earlier brain injury or a period of reversible fetal stress.

The third challenge relates to vulnerability. Preceding events may alter the fetus's ability to respond to the normal stress of labour and delivery. Safe ways of assessing vulnerability would be helpful in planning the optimal time and mode of delivery.

In summary, cerebral palsy is the most serious disabling disorder of early childhood with a devastating effect on families. Despite considerable progress

Key points for clinical practice

- Children with cerebral palsy should be fully assessed including neuro-imaging, chromosome and metabolic studies even when there is a history of birth asphyxia.

- Randomized controlled trials of therapies aimed at reducing the frequency of risk factors for cerebral palsy will not only identify effective interventions but also contribute to our understanding of the aetiology of cerebral palsy.

- An evaluation of the place of magnesium sulphate in the management of preterm labour and pre-eclampsia is needed.

- In view of the risk of CP in multiple births, the outcome of multiple pregnancy, particularly after assisted conception needs to be monitored and the information collated.

- Endocrine and metabolic imbalances appear to be risk factors for neurodevelopmental abnormalities. Maternal or fetal thyroid dysfunction has been identified as a risk for cerebral palsy.

- Before attributing cerebral palsy to a hypoxic–ischaemic intrapartum event, the following criteria need to be fulfilled:
    (i)   A major clinically identifiable hypoxic event immediately prior to or during labour.
    (ii) Severe depression of the baby at delivery
    (iii) Signs of neurological dysfunction in the neonatal period, usually with seizures
    (iv) Evidence of hypoxic damage to other organs such as myocardium, kidney, or gastro-intestinal tract.

in understanding the time of origin of brain injury which results in the clinical picture of cerebral palsy, in many children the underlying cause remains unknown. Future hypotheses about aetiology and new therapies seem likely to emerge from the fields of developmental neurobiology, neuropathology and neuroradiology.

References

Achiron R, Hamiel Pinchas O, Reichman B et al 1993 Fetal intracranial haemorrhage: clinical significance of in utero ultrasonographic diagnosis. Br J Obstet Gynaecol 100: 995–999

Ashwal S, Majcher J S, Vain N, Longo L D 1980 Patterns of fetal lamb regional cerebral blood flow during and after prolonged hypoxia. Pediatr Res 14: 1104–1110

Bhat M, Nelso K B, Cummins S K, Grether J 1992 Prevalence of developmental enamel defects in children with cerebral palsy. J Oral Pathol Med 21: 241–244

Blair E 1993 A research definition for birth asphyxia? Dev Med Child Neurol 35: 449–455

Blair E, Stanley F 1990 Intrauterine growth and spastic cerebral palsy. Am J Obstet Gynecol 162: 229–237

Coorssen E A, Msall M E, Duffy L C 1991 Multiple minor malformations as a marker for prenatal etiology of cerebral palsy. Dev Med Child Neurol 33: 730–736

Crowther C A, Hiller J E, Haslam R R, Robinson J S Actobat Study Group 1997 Australian Collaborative trial of antenatal thryrotrophin releasing hormone: Adverse effects at 12 month follow-up. Pediatrics 99: 311–317

Cummins S K, Nelson K B, Grether J K, Velie E M 1993 Cerebral palsy in four Californian counties, births 1983 through 1985. Pediatrics 123: 230–237

de Vries L S, Eken P, Rademaker K, Groenendaal F, Bruinse H 1996 Antenatal onset of haemmorhagic/ischaemic lesions in the high risk preterm infant. Paediatr Perinatol Epidemiol 10: A4–A5

den Ouden A L, Kok J H, Verkerk P H, Brand R, Verloove-Vanhorick S P 1996 The relation between neonatal thyroxine levels and neurodevelopmental outcome at age 5 and 9 years in a national cohort of very preterm and/or very low birth weight infants. Pediatr Res 31: 142–145

Edwards A D, Wyatt J S, Richardson C, Delpy D T, Cope M, Reynolds E O R 1988 Cotside measurement of cerebral blood flow in ill newborn infants by near infrared spectroscopy. Lancet ii: 770–771

Gaffney G, Sellers S, Flavell V, Squier M V, Johnson A 1994 Case-control study of intrapartum care, cerebral palsy and perinatal death. BMJ 308: 743–750

Gaffney G, Squier M V, Johnson A, Flavell V, Sellers S 1994 Clinical associations of prenatal ischaemic white matter injury. Arch Dis Child 70: F101–F106

Grether J K, Nelson K B, Emery S, Cummins S K 1996 Prenatal and perinatal factors and cerebral palsy in very low birthweight infants. J Pediatr 128: 407–414

Hillier S L, Krohn M J 1988 A case control study of chorioamnionic infection and histological chorioamnionitis in prematurity. N Engl J Med 319: 972–978

Hope P L, Gould S J, Howard S, Hamilton P A, de L Costello A M, Reynolds E O R 1988 Precision of ultrasound diagnosis of pathologically verified lesions in the brains of very preterm infants. Dev Med Child Neurol 30: 457–471

Hughes I, Newton R 1992 Genetic aspects of cerebral palsy. Dev Med Child Neurol 34: 80–86

Krageloh-Mann I, Peterson D, Hagberg G, Vollmer B, Hagberg B, Michaelis R 1995 Bilateral spastic cerebral palsy – MRI pathology and origin. Dev Med Child Neurol 37: 379–397

Kuban K C K, Leviton A, Pagano M, Fenton T, Strassfeld R, Wolff M 1992 Maternal toxaemia is associated with reduced incidence of germinal matrix haemorrhage in premature babies. J Clin Neurol 7: 70–76

Levene M 1990 Cerebral ultrasound and neurological impairment: telling the future. Arch Dis Child 65: 469–471

Leviton A 1993 Preterm birth and cerebral palsy; is tumour necrosis factor the missing link? Dev Med Child Neurol 35: 549–558

Mari G, Deter R L 1992 Middle cerebral artery flow velocity waveforms in normal and small for gestational age fetuses. Am J Obstet Gynecol 166: 1262–1270

Mercer B M, Arheart K L 1996 Antimicrobial therapy in expectant management of preterm premature rupture of the membranes. Lancet 346: 1271–1279

Murphy D J, Hope P L, Johnson A 1996 Ultrasound findings and clinical antecedents of cerebral palsy in very preterm infants. Arch Dis Child 74: F105–F109

Murphy D J, Sellers S, MacKenzie I Z, Yudkin P L, Johnson A 1995 Case-control study of antenatal and intrapartum risk factors for cerebral palsy in very preterm singleton babies. Lancet 346: 1449–1454

Nelson K B, Ellenberg J H 1986 Antecedents of cerebral palsy. Multivariate analysis of risk. N Engl J Med 315: 81–86

Nelson K B, Grether J K 1995 Can magnesium sulphate reduce the risk of cerebral palsy in very low birthweight infants? Pediatrics 95: 263–269

Pettersen B, Nelson K B, Watson L, Stanley F 1993 Twins, triplets, and cerebral palsy births in Western Australia in the 1980s. BMJ 307: 1239–1243

Pharoah P O D, Cooke T, Cooke R W I, Rosenblom L 1990 Birthweight specific trends in cerebral palsy. Arch Dis Child 65: 602–606

Pharoah P O D, Cooke T 1996 Cerebral palsy and multiple births. Arch Dis Child 75: F174–F177

Reuss M L, Paneth N, Pinto-Martin J A, Lorenz J M, Susser M 1996 The relation of transient hypothyroxinaemia in preterm infants to neurologic development at two years of age. N Engl J Med 334: 821–827

Roland E H, Hill A 1992 MR and CT evaluation of profound neonatal and infantile asphyxia. Am J Neuroradiol 13: 973–973

Romero R M K R, Mitchell M D 1989 Infection and labour. Am J Obstet Gynecol 161: 336–341

Roth S C, Edwards A D, Cady E B et al 1992 Relation between cerebral oxidative metabolism following birth asphyxia and neurodevelopmental outcome and brain growth at one year. Dev Med Child Neurol 34: 285–295

Rutherford M, Pennock J, Schieso J, Cowan F, Dubowitz L 1996 Hypoxic-ischaemic encephalopathy: early and late magnetic resonance imaging in relation to outcome. Arch Dis Child 75: F145–F151

Squier M V, Keeling J W 1991 The incidence of prenatal brain injury. Neuropathol Appl Neurobiol 17: 29–38

The Australian and New Zealand Perinatal Society 1995 The origins of cerebral palsy – a consensus statement. Med J Aust 162: 85–90

Torfs C P, vandenBerg B J, Oechsli F W, Cummins S 1990 Prenatal and perinatal factors in the aetiology of cerebral palsy. J Pediatr 116: 615–619

Truwit C L, Barkovich A J, Koch T K, Ferriers D M 1992 Cerebral palsy: MR findings in 40 patients. Am J Neuroradiol 13: 67–78

van Wassener A G, Briet J M, van Baar A L, Kok J H 1996 Thyroxine supplementation in infants < 30 weeks gestational age: neurodevelopmental outcome at age 2 years of age. Paediatr Perinatol Res 10: A13

Vyas S, Nicholiades K H, Bower S, Campbell S 1990 Middle cerebral artery flow velocity wave forms in fetal hypoxaemia. Br J Obstet Gynaecol 97: 797–803

Wladimiroff J W 1989 Fetal cerebral blood flow. Clin Obstet Gynecol 32: 710–718

Wyatt J S, Edwards A D, Azzopardi D, Reynolds E O R 1989 Magnetic resonance and near infrared spectroscopy for investigation of perinatal hypoxic-ischaemic brain injury. Arch Dis Child 64: 953–963

Ronald. W. Jones

CHAPTER 11

The diagnosis and management of vulval intra-epithelial neoplasia

The first description of the lesion which today is termed vulval intra-epithelial neoplasia (VIN) is credited to Hudelo et al in 1922, a decade following Bowen's first report of the cutaneous variety. Numerous eponyms have been applied to the disorder (Bowen's disease of the vulva, Bowenoid atypia and dysplasia, Bowenoid papulosis, erythroplasia of Querat, carcinoma in situ of the vulva, hyperplastic dystrophy with severe atypia). All these terms have now been replaced by the revised terminology of the International Society for the Study of Vulvar Disease (ISSVD) and the International Society of Gynaecological Pathologists: vulval intra-epithelial neoplasia. The ISSVD terminology includes both squamous and non-squamous varieties (Table 11.1). The latter includes Paget's disease of the vulva and melanoma in situ; the clinical significance of these lesions is quite different from the squamous lesion and they will be considered separately. The importance of VIN relates to its symptoms and potential to progress to invasive vulval carcinoma.

Until 30 years ago, VIN was a very uncommon condition, usually presenting in women in middle and later life with pruritus and a unifocal

Table 11.1 Classification of vulval intra-epithelial neoplasia

A.	Squamous intraepithelial neoplasia	
	VIN 1	mild dysplasia
	VIN 2	moderate dysplasia
	VIN 3	severe dysplasia or carcinoma in situ
B.	Non-squamous intra-epithelial neoplasia	
	Paget's disease of the vulva	
	Melanoma in situ	

Ronald W. Jones FRCSE, FRCOG, FRNZCOG, Visiting Gynaecologist/Oncologist and Clinical Reader in Gynaecological Oncology, National Womens Hospital, Auckland, New Zealand (Post: 325 Manukau Road, P.O. Box 26-090, Epsom 3, Auckland, New Zealand)

slightly raised red lesion with a well defined serpiginous margin ('Bowen's disease" of the vulva). In 1973, Woodruffe et al suggested the lesion was a 'contemporary challenge', pointing to the increasing incidence in younger women, the possible role of viral infection and the role of conservative surgery. VIN is now a relatively common disorder, seen mainly in younger women and displaying a wide range of clinical and pathological features. The dramatic increase in the incidence of the condition parallels similar trends in cervical intra-epithelial neoplasia (CIN) and both appear to be associated with changing sexual mores, human papilloma virus (HPV) infection, cigarette smoking and occasionally immunosuppression.

In our unit, the mean age in the two decades before 1980 was 52.7 years, since then it has fallen to 35.8 years. While the incidence of VIN has increased in younger women, no increase has occurred in the older population (Jones & Rowan 1994). We have also noted a substantial delay in presentation in more than half of our patients, usually because the patient or her physician mistakenly assumes the symptoms are caused by infection, such as candidiasis or genital warts. Such a delay may be crucial because the reported time for progression to invasion in both treated and untreated cases is usually within 8 years (Jones & Rowan 1994, Herod et al 1996).

PATHOLOGY AND PATHOGENESIS

The current histological classification system follows that for CIN. In VIN 1 the cellular abnormalities involve the lower one-third of the epithelium with maturation of the surface epithelium. In VIN 2, the cellular changes extend into the middle third of the epithelium and VIN 3 is a full thickness involvement previously termed carcinoma in situ. A histological diagnosis of pure VIN 1 is uncommon and should be established with caution. Most reported cases probably represent reactive or viral processes without neoplastic potential. VIN 2 is a relatively uncommon histological diagnosis and is best considered as a biological high grade abnormality. Lesions which histologically comply with the criteria for VIN 3 can be subclassified into warty (condylomatous or Bowenoid), basaloid (undifferentiated common type) and differentiated (simplex) types. Mixtures of warty and basaloid VIN are common. Warty and basaloid VIN are found adjacent to the corresponding types of invasive carcinoma in the majority of cases and are usually HPV positive. The differentiated (carcinoma in situ simplex) type of VIN 3 is usually found adjacent to the common keratinising squamous cell carcinoma seen in older women. Such lesions are usually HPV negative (Kurman et al 1990). The older terminology 'epithelial dystrophy/squamous hyperplasia with marked atypia' would now be categorised as VIN 3.

Whilst the histological classification of VIN is similar to that for CIN, there are quite marked differences in the prevalence and significance of reporting the various grades of abnormality. For example, while low grade abnormalities (CIN 1/HPV) predominate cervical pathology biopsies, VIN 3 is the predominant lesion found in biopsies of the vulval lesion. While the CIN 1 to 3 histological grading system carries an implicit inference of a biological continuum which may end with invasive carcinoma, this has not been unequivocally demonstrated with VIN. The system of grading of VIN (like CIN) should be regarded as arbitrary. From a practical perspective, the clinician usually needs to address the management and outcome in women who present initially with high grade epithelial abnormalities, usually VIN 3.

The association between VIN and neoplasia (usually CIN) elsewhere in the lower genital tract is seen in up to a half of all cases. There are few parallels between CIN and VIN in relation to the later development of invasive cancer. While convincing evidence exists to show that nearly all squamous cervical cancers are preceded by the precursor lesion CIN, there is no evidence of a single precursor lesion in vulval cancer. Vulval carcinoma most commonly arises in a field of lichen sclerosus and/or squamous hyperplasia, or VIN and occasionally in normal skin. Histologically, CIN is adjacent to 90% of squamous cervical cancers, while VIN is present in only 20 to 30% of vulval carcinomas (Leibowitch et al 1990). CIN 3 can persist for very long periods of time before progressing to invasion. By contrast, reported cases of progression of VIN 3 to invasion have generally been less than 8 years (Jones & Rowan 1994, Herod et al 1996).

Involvement of skin appendages by VIN has been reported in 28 out of 50 cases by Mene and Buckley (1985) and 18 out of 50 cases by Baggish et al (1989). Failure to eliminate disease in skin appendages will inevitably lead to recurrences following therapy. Shatz et al (1989) demonstrated sebaceous-gland and hair-follicle involvement by VIN in 21% and 32%, respectively.

HPV DNA, nearly always type 16, has been reported in 60–90% of high grade lesions (Junge et al 1995). Park et al (1991) demonstrated that HPV positive women were younger than HPV negative women and their lesions more frequently demonstrated koilocytosis. These younger women are more likely to demonstrate multifocal lesions. HPV 16 E6 protein is known to complex with p53 protein, a negative regulator of cell proliferation. This mechanism appears to occur in HPV associated vulval cancers seen in younger women. In addition, malfunction of the cellular immune response seems to be a co-factor in the genesis of HPV neoplasia in the vulva (Petry et al 1996). A monoclonal origin of VIN has been demonstrated (Tate et al 1997).

The suggestion that herpes simplex virus type 2 (HSV2) may be associated with VIN has not been confirmed; though its role as a co-factor with HPV remains a possibility (Kaufman et al 1981).

The established association between CIN and cigarette smoking can now be extended to VIN. Two studies have reported twice the expected rate of cigarette consumption in women with VIN (Wilkinson et al 1988, Jones & Rowan 1994).

Immunosuppression (congenital, acquired or iatrogenic) is associated with intra-epithelial neoplasia throughout the lower genital tract. In addition, a strong association exists between HPV infection and anogenital malignancies in women with immunodeficiency (Petry et al 1996). In such patients, the dysplastic process is more likely to recur following treatment and there is an increased risk of progression of VIN to invasion. Penn (1986) reported a 100-fold increased risk of developing in situ or squamous cell carcinoma of the vulva and anus in immunosuppressed renal transplant recipients. Disordered immune function, including human immuno-deficiency (HIV) infection, should always be considered in women with recurrent disease.

Multicentric lower genital tract neoplasia is common in women with HIV infection. one study has documented a significantly higher rate of VIN in HIV infected women (Korn et al 1995). The failure rate following treatment is also higher in this group.

NATURAL HISTORY

The natural history of VIN continues to be the subject of debate. Knight (1943) regarded the lesion as a slowly growing epithelioma, and Lewis (1956) stated that 'all true cases of Bowen's disease of the vulva progress eventually to invasive cancer'. By contrast, recent reviewers have generally considered the lesion to be of low or 'uncertain' invasive potential, suggesting that fewer than 5–10% of cases eventually progress to invasion (Singer & Monaghan 1994). Two factors appear to have influenced these latter views. Firstly, the publication of the initial large clinical studies of VIN in the 1970s and 1980s reported 'progression' in about 4% of cases (Buscena et al 1980, Benedet & Murphy 1982) and, secondly, a number of early studies stressed the potential for spontaneous regression of the lesion (Skinner et al 1973, Bernstein et al 1983). Recent studies have not commented on regression as a feature of the condition. The early studies failed to indicate that the quoted 'progression' rates reflected the outcome in treated patients, and not the natural history of the untreated lesion.

Two recent large studies provide evidence of the outcome in women treated for VIN 3. Jones and Rowan (1994) noted 4 of 105 (3.8%) treated and 7 of 8 (87.5%) untreated cases developed invasion during a 7–18 year follow-up and Herod et al (1996) reported 9 of 92 (10%) treated cases developed invasion during a mean follow-up time of 5 years. With one exception in each series, the invasion occurred within 8 years. The observation that progression occurred in nearly all cases (both treated and untreated) within 8 years suggests that the onset of invasion in a treated patient probably reflects inadequate treatment. Singer and Monaghan (1994) suggest that the 30 year interval between the mean age incidence of VIN and squamous cell carcinoma of the vulva excludes a causal relationship. This view is difficult to support in the light of the evidence that invasive carcinoma usually develops within 8 years in women with both treated and untreated VIN.

The increasing incidence of VIN seen in younger women over the past two decades and the relatively short transit time of VIN to invasion would be expected to result in an increasing frequency of invasive vulval cancer in younger women. This outcome has been demonstrated in a study examining trends in squamous cell carcinoma of the vulva which compared two groups of women separated by 2–3 decades. In the early cohort (1965–1974), only one of 56 women (1.8%) was under 50 years of age at the time of diagnosis of invasive vulval carcinoma, while 12 of 57 (21%) of a recent cohort (1990–1994) were under 50 years of age. Ten of the 13 (77%) women under 50 years of age had an HPV related warty or basaloid VIN compared with 13 of 100 (13%) of women over 50 years of age. Both cigarette smoking and multiple lower genital tract neoplasia were significantly more common in women under 50 years of age (Jones et al 1997).

The finding of occult invasion in 6–18% of treatment excisional biopsies in women in whom the initial diagnosis had shown only VIN 3, points to the invasive nature of the lesion (Chafe et al 1988, Singer & Monaghan 1994).

A key step in tumour development is the switch to an angiogenic phenotype (Bancher-Todeska 1997). Compared with VIN 1 and 2, VIN 3 lesions demonstrate a dense network of microvessels under the dysplastic epithelium and an intense expression of an angiogenic peptide (vascular endothelial growth factor).

Chronic immunosuppression is a recognised factor in the progression of VIN to invasion. Possibly too much emphasis has been placed on the role of immunosuppression and advancing age as factors in progression, because most reported cases occur in healthy women, many of whom are relatively young.

Spontaneous regression of VIN 3 is a well recognised event in women with the clinical entity of Bowenoid papulosis. Patients with Bowenoid papulosis are young, often pregnant or recently pregnant, have dark skin and the lesions are usually multifocal, papular and pigmented. Such lesions can initially be managed by biopsy and observation alone, but persistence justifies a more active approach to treatment. Caution must be exercised with Bowenoid papulosis since there are reported cases of progression to invasion in young women (Planner et al 1987).

CLINICAL FEATURES

The majority of women presenting with high grade VIN complain of pruritus. The symptom is often mistakenly considered to be chronic candidiasis. Less commonly the presenting symptoms are of vulval soreness and superficial dyspareunia. On occasions, women note a lump which may be confused both by the patient and clinician as a condyloma. VIN must always be considered when a 'condyloma' fails to respond to conventional therapy. In some cases the lesion is noted as an incidental finding during vulval inspection, particularly in women with a history of neoplasia (especially CIN) elsewhere in the lower genital tract, or in women attending a Sexual Health Clinic. In such cases, the lesion is frequently asymptomatic.

The heterogeneous nature of VIN is best illustrated by the diversity of clinical appearances of the lesion. VIN 1 is never visible macroscopically, while higher grade lesions are nearly always visible to the naked eye and usually demonstrate a relatively well defined margin. Women under 40 years most frequently demonstrate multifocal VIN, while their older counterparts more often have unifocal lesions. The lesion may be red, white or pigmented; flat or papular. A thick white keratin surface may limit the examination. In this setting the vulval dermatoses, particularly squamous hyperplasia (formerly hyperplastic dystrophy) with or without lichen sclerosus needs to be considered in the differential diagnosis. Sometimes the lesion has a papillary appearance suggestive of condyloma acuminatum. Pigmented papular lesions may be similar to naevi. The lesion frequently extends from the perineum onto the perianal skin and may also involve the skin at the external urethral meatus. If the lesion extends to the anal margin, proctoscopy is necessary because the lesion may extend into the anal canal. Failure to recognise and adequately treat periurethral and perianal intra-epithelial neoplasia may explain the apparent excess of reported cases of progression to invasion in these sites (Jones & Rowan 1994).

Up to 50% of women will have antecedent or concomitant neoplasia elsewhere in the lower genital tract, usually the cervix. Thorough colposcopic examination of the entire lower genital tract is mandatory. Colposcopic examination is an invaluable adjunct in the evaluation of vulval lesions, facilitating optimum siting of biopsies. Occult invasive disease is more likely where there is an irregular surface contour. Vessels with atypical patterns may be visible if there is absence of squamous hyperplasia or hyperkeratosis. Application of swabs soaked in 5% aqueous acetic acid for 5 min to the vulval and perianal regions may enhance the appearance of VIN, particularly those cases which lack surface keratin. A 5% acetic acid solution sometimes causes discomfort, especially if there are fissures and consideration may need to be given to using a more dilute solution, particularly in postmenopausal women. Experience is necessary in the colposcopic assessment of acetic acid enhanced vulval skin changes because clinically unimportant changes (e.g. HPV, VIN 1) may become visible. Application of 1% toluidine blue followed by washing with dilute acetic acid may also assist in defining the abnormal epithelium suitable for biopsy. This technique has been criticised and re-evaluation is necessary. Clinical photography can provide a useful basis for comparison following treatment.

Where there is no possibility of an invasive lesion, representative biopsies should be performed under local anaesthesia using a 4 mm disposable punch biopsy. Caution is necessary because small vulval biopsies may fail to identify early invasive disease. It has already been noted that unrecognised invasive carcinoma has been reported in 6–18% of women in whom pretreatment 'representative' biopsies have demonstrated VIN alone (Chafe et al 1988). The use of a colposcope facilitates the most appropriate siting of biopsies. Extensive multifocal lesions require multiple 'mapping' biopsies. Where the possibility of invasion exists, an excision type biopsy will provide a more appropriate specimen for histological assessment. The importance of such a biopsy is essential because of its relevance to the management of FIGO Stage 1A versus higher stage invasive vulval carcinoma.

TREATMENT

Treatment needs to be individualised and should be as conservative as possible with the object of the relief of symptoms, the prevention of cancer, the avoidance of vulval mutilation and the maintenance and enhancement of sexual activity. Options are dependent on the previous clinical assessment of the patient and the lesion. The possibility of psychological stress and sexual dysfunction must be taken into account when planning the treatment for women with VIN. Factors include the patient's age and sexual history, the nature and extent of the lesion, the skill of the clinician and the facilities available (e.g. laser). Extensive lesions in younger patients should ideally be managed by an experienced physician. Before treatment commences, the patient should be warned of the possibility of recurrences, the small future risk of invasive vulval cancer, and the importance of lifelong follow-up. The use of a magnifying instrument enhances the operator's ability to define accurately the lesion at the time of surgery. Effective local anaesthesia should be an integral part of all vulval operations.

Recurrences will occur in approximately 20–30% of cases following treatment. These reflect both persistent and new disease. One study using life table analysis reported the risk of recurrence to be as high as 55% over a 10 year period, though noting a low risk after 4 years of follow-up (Herod et al 1996).

Excisional techniques (cold knife or laser) do allow assessment of the specimen either by frozen section or by laboratory histopathology. Andreasson and Beck (1985) studied 49 women who had been treated by local excision and found only 1 of 23 (4.3%) patients with a clear margin developed a recurrence, compared with 11 of 19 (57.9%) with involved margins. Nine of 22 (40%) of women with multifocal disease had recurrences compared with 4 of 24 (16.7%) women with unifocal disease. The high recurrence rate in the group with multifocal disease was due to the fact that 54.6% of these patients had involved margins. Other studies (Rettenmaier et al 1987), however, have failed to predict reliably the site and frequency of recurrence by the status of the surgical margins. One must conclude that while many recurrences reflect persistent disease, some recurrences do represent new disease. New disease may develop in grafted skin and following simple vulvectomy.

Local excision

Local excision is the most universally applicable method of treatment and should be the only option where the possibility of invasion exists. It is ideal for small (especially unifocal) lesions and for the 'occasional' operator. The excision should be superficial, allowing preservation of the subcutaneous tissues. Even when large areas need to be excised, it is almost always possible to achieve primary skin closure. In these circumstances, undermining and mobilisation of the skin edges may be necessary. A vaginal advancement procedure may be required for perineal lesions. On rare occasions, a skin flap may be required. Accurate skin closure with fine absorbable suture materials produces excellent results. The excised specimen should be orientated carefully for presentation for histological assessment.

Skinning vulvectomy

When the lesion is extensive (and as an alternative to laser vaporisation), a skinning procedure with split-skin grafting can achieve satisfactory results (Rettenmaier et al 1987). Although termed 'skinning vulvectomy', the area excised would only include the area of involved skin.

Simple vulvectomy

This was the standard management technique until 30 years ago but should now be regarded as a mutilating and unnecessary operation. This radical approach is not a guarantee against future recurrences of VIN or the development of invasive cancer. On rare occasions, it may be a valid option in the elderly woman with an extensive lesion especially where the possibility exists of early invasion.

CO$_2$ laser

Treatment with laser (either ablation or excision) should only be performed by clinicians skilled in the technique. It is particularly useful in young women with extensive multifocal lesions where preservation of vulvar appearance is a priority. While some authors (Baggish et al 1981) have recommended a multi-stage procedure, the author has found an aggressive attempt to eliminate as much disease at the primary procedure is preferable, followed by smaller secondary procedures if required.

The technique involves a detailed knowledge of the anatomy of the vulvar skin and the histopathology of VIN, in particular the involvement of skin appendages (Reid 1985, Shatz 1989, Baggish 1989). It should only be performed by an experienced operator. On the basis of Shatz's (1989) observations, the depth of destruction of VIN affecting non-hairy skin should be 1 mm and in hairy skin 2 mm. In general, laser vaporisation achieves better results in non-hairy skin because of the lack of occult disease in hair follicles. The prevention of postoperative pain and urinary difficulties is a vital part of management. Patients need to be warned that complete skin healing usually takes some weeks.

Electrocoagulation, loop excision, cryosurgery and ultrasonic aspiration techniques are also described, but none appear to have significant advantages over the methods described above.

Special sites

The clitoris, external urethral meatus and perianal skin present particular difficulties in management. The apparent excess of invasive cancers noted in some studies at these sites in women who have previously been treated for VIN probably reflects persistent disease (Jones & Rowan 1994). Thorough pre-operative assessment of these sites is vital if effective treatment is to be performed.

Laser treatment to the clitoris is theoretically appealing but the irregular surface topography of the small organ creates difficulty with optimum laser application. Residual islands of VIN create the potential for later invasive disease. Complete skinning of the glans clitoris with a scalpel (sometimes with grafting) without removal of the body of the clitoris avoids this possibility.

Perineal involvement with VIN should always raise the possibility of perianal or anal canal involvement. The laser has no place in the treatment of perianal or anal canal disease and complete excision is the preferred management. Similarly, involvement of the epithelium at the external urethral meatus demands an excisional procedure, with care being taken to ensure that the margins of the specimen are normal.

Medical therapy

Attempts to treat VIN with topical 5-fluorouracil (5-FU) have largely been abandoned. In a review of 17 papers, including 68 patients, Sillman et al (1985) recorded remissions in only 34% and failures in 59%. They noted that the endpoint was 'determined more by patient intolerance than by tumour clearance'. Topical immunotherapy has also been investigated. While theoretically appealing, treatment again appears to be limited by patient tolerance and there are no reports on long term effectiveness. Spirtos et al (1990) report a complete response lasting at least 1 year in 50% of 21 patients with VIN 3 treated with topical alpha interferon. In this study, 2 of 21 (9%) women had to be withdrawn because they were found to have invasive vulval carcinoma. Topical and intradermal bleomycin also appear to be ineffective. In summary, all of the medical therapies studied to date have been associated with both significant local discomfort and unproven long term effectiveness.

Follow-up

Life-long surveillance of all women who have had a previous diagnosis of VIN 2–3 is essential. Whilst most recurrences occur in the early years following initial treatment, recurrences of VIN and the development of invasive vulval cancer can occur decades later. The follow-up examination must include annual cervical cytology, together with colposcopic assessment of the entire lower genital tract. The initial follow-up intervals of between 3 and 6 months may be relaxed to annual examinations when the risk of recurrence is considered to be low; the immunosuppressed patient requires at least 6 monthly follow-up for life. The onset of vulval symptomatology warrants urgent re-assessment in all patients with a history of VIN.

The concept of screening for VIN and other vulval dermatoses with the potential for neoplastic transformation has yet to be explored. Women with a history of multiple lower genital tract neoplasia are an 'at risk' group in whom regular and detailed inspection by a clinician is necessary. Finally, all women should be encouraged to inspect the vulva regularly with the assistance of a mirror.

PAGET'S DISEASE OF THE VULVA

Extramammary Paget's disease of the vulva is an intra-epithelial neoplasia associated with proliferation of atypical glandular cells of apocrine type. It is primarily seen in postmenopausal women. Unlike its counterpart in the breast which is invariably associated with an underlying ductal carcinoma, only 20% of women with vulval Paget's disease have an underlying carcinoma. Such adenocarcinomas most commonly arise from the Bartholin's gland or adjacent sweat gland skin appendages. Perianal Paget's disease is commonly associated with underlying rectal adenocarcinoma.

Paget's disease is characterised by distinctive large Paget's cells which are present singly or in clusters throughout the epithelium. Histochemical staining (especially PAS or mucicarmine) will assist in excluding melanoma in situ or VIN. Unlike VIN, where the histological extent of the disease correlates closely with the macroscopoic lesion, Paget's cells usually extend well beyond the gross lesion. However, there is an insignificant risk of an underlying adenocarcinoma in the clinically normal skin peripheral to the Paget's disease.

Most patients have long-standing pruritus or soreness and classically present with moist erythematous areas interspersed with areas of white epithelium. Careful palpation of the lesion is important because underlying carcinomas may be present. Extravulval carcinomas are reported in up to 30% of cases and appropriate evaluation of all patients is necessary.

When there is no evidence of an underlying carcinoma, the management of choice is wide local excision to the fascia with a 2–3 cm margin. Frozen section is often not clinically useful. Long term follow-up is necessary because in situ recurrences are not uncommon. These are best treated with local re-excision.

Intraepithelial melanoma

Intraepithelial melanoma (melanoma in situ) is an uncommon and usually incidental finding in patients who have had excision of a pigmented lesion. The clinical presentation is a flat lesion with an irregular border and variable pigmentation. The histology is characterised by atypia of basal melanocytes without involvement of the underlying dermis. The atypical melanocytes proliferate as single cells or as clusters and migrate through the epidermis similar to Paget's disease. It corresponds with Clark and Chung's classification level 1 malignant melanoma (Kurman et al 1990).

EARLY INVASIVE VULVA CARCINOMA

In 1995, FIGO included a substage (FIGO Stage 1A) of vulval cancer which includes solitary squamous carcinomas of 2 cm or less in diameter with a depth of invasion of 1 mm or less. These tumours are also termed 'superficially invasive carcinoma' (SICa). In this situation, the most common surface epithelial finding is VIN. These early invasive carcinomas may be more frequent than previously recognised.

The importance of recognising this lesion relates to management. In large series where the depth of invasion has been well defined, lymph node metastasis with invasion to a depth of 1 mm or less is nil. Such lesions can, therefore, be managed by local excision alone.

References

Andreasson B, Bock J E 1985 Intraepithelial neoplasia in the vulvar region. Gynecol Oncol 21: 300–305
Baggish M S, Dorsey J H 1981 CO$_2$ laser for the treatment of vulvar carcinoma in situ. Obstet Gynecol 57: 371–375
Baggish M S, Sze E H, Adelson M D et al 1989 Quantitative evaluation of the skin and accessory appendages in vulvar carcinoma in situ. Obstet Gynecol 74: 169–173
Bancher-Todesca D, Obermair A, Bilgi S et al 1997 Angiogenesis in vulvar intraepithelial neoplasia. Gynecol Oncol 64: 496–500
Benedet J L, Murphy K J 1982 Squamous carcinoma in situ of the vulva. Gynecol Oncol 14: 213–219
Bernstein S G, Kovacs B R, Townsend D E et al 1983 Vulvar carcinoma in situ. Obstet Gynecol 61: 304–307
Buscema J, Woodruffe J D, Parmley T H et al 1980 Carcinoma in situ of the vulva. Obstet Gynecol 55: 225–230

Key points for clinical practice

- The VIN terminology has now replaced all previous terminology.

- There has been a significant increase in the incidence of the disease in younger women over the past 2–3 decades. The majority of these cases are associated with HPV 16 infection.

- A histological diagnosis of pure VIN 1 is uncommon. Most cases probably represent viral or reactive changes, are without neoplastic potential, and do not require treatment.

- VIN 2–3 is a heterogeneous condition with a range of clinical and pathological features. The pruritus associated with VIN is often mistakenly considered to be chronic candidiasis and 'lumps' may be confused with condyloma. VIN may be asymptomatic. Up to one-half of all cases are associated with CIN or invasive cervical cancer and cigarette smoking.

- The 'low' progression rate of VIN to invasive vulvar cancer (4–10%) quoted by many authors represents the outcome in treated cases. Untreated cases in women of all ages appear to have a significant risk of progression to invasion within 8 years. A small clinically defined subset of VIN 2–3 (Bowenoid papulosis) may sometimes spontaneously regress.

- Treatment needs to be individualised, with the exclusion of invasive cancer a priority. Local surgical excision is the mainstay of management. Extensive lesions should be referred to specialist centres.

Chafe W, Richards A, Morgan L et al 1988 Unrecognized invasive carcinoma in vulvar intraepithelial neoplasia. Gynecol Oncol 31: 154–162

Herod J J, Shafi M I, Rollason T P et al 1996 Vulvar intraepithelial neoplasia: long term follow up of treated and untreated women. Br J Obstet Gynaecol 103: 446–452

Hudelo M M, Oury et Cailliau 1922 Dyskeratose erythroplasiforme de la muqueuse vulvaire. Bull Soc Franc de Dermat et Syph 29: 139–142

Jones R W, Rowan D M 1994 Vulvar intraepithelial neoplasia III. A clinical study of the outcome in 113 cases with relation to the later development of invasive vulvar carcinoma. Obstet Gynecol 84: 741–745

Jones R W, Baranyai J, Staples S 1997 Trends in squamous cell carcinoma of the vulva: the influence of vulvar intraepithelial neoplasia. Obstet Gynecol 90: 448–452

Junge J, Poulsen H, Horn T et al 1995 Human papillomavirus in vulvar dysplasia and carcinoma in situ. APMIS 103: 501–510

Kaufman R H, Dreesman G R, Burek J et al 1981 Herpes virus induced antigens in squamous cell carcinoma in situ of the vulva. N Engl J Med 305: 483–488

Knight R van D 1943 Bowen's disease of the vulva. Am J Obstet Gynecol 46: 514–524

Korn A P, Abercrombie P D, Foster A 1996 Vulvar intraepithelial neoplasia in women infected with human immunodeficiency virus-1. Gynecol Oncol 61: 384–386

Kurman R J, Norris H J, Wilkinson E J 1990 Tumours of the cervix, vagina and vulva In: Atlas of Tumor Pathology, 3rd series. Washington: Armed Forces Institute of Pathology

Leibowitch M, Neill S, Pelisse M 1990 The epithelial changes associated with squamous cell carcinoma of the vulva: a review of the clinical, histological and viral findings in 78 women. Br J Obstet Gynaecol 97: 1135–1139

Lewis T L 1956 Progress in Clinical Obstetrics and Gynaecology. London: J & A Churchill, 541–562

Mene A, Buckley C H 1985 Involvement of the vulval skin appendages by intraepithelial neoplasia. Br J Obstet Gynaecol 92: 634–638

Park J S, Jones R W, McLean M R et al 1991 Possible etiologic heterogeneity of vulvar intraepithelial neoplasia. Cancer 67: 1599–1607

Penn I 1986 Cancers of the anogenital region in renal transplant recipients. Cancer 58: 611–616

Petry K U, Kochel H, Bode U et al 1996 Human papillomavirus is associated with the frequent detection of warty and basaloid high grade neoplasia of the vulva and cervical neoplasia among immunocompromised women. Gynecol Oncol 60: 30–34

Planner R S, Andersen H E, Hobbs J B et al 1987 Multifocal invasive carcinoma of the vulva in a 25 year old woman with Bowenoid papulosis. Aust NZ J Obstet Gynaecol 27: 291–295

Reid R 1985 Superficial laser vulvectomy. A new surgical technique for appendage-conserving ablation of refractory condylomas and vulvar intraepithelial neoplasia. Am J Obstet Gynecol 152: 504–509

Rettenmaier M A, Berman M L, DiSaia P J 1987 Skinning vulvectomy for the treatment of multifocal vulvar intraepithelial neoplasia. Obstet Gynaecol 69: 247–250

Shatz P, Bergeron C, Wilkinson E J et al 1989 Vulvar intraepithelial neoplasia and skin appendage involvement. Obstet Gynecol 74: 769–774

Sillman F H, Sedlis A, Boyce J G 1985 A review of lower genital tract neoplasia and the use of topical 5-fluorouracil. Obstet Gynecol Surv 40: 190–220

Singer A, Monaghan J M 1994 Vulvar intraepithelial neoplasia. In: Singer A, Monaghan J M (eds) Lower Genital Tract Precancer. Boston: Blackwell, 177–223

Skinner M S, Sternberg W H, Ichinose H 1973 Spontaneous regression of Bowenoid atypia of the vulva. Obstet Gynecol 42: 40–46

Spirtos N M, Smith L H, Nelson N H 1990 Prospective randomised trial of topical alpha interferon for the treatment of vulvar intraepithelial neoplasia 111. Gynecol Oncol 37: 34–38

Tate J E, Mutter G L, Boynton K A et al 1997 Monoclonal origin of vulvar intraepithelial neoplasia and some vulvar hyperplasias. Am J Pathol 150: 315–322

Wilkinson E J, Cook J C, Friedrich E G et al 1988 Vulvar intraepithelial neopolasia: association with cigarette smoking. Colposc Gynecol Laser Surg 4: 153–159

Woodruffe J D, Julian C, Puray T et al 1973 The contemporary challenge of carcinoma in situ of the vulva. Am J Obstet Gynecol 115: 677–686

Paul Donnellan David Fennelly

Advances in the treatment of ovarian cancer with paclitaxel

The incidence of ovarian cancer is high in North America and Northern Europe. In the US, approximately 1 woman in 70 will develop ovarian cancer (Green et al 1984) and this accounts for approximately 13 000 deaths each year. In Ireland, ovarian cancer is responsible for about 200 deaths each year. The death rate from ovarian cancer surpasses the death rates from cervical and endometrial cancer combined.

The primary treatment for early stage ovarian cancer is surgery which should entail a total abdominal hysterectomy in addition to bilateral salpingo-oophorectomy, and complete surgical staging. In situations of borderline ovarian tumours where future fertility is important, a unilateral oophorectomy may be an option. For these patients and patients with stage IA well differentiated tumours, no additional therapy is indicated. These patients have a 10 year relapse rate of only 10% (Ozols et al 1992). All other patients with early stage ovarian cancer should receive adjuvant therapy as these have a 10 year relapse rate of 30–40%.

More than two-thirds of cases are advanced at the time of diagnosis, i.e. stage III/IV (Nejit 1992) and these patients cannot be cured with surgery alone. Consequently, systemic chemotherapy has become the major treatment modality for this cancer. Cyto-reductive surgery to reduce the diameter of the largest residual mass to less than 2 cm results in a better response to chemotherapy.

Platinum-based chemotherapy, initially cisplatin and more recently carboplatin, has been the cornerstone of combination chemotherapy for advanced ovarian cancer since the late 1970s. Platinum-based combination chemotherapy yields overall response rates in the region of 70%, with a complete response rate of 20%. Meta-analysis has demonstrated the superiority of

Dr Paul Donnellan MSc MB MRCP(I), Research Fellow in Medical Oncology, St Vincent's Hospital, Elm Park, Dublin 4, Ireland

Dr David Fennelly MSc MB MRCP(I), Consultant Medical Oncologist, St Vincent's Hospital, Elm Park, Dublin 4, Ireland

platinum based combination chemotherapy when compared with non-platinum single-agent therapy, when compared with non-platinum containing combination therapy and finally when compared with single-agent platinum therapy (Advanced Ovarian Cancer Trialists' Group 1991). However, despite improved response rates, platinum-based combinations appear not to confer any additional advantage in terms of survival compared to single-agent platinum.

With 'standard' cisplatin and cyclophosphamide treatment, long-term disease control may be expected in less than 10% of women with incompletely resected stage III, and less than 5% of women with stage IV disease (Sutton et al 1989). The prognosis for patients with advanced ovarian cancer remains poor with reported 5-year survival rates ranging between 15–20% (Wingo 1995). In view of this, it is apparent that adequate disease control requires regimens containing new drugs.

TAXANES

The taxanes, comprise a new class of chemotherapy agents that have a totally different chemical structure as well as a unique mechanism of action. Taxanes were originally obtained from the bark of the uncommon and slow-growing Pacific yew (*Taxus brevifolia*). The crude extract from this plant was noticed to have anti-cancer activity in 1963, following a National Cancer Institute screening of thousands of plants for such activity. Paclitaxel, the first taxane to be studied in clinical trials, was identified as the active component and purified from the plant in 1971. Initially development was slow, partly because of difficulty obtaining large amounts of the drug from such a scarce resource, and also because of solubility problems. The solubility problems were later overcome with the use of a polyethylated castor oil vehicle (Cremophor).

In contrast to the vinca alkaloids, which were known to interfere with the assembly of tubulin subunits into microtubules, paclitaxel was found to actually promote the assembly of tubulin subunits, as well as enhancing the stability of the microtubules once formed. This interferes with the normal turnover of the cytoskeleton components and thus reduces intracellular transport and cell division. The cell cycle is halted at a crucial phase of division resulting in so-called 'meta-phase arrest'. This is also the phase of the cell cycle during which the cell is most sensitive to ionising radiation and may explain the observed activity of paclitaxel as a radiosensitiser. Paclitaxel also promotes the expression of the gene for tumour necrosis factor α, although the mechanism and significance of this are unclear.

Early clinical trials

Early phase I trials with paclitaxel were hampered by hypersensitivity reactions to the extent that its future looked in doubt. The hypersensitivity reactions were mostly type I and occurred in over one-quarter of patients. The Cremophor carrier was thought to be responsible as it was shown to induce histamine release and similar reactions in animal studies. Phase I studies were made possible by employing a prolonged (24 h) infusion of paclitaxel following premedication with corticosteroids, and histamine H_1 and H_2 antagonists. With premedication the incidence of hypersensitivity has been reduced to less than 3% (Rowinsky et al 1993).

Paclitaxel toxicity

The phase I studies revealed neutropenia to be the principal toxicity of paclitaxel. With doses of paclitaxel, of 200–250 mg/m^2, granulocyte colony stimulating factor (G-CSF) is usually given to prevent neutropenic complications. The maximum tolerated dose without G-CSF support appears to be in the range of 175-200 mg/m^2.

Paclitaxel also commonly causes paraesthesia which is usually mild, symmetrical and in a 'glove and stocking' distribution. Symptoms usually come on gradually after multiple cycles at conventional doses (135–250 mg/m^2). Rarely, the neuropathy may manifest as a motor or autonomic dysfunction or as optic nerve symptoms such as scotomata.

Other side effects of paclitaxel include transient myalgia, asymptomatic bradycardia and, rarely, cardiac conduction defects and dysrhythmias. Paclitaxel has limited gastrointestinal tract toxicity with vomiting and diarrhoea being infrequent. Mucositis may occur with prolonged infusions. Alopecia occurs in practically all patients treated with paclitaxel though this is reversible.

Paclitaxel anti-tumour activity

Early phase I (Sarosy et al 1992) and phase II (McGuire et al 1989, Thigpen et al 1994, Einzig 1992, Kohn et al 1994) studies of single agent paclitaxel in patients with advanced or platinum-refractory ovarian cancer, involving a total of 171 patients demonstrated an overall response rate (ORR) of 38% in platinum-sensitive and 32% in platinum-refractory patients (Rowinsky & Donehower 1995). The doses of paclitaxel used in these studies were substantially lower than the maximum tolerated dose for that drug. All of these studies employed paclitaxel as a 24 h infusion. Such response rates had not been seen with any other drug in ovarian cancer since the advent of cisplatin. Based on early results from these trials, paclitaxel was approved by the Food and Drug Administration in 1992, at a dose of 135 mg/m^2 on a 24 h schedule, for the treatment of women with refractory or recurrent epithelial ovarian cancer.

Following this, the National Cancer Center instituted a treatment-referral-center program to facilitate the compassionate use of paclitaxel in women whose ovarian cancer had progressed after treatment with two or more different regimens (Trimble et al 1993). The women who enrolled on this program were treated with paclitaxel 135 mg/m^2 over 24 h. Of the first 1000 of these heavily pre-treated, poor-prognosis patients, 22% had a major response. The median time to progression was 7 months and the median survival was 9 months. The toxicity profile was acceptable and, unlike other chemotherapeutic agents, did not appear to be cumulative.

Paclitaxel dose and scheduling

Following the encouraging early results with moderate doses of paclitaxel, phase II trials of higher doses with G-CSF support were conducted. One such trial from the National Cancer Institute (Kohn et al 1994), using paclitaxel 250 mg/m^2 in patients with platinum-resistant recurrent ovary cancer, obtained an ORR of 48%, indicating a possible dose-response relationship. However, median survival time (11.5 months) and relapse free survival time (6.2 months) were similar to those reported in the earlier trials using lower doses. Following this study, the Gynecologic Oncologic Group (GOG) is performing a prospective randomised trial comparing paclitaxel at 135, 175 and 250 mg/m^2 with G-CSF support in patients with platinum-refractory ovarian cancer. In fact, the lowest dose arm in this study has been discontinued due to reduced accrual once paclitaxel became commercially available.

In a further randomized study of paclitaxel at 175 mg/m^2 versus 250 mg/m^2 in patients with platinum pretreated advanced ovarian cancer, improved response rates (36% versus 27.5%) were demonstrated for the higher dose arm, but again no significant benefit in either progression-free survival or overall survival (Omura et al 1996).

In an effort to increase the intensity of paclitaxel exposure, many investigators have evaluated the potential for weekly paclitaxel administration. Fennelly and colleagues (1995) have reported on the efficacy and feasibility of weekly 1 h paclitaxel schedules in patients with recurrent ovarian cancers. A phase II dose of 80 mg/m^2 was established in this population of heavily pretreated patients. Similar results have been reported by other investigators (Loeffler et al 1995, Klassen et al 1996).

A 2 × 2 study from the National Cancer Institute of Canada Clinical Trials Group compared paclitaxel in two different doses (135 versus 175 mg/m^2) and infusion schedules (24 h versus 3 h) in patients with relapsed ovarian cancer. Though a difference was found in disease-free survival between the higher and lower dose groups, no significant difference was seen in overall survival between either of the dose or schedule groups.

Regarding toxicity, this study showed that, with standard premedication, the incidence of hypersensitivity is similar in the 24 h infusion (1%) to the 3 h infusion (2.1%) schedule (Eisenhauer et al 1994). Interestingly, the neutropenia was found to be more dependent on scheduling than dose. The severity of the neutropenia appears to be directly related to the duration that the plasma concentration is greater than the biologically active concentration and, as a result, the neutropenia is more severe following 24 h infusion than 3 h infusion schedule. On the other hand, the neuropathy was more dose-related than schedule-related. Based on this study paclitaxel was approved in doses of up to 175 mg/m^2 for infusion over 3 h.

The shorter infusion schedule has the obvious advantage in terms of milder neutropenia, convenience and expense. However, it is not yet known if 3 h paclitaxel is as active against cancer as the longer 24 h infusion schedule.

Paclitaxel/cisplatin combination versus standard treatment

A phase I study of paclitaxel administered over 24 h, followed by cisplatin, showed that this combination was feasible (Rowinsky et al 1991). The combination of paclitaxel 135 mg/m^2 followed by cisplatin 75 mg/m^2 was found to be safe for further evaluation in previously untreated patients with advanced ovarian cancer.

This paved the way for the Gynecologic Oncology Group randomised phase III trial (GOG 111) comparing the new combination of paclitaxel (135 mg/m²) and cisplatin (75 mg/m²) versus the best available treatment at the time, i.e. cisplatin and cyclophosphamide, as first line chemotherapy in women with suboptimally debulked stage III or stage IV ovarian cancer. Patients were treated 3 weekly for 6 cycles.

Final analysis of the data from the GOG 111 study ($n = 410$) demonstrated a significantly higher major response rate (77% versus 62%), a higher complete response rate (25% versus 19%), and a 14 month overall survival advantage in favour of the paclitaxel-containing arm. (McGuire et al 1996). Patients treated with paclitaxel had a higher incidence of neutropenia but septic complications were equally uncommon (3%) in both arms. Peripheral neurotoxicity was common in the paclitaxel arm but was mild. On the basis of this study, the GOG recommended cisplatin and paclitaxel as the standard treatment for patients with advanced ovarian cancer. A confirmatory study, with paclitaxel administered over 3 h, is being conducted in Europe and Canada and has currently enrolled 680 patients.

The improved outcome for patients with sub-optimal disease, who are treated with cisplatin and paclitaxel combination, led the GOG to study this combination in patients with optimal disease. GOG 114 randomised patients who had optimally debulked stage III ovarian cancer to receive either cisplatin and cyclophosphamide (standard), cisplatin and paclitaxel, or 2 cycles of high-dose carboplatin followed by intraperitoneal cisplatin and intravenous paclitaxel. The standard arm of this protocol had to be discontinued, once the results of GOG 111 emerged. This study has now closed and final analysis is ongoing.

Paclitaxel/cisplatin combination versus single agent paclitaxel

It remains unclear, whether the cisplatin/paclitaxel combination is more effective than paclitaxel alone. This question is being addressed in a three arm study (GOG 132), again involving women with sub-optimally debulked stage III or stage IV ovarian cancer. In this study, patients are randomised to receive the standard combination of cisplatin 75/paclitaxel 135, or single agent cisplatin 100 or single agent paclitaxel 200. Recently published results from this study (Muggia et al 1997) ($n = 648$) indicate that overall response rates are significantly lower in the paclitaxel alone arm compared with the other two arms (46% compared with 72% and 74%). The duration of progression free survival (PFS) is also shorter in the paclitaxel arm (11.4 months) compared with the cisplatin arm (16.4 months) and the combination arm (14.1 months). Despite the differences in PFS, no statistically significant difference was found in the overall median survival between the three groups. The cross-over design of the study may account for this. This study will also examine whether sequential therapy with cisplatin followed by paclitaxel at the time of recurrence is equivalent to initial treatment with the cisplatin/paclitaxel combination.

Paclitaxel carboplatin combination

We have already alluded to the possibility that the anti-cancer activity of paclitaxel may be dose-dependent. Platinum dose-intensification also appears to increase response rates though its impact on survival is uncertain (Ozols et al 1993a). High-dose investigations of the paclitaxel/cisplatin combination are not feasible in view of the overlapping dose limiting toxicities, in particular the peripheral neuropathy. However, the cisplatin analogue carboplatin has a more favourable toxicity profile and is commonly used in high-dose regimens. Though myelosuppression is observed more frequently with carboplatin than cisplatin, the other non-haematological toxicities such as nausea, vomiting, peripheral neuropathy, ototoxicity, and renal toxicity, are considerably less frequent (Williams et al 1992). The dose of carboplatin is given on an area under the curve (AUC) basis and is adjusted according to renal function by means of the Calvert formula:

$$\text{Carboplatin dose (mg)} = \text{Target AUC} \times [\text{GFR} + 25]$$

An AUC of 4–6 or 6–8 is generally recommended for previously treated and previously untreated patients, respectively. In order to achieve higher doses of carboplatin, the dose-limiting myelosuppression must be overcome with G-CSF ± blood 'stem-cell' support. Stem-cells are haematopoietic progenitor cells which normally reside in the bone marrow and produce white blood cells. They are obtained either from autologous bone-marrow or by the newer technology of peripheral blood leukapheresis.

The maximum tolerated dose of paclitaxel with carboplatin was studied in a GOG phase I/II trial (Ozols et al 1993b). In part 1 of this study, patients with previously untreated advanced ovarian cancer were enrolled to receive fixed-dose paclitaxel 135 mg/m^2 with increasing doses of carboplatin (AUC 5, 7.5, 10) and G-CSF support. The MTD of carboplatin was found to be AUC 7.5. In part 2 of this study, patients received carboplatin fixed at AUC 7.5 with paclitaxel at increasing doses (135, 175 or 225 mg/m^2). In fact, it was not possible to increase the dose of paclitaxel in this part of the study above 135 mg/m^2 because of chronic neutropenia requiring cycle-delays and dose reductions. Part 3 of the study was similar to part 2 except that the paclitaxel was administered over 3 h instead of 24 h. The shorter infusion schedule allowed a dose of paclitaxel 175 mg/m^2 to be administered safely in combination with carboplatin (AUC 7.5), even without G-CSF, though G-CSF was administered to patients who developed chronic neutropenia (Bookman et al 1995). Hospitalisation for neutropenic sepsis in this phase I/II study occurred following less than 3% of cycles and a similar number of cycles resulted in the requirement for platelet transfusion. In these patients with previously untreated disease, the combination has an overall major response rate of 75%, clinical complete response rate of 67%, and a median duration PFS of 15 months. The phase I dose-escalation part of this study, therefore, recommended paclitaxel 175 infused over 3 h followed by carboplatin AUC 7.5 (median equivalent dose 471) every 3 weeks without immediate use of G-CSF, for further investigations.

European investigators have also investigated the feasibility of substituting carboplatin for cisplatin in combination with paclitaxel (Meerpohl et al 1995). The reported maximum tolerated dose in this study was paclitaxel 185 in a 3 h schedule, followed by carboplatin AUC 6. This was a small study ($n = 30$) but, nonetheless, the results appear to confirm those of the GOG study.

Table 12.1 Current and planned GOG randomised studies of paclitaxel and a platinum compound in patients with previously untreated ovarian cancer

Patients	Randomisation
Stage II, Stage IC, or Stage IA/IB with poorly differentiated histology	Paclitaxel 175 (3 h) + carboplatin (AUC 7.5) × 6 *versus* Paclitaxel 175 (3 h) + carboplatin (AUC 7.5) × 3
Stage III optimally debulked	Paclitaxel 135 (24 h) + cisplatin 75 × 6 versus Paclitaxel 120 (96 h) + cisplatin 75 × 6 *versus* Paclitaxel 175 (3 h) + carboplatin (AUC 7.5) × 6
Stage III sub-optimally debulked Stage IV	Paclitaxel 135 (24 h) + cisplatin 75 × 6 *versus* Paclitaxel 135 (24 h) + cisplatin 75 × 3 *interval debulking* Paclitaxel 135 (24 h) + cisplatin 75 × 3

Paclitaxel/cisplatin versus paclitaxel/carboplatin

A phase III European study, compared the combinations of paclitaxel 175 (3 h) and either cisplatin 75 or carboplatin AUC 5. Previously untreated patients with advanced ovarian cancer ($n = 190$) have been enrolled on this study and the interim analysis of the first 148 patients has recently been reported (Neijt et al 1997). No significant differences were found in terms of efficacy between the two regimens and the authors conclude that the paclitaxel/carboplatin regimen is feasible and more convenient.

Preliminary analysis of another European phase III study is also available (du Bois et al 1997). This trial compared paclitaxel 185/cisplatin 75 versus paclitaxel 185/carboplatin AUC 6. The toxicity was found to be acceptable and overall response rate 59% was obtained (25% complete response).

This combination of paclitaxel 175 mg/m^2 and carboplatin AUC 7.5 is now being evaluated in GOG phase III trials (Ozols 1995) (Table 12.1). Since the European Organisation for the Research and Treatment of Cancer (EORTC) trial showed that survival of patients with suboptimally debulked stage III and stage IV ovarian cancer could be prolonged by 'interval debulking' (van der Burg et al 1993), this has been incorporated into current trials. A major difference between the EORTC and GOG studies, however, is that patients on the GOG study will receive cisplatin and paclitaxel as standard.

Paclitaxel in high dose chemotherapy

Paclitaxel is being incorporated into stem-cell supported high dose chemotherapy protocols for patients with advanced ovarian cancer. The pilot phase of one such study involves a mobilising regimen of etoposide and cyclophosphamide with G-CSF, peripheral stem-cell harvesting, and then 2 cycles of high dose paclitaxel 250 and carboplatin AUC 12, each followed by stem-cell reinfusion.

Investigators in Dublin are exploring the role of sequential carboplatin based high dose treatment, followed by tandem high dose alkylating agent therapy. This ongoing Phase I study follows a similar design to the current GOG study for patients with optimal disease.

OTHER TAXANES

Another taxane, docetaxel, which has shown response rates of over 20% in relapsed ovarian cancer is currently being studied in combination with cisplatin in clinical trials. One phase I/II study in previously untreated advanced ovarian cancer reports the feasibility of docetaxel 75–85 with cisplatin 75 and a preliminary clinical complete response rate of 58% ($n = 33$). Preliminary studies have been complicated by fluid retention and oedema.

Key points for clinical practice

- Ovarian cancer remains a major cause of female morbidity and mortality throughout the world.

- Currently, the addition of paclitaxel has significantly improved the management of this disease.

- For advanced ovarian cancer, current front-line management should include paclitaxel in addition to a platinum compound.

- The optimum dose, schedule and number of cycles of paclitaxel remains to be clarified. The role of high-dose chemotherapy containing paclitaxel also requires further investigation.

- Current clinical trials are addressing these issues to enable patients to derive maximum benefit from paclitaxel.

References

Advanced Ovarian Cancer Trialists' Group 1991 Chemotherapy in advanced ovarian cancer: an overview of randomised clinical trials. BMJ 303: 884–893

Bookman M A, McGuire W P, Kilpatrick D 1995 Phase I Gynecologic Oncology Group (GOG) study of 3-h and 24-h paclitaxel with carboplatin as initial therapy for advanced epithelial ovarian cancer. Proc Am Soc Clin Oncol 14: 755

du Bois A, Nitz U, Schroder W et al 1997 Cisplatin/paclitaxel versus carboplatin/paclitaxel as first-line chemotherapy in ovarian cancer; interim analysis of an AGO Study Group trial. Proc Am Soc Clin Oncol 16: 357

Einzig A I, Wiernik P H, Sasloff J, Runowicz C D, Goldberg G L 1992 Phase II study and long-term follow-up of patients treated with taxol for advanced ovarian adenocarcinoma. J Clin Oncol 10: 1748–1753

Eisenhauer E A, ten Bokkel Huinink W W, Swenerton K D et al 1994 European–Canadian randomized trial of paclitaxel in relapsed ovarian cancer: high-dose versus low-dose and long versus short infusion. J Clin Oncol 12: 2654–2666

Fennelly D, Shapiro F, Spriggs D et al 1995 Efficacy and feasibility of weekly taxol administration in patients with refractory ovarian cancer: a phase I study. Proc Am Soc Clin Oncol 14: 272

Green M H, Clark J W, Blaynew D W 1984 The epidemiology of ovarian cancer. Semin Oncol 11: 209

Klassen U, Wilke H, Strumberg D, Eberhardt W, Korn M, Seeber S 1996 Phase I study of a weekly 1-h infusion of paclitaxel in heavily pretreated patients with metastatic breast and ovarian cancer. Eur J Cancer 32: 547–549

Kohn E C, Sarosy G, Bicher A et al 1994 Dose intense taxol: high response rate in patients with platinum-resistant recurrent ovarian cancer. J Natl Cancer Inst 86: 18–24

Loeffler T M, Freund W, Lipke J et al 1995 Schedule and dose intensified paclitaxel as a weekly 1-hour infusion: evidence for an improved toxicity profile and response activity in pre-treated solid tumors. Proc Am Soc Clin Oncol 14: 1522

McGuire W P, Rowinsky E K, Rosenschein N B et al 1989 Taxol: a unique anti-neoplastic agent with significant activity in advanced ovarian epithelial neoplasms. Ann Intern Med 111: 273–279

McGuire W P, Hoskins W J, Brady M F et al 1996 Cyclophosphamide and cisplatin compared with paclitaxel and cisplatin in patients with stage III and stage IV ovarian cancer. N Engl J Med 334: 1–6

Meerpohl H-G, du Bois A, Kuhnle H et al 1995 Paclitaxel combined with carboplatin in the first-line treatment of advanced ovarian cancer. Semin Oncol 22 (Suppl 15): 7–12

Muggia F M, Braly P S, Brady M F et al 1997 Phase III study of cisplatin or paclitaxel versus their combination in suboptimal stage III and IV epithelial ovarian cancer: Gynecologic Oncology Group (GOG) study #132. Proc Am Soc Clin Oncol 16: 352

Nejit J P 1992 Treatment of advanced ovarian cancer: 10 years of experience. Ann Oncol 3: 17–27

Neijt J P, Hansen M, Hansen S W et al 1997 Randomized phase III study in previously untreated epithelial ovarian cancer FIGO stage IIB, IIC, III, IV, comparing paclitaxel-cisplatin and paclitaxel-carboplatin. Proc Am Soc Clin Oncol 16: 352

Omura G A, Brady M P, Delmore J E et al 1996 A randomised trial of paclitaxel at 2 dose-levels and filgrastim (GCSF) at 2 doses in platinum pretreated epithelial ovarian cancer. Proc Am Soc Clin Oncol 15: 280 (abs 755)

Ozols R F, Rubin S C, Dembo A J et al 1992 Epithelial ovarian cancer. In: Hoskins W J, Perez C A, Young R C (eds) Principles and Practice of Gynecologic Oncology. Philadelphia: JB Lippincott, 731–781

Ozols R F, Thigpen J T, Dauplat J et al 1993a Dose intensity. Ann Oncol 4: S49–S56

Ozols R F, Kilpatrick D, O'Dwyer P et al 1993b Phase I and pharmacokinetic study of taxol and carboplatin in previously untreated patients with advanced epithelial ovarian cancer: a pilot study of the Gynecologic Oncology Group. Proc Am Soc Clin Oncol 12: 259

Ozols R F 1995 Combination regimens of paclitaxel and the platinum drugs as first line regimens for ovarian cancer [review]. Semin Oncol 22 (Suppl 15): 1–6

Rowinsky E K, Gilbert M, McGuire W P et al 1991 Sequences of taxol and cisplatin: a phase I and pharmacologic study. J Clin Oncol 9: 1692–1703

Rowinsky E K, Eisenhauer E A, Chaudhry V, Arbuck S G, Finley A 1993 Clinical toxicities encountered with paclitaxel (Taxol). Semin Oncol 20 Suppl 3: 1–15

Rowinsky E K, Donehower R C 1995 Paclitaxel (taxol). N Engl J Med 332: 1004–1014

Sarosy G, Kohn E, Stone D A et al 1992 Phase I study of Taxol and granulocyte colony stimulatimg factor in patients with refractory ovarian cancer. J Clin Oncol 10: 1165–1170

Sutton G P, Stehman F B, Einhorn L H, Roth L M, Blessing J A, Ehrlich C E 1989 Ten-year follow-up of patients receiving cisplatin, doxorubicin, and cyclophosphamide chemotherapy for advanced epithelial ovarian carcinoma. J Clin Oncol 7: 223–229

Thigpen J T, Blessing J A, Ball H, Hummel S J, Barrett R J 1994 Phase II trial of paclitaxel in patients with progressive ovarian carcinoma after platinum-based chemotherapy: a Gynecological Oncology Group study. J Clin Oncol 12: 1748–1753

Trimble E L, Adams J D, Vena D et al 1993 Paclitaxel for platinum-refractory ovarian cancer: J Clin Oncol 11: 2405–2410

van der Burg M E L, van Lent M, Kobierska A et al 1993 Intervention debulking surgery does improve survival in advanced epithelial ovarian cancer: an EORTC Gynecological Cancer Cooperative Group study. Proc Am Soc Clin Oncol 12: 258

Williams C J, Stewart L, Parmar M et al 1992 Meta-analysis of the role of platinum compounds in advanced ovarian cancer. Semin Oncol 19: 120–128

Wingo P A, Tong T, Bolden S 1995 Cancer Statistics. CA Cancer J Clin 45: 8–30

Ray Garry

Complications of laparoscopy and how to avoid them

Advances in electronics, optics and engineering have made it possible to perform almost every intra-abdominal operation by minimal access surgery. The laparoscopic approach offers the potential for surgery which causes less pain, less scarring and is associated with quicker recovery than can occur after conventional laparotomy.

Every surgical procedure, however, has complications. Laparoscopic surgery is associated both with risks inherent in the specific operation, and also with risks of the laparoscopic mode of access which would not have occurred if conventional surgery had been selected. When, for example, a hysterectomy is performed there is an inherent risk of ureteric damage no matter whether the uterus is removed by the abdominal, vaginal or laparoscopic approach. Clinical studies must be performed to determine the relative risks of such complications with different surgical approaches but each approach will have an incidence of complications.

The laparoscopic approach uniquely involves perforating the abdominal wall with a number of conduits to facilitate minimal access surgery. Gaining laparoscopic access is, therefore, associated with a number of specific risks which would not occur if the abdominal or vaginal route had been chosen. This chapter concentrates on defining these complications which are specific to minimal access surgery and seeks to identify strategies which will minimise their occurrence.

INCIDENCE OF COMPLICATIONS

Prior to the development of advanced laparoscopic surgery, the incidence of death associated with minor laparoscopic procedures was reported as being

Ray Garry MD FRCOG, Consultant Gynaecologist and Medical Director, The Women's Endoscopic Laser Foundation, South Cleveland Hospital, South Tees Acute Hospitals NHS Trust, Marton Road, Middlesbrough, Cleveland TS4 3BW, UK

between 0.08 and 0.2 per 1000 procedures (Mintz 1977, Chamberlain 1978). More recently Querleu et al (1993), in a multi-centre study from a number of leading French centres undertaking advanced endoscopic surgery reported a death rate of 0.057 per 1000 and an incidence of severe complications sufficient to require laparotomy of 4.2 per 1000. Complications were more frequent after advanced laparoscopic surgery than after diagnostic and sterilisation procedures. In a recent prospective study from 72 hospitals in Holland (Jansen et al 1997), the overall complication rate in 25 764 laparoscopies was 5.7 per 1000 cases but the rate was significantly higher after advanced procedures at 17.9 per 1000 compared to 2.7 per 1000 after diagnostic and 4.5 per 1000 after sterilisation procedures. This study indicated that the risk of complications was related to the experience of the operator. A prior laparotomy also increased significantly the risks of subsequent laparoscopy.

These studies provide a selected or partial view of complication rates. A more comprehensive review of all the complications of laparoscopic surgery occurring in a single country over a 5 year period has been reported by Harkki-Siren and Kurki (1997). There were no deaths associated with 70 607 laparoscopies and the rate of major complications was 3.6 per 1000 procedures.

These figures provide some reassurance that severe complications associated with laparoscopic surgery are rare. The complications may, however, be life threatening and the consequences of damage to major vessels or bowel are so potentially catastrophic that every effort must be made to avoid them. This can only be achieved by strict attention to the techniques used to enter the abdomen. With a major complication rate of only 4 per 1000, an individual gynaecologist will rarely encounter a major complication. This is fortunately true even if the technique employed is sub-optimum. Almost every gynaecologist performs laparoscopy and almost all believe that their personal technique is perfect. Many feel that their personal experience adequately shows that they have no need to change their long practised techniques. This comfortable feeling is not shared by those of us who are asked to give opinions in litigation cases. An uncomfortable number of major disasters occur every year related to the use of the laparoscopic mode of access. In the UK in 1994, there were 124 548 gynaecological laparoscopies performed. This could be expected to give rise to about 500 serious complications each year of whom a proportion will be critically ill and a number may die. Each of these adverse outcomes can lead to considerable physical and emotional suffering for patient, relatives and doctors as well as vast financial costs and almost inevitably to litigation.

Many different techniques are proposed for safe laparoscopic entry, but it is unlikely that all the suggested approaches are equally safe. To demonstrate the superiority of one approach above another would require a randomised trial of enormous size and one with so many practical difficulties that it is unlikely ever to be undertaken. In this chapter I will review the approaches available, discuss the evidence, such as it is, in favour of each approach and give my personal view.

The complications of direct concern to the gynaecologist are: (i) failure to gain access to the abdominal cavity; (ii) damage to a major retro-peritoneal blood vessel; (iii) damage to the gastro-intestinal tract; (iv) damage to the vessels of the abdominal wall; and (v) post-laparoscopic bowel herniation through the entry scars.

Each technique will be evaluated to determine how effective each of the procedures seems to be in avoiding the above complications. In particular we **must avoid damage to the major intra-abdominal blood vessels and the bowel.** The bowel may be damaged in two different circumstances. Bowel may be injured when lying in its normal position with no adhesions and quite mobile. Damage in this circumstance almost always reflects poor technique. Bowel is more vulnerable to damage in the presence of pre-existing intra-abdominal adhesions. If the bowel is firmly adherent to the undersurface of the abdominal wall at the site of entry, then damage will only be avoided by developing techniques which will detect this situation and allow the use of an appropriate alternative entry site.

It is widely accepted that the most dangerous moment in laparoscopic surgery is during the insertion of the sharp primary trocar which is almost invariably performed in a blind fashion (Hill 1995). This step is preceded in most techniques by the induction of a CO_2 pneumoperitoeum via a Veress needle. In what can be perhaps called the classic technique the following steps are employed:

1. A skin incision is made just caudal to the umbilicus.

2. The abdominal wall is elevated.

3. A Veress needle is grasped high up on the shoulder of the shaft and inserted through the skin incision along a line through the abdominal wall aimed at the centre of the pelvis and directed in the mid line at an angle of 45 degrees.

4. The satisfactory positioning of the needle is checked by moving the handle of the needle to ensure that it moves freely in all directions.

5. When the position of the Veress appears correct, CO_2 is insufflated into the abdominal cavity. A volume of 2–3 l is usually thought to be appropriate and the volume required is often recorded.

6. The primary trocar is then inserted. A trocar with a long shaft with 10 cm or more below the gas inlet mechanism is selected and inserted again at a 45 degree angle directed in the midline.

Most complications follow use of this 'classical' approach to laparoscopic entry and so a number of alternative strategies have been developed in attempts to reduce these problems.

DIRECT INSERTION

One approach has been to avoid the use of CO_2 pneumoperitoneum completely and insert the primary trocar in a 'direct approach'. This technique is advocated by a number of highly experienced laparoscopists (Phipps 1995). The approach avoids the use of the Veress needle and, therefore, any complication associated with it. In this technique, the abdominal wall is elevated by the surgeon's hand. This creates a negative pressure in the closed abdominal cavity. The 10 mm trocar is thrust through all the layers of the abdominal wall in the midline subumbilically. It is important with this technique to ensure that the gas tap is in the open position when introducing the trocar so that the negative pressure will be released as soon as the abdominal cavity is entered so allowing the bowel to fall away. The laparoscope is then immediately introduced and the tissue lying at the end of the sheath inspected. If bowel serosa or intraperitoneal fat is seen then correct location is immediately confirmed. This is a rapid technique which avoids the use of a Veress needle but, in my opinion, is rather inelegant and allows no strategy to avoid bowel which may be adherent to the undersurface of the abdominal wall. In such circumstances, a 10 mm lesion in the bowel is inevitable and an unrecognised complete penetration through anterior and posterior walls is a real possibility. If this technique is selected, it is essential both to rotate the laparoscope around 360 degrees to inspect the whole of the abdominal cavity at the beginning of the operation and at its completion to ensure that the laparoscope is withdrawn under direct vision to detect any through and through bowel injury. A study in France has shown, in a rabbit model, that the direct insertion technique is associated with more bowel injuries than a conventional pneumoperitoneal approach, particularly in the presence of intra abdominal adhesions (Querleu et al 1993).

OPEN LAPAROSCOPY

To avoid the risks inherent with the use of sharp instruments in the introduction of the primary trocar, a technique using only blunt instruments has been described by Hasson (1980). In this technique, the skin and rectus sheath of the abdominal wall is incised under direct vision in the manner of an umbilical mini laparotomy incision. When the rectus sheath is divided, two firm stay sutures are placed through the rectus sheath. These sutures are kept long to enable subsequent anchorage of the Hasson cannula. The peritoneum is entered using blunt ended forceps, the cannula fixed in place and the abdomen distended in the standard way. It is essential to ensure that the cone is firmly wedged in position to maintain the pneumoperitoneum. By entering the cavity under direct vision with blunt instruments, damage to the intra abdominal structures may be avoided. Such an approach should certainly reduce the risks of major blood vessel damage but, unfortunately, seems to do very little to reduce the risk of bowel injury. In a membership survey conducted by the American Association of Gynecologic Laparoscopists (Hulka et al 1995), 10% of 80,031 cases had an open laparoscopic approach and these were associated with an incidence of bowel damage of 1.2% compared to an incidence of 0.15% associated with those who had the conventional closed approach. This significantly increased incidence of bowel injury is probably explained by case selection as this approach was frequently selected for use in higher risk cases. Clearly, however this route (as with open laparotomy) does not avoid the risk of injury to bowel adherent to the abdominal wall.

GASLESS LAPAROSCOPY

Another method of avoiding the risks of inducing a pneumoperitoneum is to distend the abdominal cavity by mechanical means and avoid the pneumoperitoneum entirely. There is little data about the risks associated with the entry techniques required for gasless laparoscopy. In the most widely used approach, the initial incision is similar to that required by the open Hasson's approach and the morbidity would be expected to be the same. Intra-abdominal adhesions and bowel adherent to the abdominal wall are relative contra-indications to this approach and it is essential to palpate digitally the inner peritoneal surface of the abdominal wall before inserting the supporting mechanism into the cavity. This approach is unlikely to reduce the risk of bowel injury and may, in fact, increase it.

INSERTION UNDER DIRECT VISION

A number of approaches have been described to get around the problem of blind insertion. Semm (1979) described a technique of entering the cavity under direct vision by routinely incising the skin and rectus sheath and then inserting a 5 mm telescope down to the level of the peritoneum. He describes the use of the light reflex. If the area beneath the peritoneum is clear of bowel, there will be a dark area. If bowel or adhesions are present, they will reflect the light of the laparoscope and appear as a brighter area. He recommends that the laparoscope tip is used to penetrate the peritoneum only in a dark area. If this technique is followed, the incidence of bowel damage should be reduced, but I know of no data to confirm that this is true in practice.

Some of the major equipment manufacturers have produced sophisticated devices which allow the laparoscope to be inserted through the abdominal wall under direct vision. These devices allow each layer to be seen as it is being divided and the moment of entry into the cavity can be clearly seen. There is, as yet, no evidence that these devices reduce entry risks; they are expensive disposable products and the quality of the view obtained is less than optimum. Obviously, safety with such devices will improve with experience and they could perhaps be most beneficial in high risk patients. Further work with this type of approach is needed.

A recent development is to utilise the vastly improved optics of the so called micro-laparoscopic equipment to produce a laparoscope small enough to fit down a standard size Veress needle. Such equipment is being evaluated and, by passing the Veress needle under direct vision, it may be possible to ensure that both the Veress needle and the trocar are always inserted into a safe space. An associated development is the use of radial expanding trocar sleeves. Sleeves fitting around a Veress needle are introduced in the standard manner. These sleeves are designed in such away that they can progressively be dilated without being removed so that a standard 10 mm telescope can be introduced down a sleeve that was introduced around a 1.5 mm Veress needle. Such an approach will also have significant cost implications but it can achieve the blunt introduction of a 10 mm device through an incision of 1.5 mm and may avoid many cases of inadvertent bowel and vessel damage.

Complications of laparoscopy and how to avoid them

In my opinion, the classical closed approach with a CO_2 pneumoperitoeum will remain the most important mode of access for laparoscopic surgery for some time to come. I believe that it can be made much safer by paying more attention to the details of the technique and by challenging a few basic practices.

Initial skin incision

Most gynaecologists choose a sub-umbilical site for their primary laparoscopic incision. An intra-umbilical incision in the base of the umbilicus is to be preferred for the following reasons:

1. The abdominal wall is thinnest in this area with the least distance for the trocar to penetrate. In most people, the thickness of the abdominal wall is less than 1 cm at the base of the umbilicus. Even in the very obese, the distance between the outer skin and inner peritoneal surface is much less than the distance only a short distance away in the sub-umbilical area.

2. The parietal peritoneum is only loosely attached to the abdominal wall **except** around the umbilicus. If entry is attempted where the peritoneum is most firmly attached, the trocar is least likely to come to rest in the pre-peritoneal space and is most likely to enter the cavity.

3. The scar is usually least obtrusive and most acceptable in this area.

Elevation of the abdominal wall

The abdominal wall is lifted to create a space between the abdominal wall and abdominal contents in which to insert the trocar. Lifting the abdominal wall does not necessarily also lift the underlying peritoneum and entry into the pre-peritoneal space is all to easy with this approach. Conversely, if bowel is firmly adherent to the abdominal wall, no amount of elevation will create a space to permit safe trocar insertion.

Insertion of the Veress needle

The Veress needle has a sharp outer sheath below which protrudes an inner blunt ended gas carrying shaft. The blunt end is pushed behind the sharp needle during its travel through the abdominal wall and springs out immediately the resistance provided by the abdominal wall structures is removed. If the needle functions correctly, it is very difficult to penetrate the walls of a major blood vessel with the blunt end. Care must be taken to ensure that the Veress is as sharp as possible to pass through the abdominal wall with the least possible force and that the mechanism of the inner retractable tip is free running. Many, including the author, feel that these two requirements justify the extra cost of using a single use disposable trocar. It is only necessary to insert the Veress through the layers of the abdominal wall into the cavity. Once in the cavity, there is no benefit to inserting several more centimetres of metal shaft just 'to be sure', because the only consequence of this is to increase the risk of inadvertent damage to the surrounding structures.

Great care should, therefore, be undertaken to insert only as much shaft of the Veress needle as is needed to enter the cavity. This can be ensured by inserting the needle through the previously cut skin. The Veress needle must then pass through the rectus sheath and the peritoneum to enter the cavity. These two structures can be identified by the two distinct layers of resistance to entry into the cavity. If the needle is held low on the shaft (many think you need to hold the moving shoulder piece for the mechanism to work but this is not the case) and advanced carefully, entry through the two layers can be sensed and, if the Veress needle has a ball valve mechanism, a distinct double click will be both heard and felt.

Checking the position of the Veress needle

When the needle has entered the abdominal cavity, it should not be moved around to check that it is free in the cavity. Rather, the correct sighting of the needle should be confirmed with the following two tests. The first was described by the French pioneer of laparoscopic surgery Palmer. His test requires a 20 ml syringe half filled with normal saline. The syringe is attached to the Veress and the plunger is first drawn back. Failure to aspirate blood or bowel contents suggests the needle is not in a major splanchnic structure. When this is confirmed the saline is flushed into the cavity. This should be done easily without resistance. The final phase of the test is to withdraw the plunger again. When the needle is correctly situated no fluid with be sucked back into the syringe, when the tip is lying in adhesions or in the abdominal walls the saline will have collected as a pool and can be drawn back.

The correct location of the Veress needle can be confirmed by carefully setting the CO_2 insufflator. If a flow rate of 1 l/min is selected, this flow should be achieved and the recorded intra abdominal pressure (IAP) should be low (> 10 mmHg). The combination of good flow with low pressure suggests correct placement, the alternative of low flow rates and high and rapidly increasing IAP suggests an incorrectly situated needle.

Both these tests can be performed without moving the tip of the Veress needle around the abdominal cavity. This is important, for if the needle has been cleanly, but inadvertently, inserted into an important abdominal structure and this is recognised, the needle can simply be withdrawn and no further action may be required. If the needle is moved about violently in the abdomen not only will this action increase the risk of structural damage but it will also convert a small needle hole into a large linear tear which will inevitably require more extensive surgical repair.

CO_2 insufflation

Once the position of the Veress needle is deemed satisfactory, the CO_2 can be insuflated as rapidly as possible. The diameter of the needle usually limits this to about 3 l/min no matter what the insufflation rate is set at. It is traditional to use 2–3 l of CO_2 to distend the abdomen. Larger volumes than this are considered by many to be inappropriate and by some to be frankly dangerous. The abdominal cavity is being distended to elevate the abdominal wall away from the underlying structures so that the sharp trocar can be inserted safely into the gas space which has been created. What is the safest size of gas space we can achieve? Why is 2 or 3 l considered by most to be the optimum volume? We have investigated this matter in detail in order to determine what are the optimum conditions for safe insertion of the primary trocar.

The first fact which became clear to us is that measuring by volume is inappropriate. There may be a leak in the tubing or delivery system and all of the indicated gas may not have entered the abdominal cavity. More importantly, the capacity of the abdominal cavity varies as much as any other human vital statistic and a single arbitrary volume of gas will not produce a similar degree of distension in all shapes and sizes of patient. Attention should be directed instead to the level of intra-abdominal pressure produced by the gas: 3 l of CO_2 produces an intra-abdominal pressure (IAP) of about 10 mmHg in the average size woman.

We have found that increasing the IAP increases the size of the gas space. We believe it is self evident that the larger the gas space, the safer will be the insertion of the trocar, because there is a greater distance between the abdominal wall and the underlying structures. In a series of studies in which we measured the distance between the abdominal wall and the bowel at different intra-uterine pressures, we found that the mean distance at 10 mmHg pressure was 7 cm whilst at 25 mmHg it was 10 cm. More importantly, we have found that the higher the IAP the more the abdominal wall is splinted by the contained gas and the less it is deformed by downward pressure. It has been estimated that a difficult trocar insertion requires 4–5 kg of force. If a standardised force of 4 kg is applied vertically down onto the umbilical area of a patient with an IAP of 10 mmHg then the umbilicus will touch the underlying structures making them very vulnerable to damage. When the procedure is repeated at an IAP of 25mmHg the force applied indents the abdominal wall in such a way that there is still a gas bubble of at least 5 cm between the abdominal wall and the underlying bowel.

Many doctors are concerned that the use of such a high IAP will produce adverse effects on the cardiac or respiratory systems. We have investigated this and have demonstrated that, at least in anaesthetised and ventilated patients, the only parameter to change was the compliance of the lungs. The increase in compliance required the ventilator to work harder. The work the ventilator was required to do increased proportionally to the level of the IAP but never went outside the safe working range of the equipment. All the cardiac and respiratory parameters we tested remained completely unchanged and there was no detectable effect of this higher IAP on cardio/respiratory function. We recommend that the IAP is retained at 25 mmHg only for the period of the trocar insertions and once all the trocars have been safely inserted this pressure is lowered to the more conventional 15 mmHg for the remainder of the procedure.

Primary trocar insertion

A long trocar is usually inserted at an angle of 45 degrees in the direction of the pelvis in the midline in order to enter the cavity in a direction away from the aorta and iliac vessels. In the Finnish study (Jansen 1997) the iliac vessels were damaged 6 times and the aorta once. This widely recommended method of trocar insertion requires the trocar to travel a considerable, but variable, distance through the abdominal wall. The distance travelled will depend on the thickness and adiposity of the abdominal wall and in the very obese can be many centimetres. The main difficulty with this route of insertion is the unpredictability of the length of travel required and the need to use long shafted trocars. Clearly, the greater the length of trocar inserted into the abdominal cavity, the greater the risk of damaging an abdominal structure.

To improve safety, several of the major equipment companies have developed trocars with guarded tips, similar in principle to the design of the Veress needle. These devices are long, have effective but elaborate valve mechanisms and they have plastic or metal guards which protect the sharp point of the device until they are pushed out of the way during insertion through the abdominal wall. These shields should springback to recover the tip immediately after entry into the abdominal cavity before meeting any other structure. They were originally designated 'safety shields' but the name has been withdrawn because they are demonstrably no safer than other trocars and I personally believe their clumsy design may make insertion more dangerous. Certainly, many cases of damage to both bowel and major blood vessels have occurred with these devices. Querleu's team in an animal model demonstrated that, in the absence of intra-abdominal adhesions (which is when we least expect clinical problems), these devices may been of some value in reducing bowel damage but, in the presence of intra-abdominal adhesions, they were of no benefit (Mintz 1997). They are also very expensive, in fact in my opinion unacceptably expensive, and their complex design prohibits re-use. A set of 4 such trocars required for most advanced procedure would add £200 costs to each procedure. In my unit where we undertake about 1250 laparoscopic surgical procedures per year, the extra unnecessary costs would amount to about £250 000.

I have sought to develop a technique to minimise the risks of primary entry based on the recommendations of the American pioneers of laparoscopic surgery Hulka and Reich (1995). To be effective the entry technique should be safe, rapid and as economical as possible.

The trocar should be inserted through the abdominal wall at its thinnest and most constant thickness point. This is obviously in the base of the umbilicus and this site is strongly recommended for primary trocar insertion. The shortest path is also the most vertical one and the path of insertion should be at right angles to the skin, although once the whole thickness of the abdominal wall is traversed the direction of thrust should be rotated up into the direction of the fundus of the uterus. When this short route is selected, a much shorter length trocar can be used. The advantage of using a short length trocar is that such an instrument appears to give better control and a safer entry. When the insertion is made at the base of the umbilicus, the distance through the abdominal wall will seldom be more than 1 cm even in very obese patients.

The use of a short trocar allows even those with small hands to cup the top of the trocar in the palm of the hand and extend the index finger down the shaft of the trocar. When the trocar is 'palmed' in this way, no more than 1 cm of point is exposed and so this is the greatest depth of the sharp metal trocar point which can enter the abdominal cavity in the initial thrust.

If this insertion technique is combined with the production of an IAP of 25 mmHg, which ensures a minimum gas space depth of 5 cm even when exposed to considerable downward thrust, then the sharp tip of the trocar should always be well clear of the vulnerable underlying structures.

SUMMARY OF PRIMARY TROCAR INSERTION TECHNIQUE

The primary incision should be a 1 cm vertical incision made in the base of the umbilicus. A sharp Veress needle should be grasped down the barrel and carefully inserted vertically through the rectus sheath fascia and peritoneum. Once inside the abdomen, it should not be moved about but its correct position should be confirmed with Palmer's test and by observing the rate of gas flow and IAP. The pneumoperitoneum should be continued until an IAP of 25 mmHg is obtained. A short barrelled sharp trocar should be palmed and all but the distal 1 cm guarded by the extended index finger. The trocar should be inserted vertically through the abdominal wall until the cavity is reached and then the trocar immediately withdrawn leaving the sheath in the correct position.

It must be emphasised that the most important step in this approach is the production of an IAP of 25 mmHg. A vertical thrust of the trocar must **never** be performed at pressures lower than this for, in such circumstances, the bowel and aorta are very vulnerable.

ALTERNATIVE PRIMARY ENTRY SITES

This approach should prevent damage to the major vessels and the normally situated vessels on a consistent and predictable basis and also permits a strategy to detect bowel adherent to the abdominal wall. If bowel adhesions in the region of the umbilicus are suspected, then an alternative primary entry site should be selected. A number of authorities recommend a supra pubic entry or inserting a Veress needle up the posterior vaginal fornix. As both these areas are commonly involved with pelvic adhesions and endometriosis, they cannot be recommended as an entry site for those at high risk. I prefer the site first suggested by Palmer which is in the left hypochondrial area of the abdomen just below the 9th rib in the mid-clavicular line. The left hypochondrial area of the abdomen is the area least likely to be associated with intra-abdominal adhesions and, therefore, the area of greatest safety for blind insertion. In this area, a skin incision is made and a Veress needle is carefully inserted at right angles to the skin until the cavity is just entered. A 5 mm trocar is then inserted down which a 5 mm laparoscope is then inserted and the umbilical area is inspected. If it is clear of adhesions, the standard trocar is inserted under direct vision. If adhesions are present, extra ports are inserted to free the adhesions and, when the whole area is clear, the umbilical trocar can then be safely inserted into the abdomen at an IAP of 25 mmHg.

SECONDARY TROCAR INSERTIONS

The first requirement for the correct insertion of secondary trocars is to ensure that they are located in the optimum position to facilitate the type of surgery being undertaken. The position selected will, therefore, vary according to the pathology, the procedure, the size of the patient, etc. Wherever is selected, it is essential that the site chosen is also safe. The principle structure that can be damaged in the lower abdominal wall are the inferior epigastric vessels. In the study of Jansen (1997), injury of these vessels was the most common major complication and, indeed, caused the death of a 25-year-old patient with testicular feminisation.

The inferior epigastric vessels ascend the sub-umbilical wall on the undersurface of the rectus muscle. In women of average or greater build, the line of the rectus muscle cannot be clearly defined and the vessels often cannot be seen by the technique of transillumination. Indeed transillumination alone may be misleading for it will often demonstrate significant superficial vessels which, if carefully avoided, may inadvertently direct the surgeon onto the deeper more major vessels. In almost every case, however, the deep epigastric vessels can be identified on laparoscopic inspection of the abdominal wall. The course of the vessels should be identified and marked so that the trocars can be safely inserted lateral to them. The combination of direct visualisation with transillumination in a darkened operating theatre should ensure that the vessels are readily avoided.

REPAIR OF ABDOMINAL INCISIONS

In my own practice, I seldom use any instrument greater than 5 mm down a secondary port. Such 5 mm incisions can usually safely be secured with simple skin sutures, clips or skin adhesives. There have been a large number of reports of incisional and Richter's herniation with associated intestinal obstruction following the use of larger ports. When such incisions are used, they should be formally closed with a suture through the sheath. This cannot be readily done with conventional instruments from the outside. A series of devices for introducing sutures through the wound have been developed. Each seek to ensure that the suture is passed through the subcutaneous tissues, the rectus sheath and peritoneum on one side of the incision and is passed under laparoscopic vision out through the same structures on the other side of the incision. It is now considered essential practice to perform this type of repair and, from a medico-legal point of view, record that such a repair has been performed.

One of the most important benefits of laparoscopic surgery is that the convalescent time is usually very short and relatively pain free. This should be the expected recovery pattern. Every patient failing to improve rapidly after laparoscopy should be suspected of having sustained damage to an important intra-abdominal structure. The next best thing to preventing a complication is to diagnose and manage the complication rapidly. It is absolutely essential that a perforated bowel is detected and managed speedily. All surgeons undertaking laparoscopic procedures should become aware of the non-specific nature of the signs and symptoms of peritonitis developing after laparoscopy. An ill patient after laparoscopic surgery = peritonitis = bowel damage (or haemorrhage) and must be investigated and treated urgently.

Key points for clinical practice

- Laparoscopic surgery is associated with several specific complications related to the nature of the surgical mode of entry into the abdominal cavity.

- Great efforts should be made to limit these potentially devastating complications.

- The primary incision should be in the base of the umbilicus.

- The Veress needle should be inserted with care and its position checked without moving the point.

- The CO_2 pneumoperitoneum should be maintained at 25 mmHg pressure whilst the trocars are being inserted before being brought down to the conventional 15 mmHg for the remainder of the procedure.

- A short trocar should be palmed and inserted vertically through the umbilicus.

- Secondary trocars should be inserted under direct vision lateral to the inferior epigastric vessels.

- Patients after laparoscopic surgery should improve rapidly. Failure to do so should suggest major intra-abdominal complications and damaged bowel or intra-abdominal vessels should be suspected until diagnosis is completely excluded.

References

Chamberlain G, Brown J D 1978 Gynaecological Laparoscopy Report on the Confidential Enquiry into Gynaecological Laparoscopy. London: RCOG Press
Harkki-Siren P, Kurki T 1997 A nationwide analysis of laparoscopic complications. Obstet Gynecol 89: 108–112
Hasson H M 1980 Window for open laparoscopy. Am J Obstet Gynecol : 137: 869–870
Hill D J 1995 Complications of the laparoscopic approach. Baillières Clin Obstet Gynaecol 8: 865–879
Hulka J, Peterson H, Phillips J, Surrey M 1995 Operative Laparoscopy. American Association of Gynecologic Laparoscopists 1993 membership survey 2: 133–136
Hulka J, Reich H (eds) 1994 Abdominal Entry in Textbook of Laparoscopy. Philadelphia: WB Saunders, 86–102
Jansen F W, Kapiteyn K, Trimbos-Kemper T, Hermens J, Trimbos J B 1997 Complications of laparoscopy: a prospective multicentre observational study. Br J Obstet Gynaecol 104: 595–600
Mintz M 1997 The risks and prophylaxis in laparoscopy. A survey of 100,000 cases. J Reprod Med 18: 269
Phipps J H 1995 Complications of laparoscopic surgery. Avoidance and management. In: Studd J (ed) Yearbook of the Royal College of Obstetrics and Gynaecology. London: RCOG, 67–78)
Querleu D, Chevallier L, Chapron C, Bruhat M A 1993 Complications of gynaecological laparoscopic surgery. A French collaborative study. Gynaecol Endosc 2: 3–6
Semm K 1979 New methods of pelviscopy for myomectomy, ovariectomy, tubectomy, adenectomy. Endoscopy 2: 85

Hugh O'Connor Adam Magos

How to avoid complications at hysteroscopic surgery

Endoscopic surgery is one of the major surgical advances of the past century and its safe introduction into routine clinical practice is a significant challenge. High profile medico-legal cases have cast some doubt on the benefits of this new technology. However, when practiced by experienced surgeons on carefully selected patients, the advantages to the patient over conventional open surgery are substantial (O'Connor et al 1997).

Avoiding complications at hysteroscopic surgery requires appropriate patient selection and counselling, good equipment and surgical skill in endoscopy. Foremost the surgeon must be skilled in diagnostic hysteroscopy before proceeding to operative hysteroscopy (Garry 1995). This involves attending training courses and, where feasible, a period of close supervision. Increasingly, national endoscopy societies are becoming concerned with the issues of training, recognition of endoscopic courses and in some instances, certification of gynaecologists.

TRAINING

The ideal training course combines a number of modules including lectures, videos and practice sessions. There are a few courses that offer hands-on training. This is the ideal, but not always possible.

Lectures should be interactive and cover the equipment used, indications for surgery, patient selection, surgical technique and results. Practical and hands on sessions should form the bulk of the course. Candidates should have

Hugh O'Connor BA DCH MRCP(I) MRCOG, Consultant Obstetrician and Gynaecologist, The Coombe Women's Hospital, Dublin 8, Ireland

Adam Magos BSc MD MRCOG, Consultant Obstetrician and Gynaecologist, Minimally Invasive Therapy Unit and Endoscopy Training Center, University Department of Obstetrics and Gynaecology, The Royal Free Hospital, London NW3 2QG, UK

Recent Advances in Obstetrics and Gynaecology 20

one-to-one tuition when practicing on models. These sessions serve to reinforce the theory discussed during lectures.

Practical sessions explaining the instruments and their capabilities are important. Surgeons have a tendency to use equipment before being completely familiar with it. Endoscopic surgery relies heavily on technology, and an understanding of the camera, insufflator, video systems and electrosurgical generator is vital in order to avoid problems.

An endotrainer (Wallwiener et al 1994) or models such as a potato, or a pepper can be used to practice resection and directed biopsy. Uteri from hysterectomies can be mounted after removal and used to practice resection.

In a perfect world, the gynaecologist would perform a number of cases under the supervision of an expert before operating solo. This is not always possible and, in such instances, it may be acceptable, with the patient's consent, to perform an ablation on a patient undergoing hysterectomy. The uterine specimen should be opened after hysterectomy and the depth of resection assessed. In such instances, the fundal and cornual regions should be rollerball ablated, the endometrium in the body of the uterus can then be resected. Alternatively, early cases could be performed under laparoscopic guidance.

The report of the RCOG (Royal College of Obstetricians and Gynaecologists) working party on training in gynaecological endoscopic surgery (1994) stratifies hysteroscopic procedures into three levels. Levels one and two include diagnostic hysteroscopy with target biopsy to removal of a pedunculated fibroid, and should be part of general specialist training. Endometrial ablation is a level three procedure and the trainee should attend a formal course. Certification in level three procedures may be required in the future.

COUNSELLING/CONSENT

The procedure, complications and outcome should be discussed in the clinic rather than on the pre-operative ward round. A leaflet explaining the intended hysteroscopic procedure, its advantages and disadvantages over conventional surgery, is useful. This type of data will become more important as hospitals improve their risk management. A plan of action should be agreed in the event of an intra-operative complication; for instance in the event of a laparotomy being necessary because of a perforation, should the surgeon proceed to hysterectomy?

Patient expectation is an important determinant of a successful outcome. The patient having an endometrial ablation can expect a 40% amenorrhoea rate, and 95% are improved following surgery. Overall, approximately 90% will avoid hysterectomy, but another 5–8% will need a further procedure such as repeat endometrial ablation (O'Connor et al 1996). Clearly, if amenorrhoea is the only outcome that will satisfy the patient, then endometrial ablation may not be the procedure of choice. Submucosal fibroids can be resected with good results (Magos et al 1991, Indman 1993) . However, fibroids that are intramural or subserosal are not treated by this operation, and symptoms referable to such myomas will not improve. Polyps may re-occur following resection as this does not alter the underlying cause.

Menorrhagia is one of the most common complaints in otherwise healthy women, affecting some 22% of the female population and accounting for 21% of referrals to gynaecological outpatients. Approximately 73 000 hysterectomies are performed annually in the UK, of which 35–64% are for menorrhagia. In up to 50% of these cases, no pathology will be found on histological examination of the uterus. Such patients are ideal candidates for endometrial ablation, but identifying them can be difficult. There are few absolute contra-indications to endometrial ablation, endometrial cancer being one, however, certain factors affect outcome and these must be considered in making a recommendation for surgery (Raiga et al 1995). The randomized trials reported to date, comparing ablation and hysterectomy, have sought to exclude those women with extra-uterine pelvic pathology from the studies (O'Connor et al 1997, Pinion et al 1994, Dwyer et al 1993). Despite this, 14–23% of the enrolled patients had pathology such as endometriosis, ovarian cysts or adhesions when they came to surgery. The more selected the population offered hysteroscopic surgery, the better the outcome. Endometrial ablation is not definitive in the way that hysterectomy is, the uterus is preserved and may develop further pathology.

The ideal patient for endometrial ablation is over 40 years old, family complete, with regular, heavy periods, menses lasting for no more than a week and a diagnosis of dysfunctional uterine bleeding. Although restrictive, these are the most suitable patients and should have the best outcome. That is not to say that patients with enlarged uteri, prolonged or irregular uterine bleeding cannot be offered endometrial ablation. The results in this latter group are not as good as in the dysfunctional uterine bleeding group, but the difference is small, becoming more divergent the greater the pathology.

Endometrial ablation is also an alternative to hysterectomy in the presence of significant medical problems. In 1987, DeCherney et al described the use of the resectoscope to ablate the endometrium of 21 women, 14 of whom had blood dyscrasias, four were poor anaesthetic risks and three had refused hysterectomy. Three patients died within 6 months of their original disease, but 18/19 had no further bleeding and 1/19 had spotting.

Hysteroscopic surgery may enhance fertility when intra-uterine adhesions in the case of Asherman's syndrome or Mullerian defects such as uterine septa are divided. Difficult adhesiolysis should be performed under laparoscopic or ultrasound control. In the case of septa, a prior laparoscopy to inspect the serosal surface of the uterus is necessary.

Intra-cavity myomata should be assessed hysteroscopically (Wamsteker et al 1993) and with ultrasound before resection. The angle that the fibroid makes

Table 14.1 Classification of fibroids

Type	
Type 0	Pedunculated
Type 1	< 50% intra-mural
Type 2	> 50% intra-mural

with the endometrium gives an idea as to the proportion of the fibroid that is in the cavity and that which is in the myometrium. Only those fibroids that are predominantly intra-cavity are suitable for resection (Table 14.1). As with all rules in medicine there are exceptions, but only those who are truly expert in hysteroscopic surgery should attempt type 2 fibroids, and then in selected cases. The patient should also be warned that more than one procedure may be required.

ENDOMETRIAL PREPARATION

Endometrial thickness varies throughout the menstrual cycle. Post menstrual endometrium is 1 mm thick, but it is over 12 mm in the late secretary phase. Nd:YAG laser will penetrate to a depth of 5–6 mm, rollerball similar and the resection loop has a radius of 4 mm. Thicker endometrium increases the likelihood that more than one pass will be necessary for a complete ablation. The risk of complications, in particular perforation and fluid absorption, is greater. In addition, endometrial debris obscures the view.

The endometrium is thinnest during menstruation, but it is not feasible to schedule cases in a busy institution by reference to the patient's menstrual cycle. Mechanical preparation of the endometrium with suction curettage has been reported (Gimpelson et al 1992, Lefler et al 1991) but pharmacological thinning with GnRH analogues or danazol is more commonly used (Fraser et al 1996). There is little to chose between these agents. Studies comparing analogue or danazol with placebo report a better outcome with pharmacological preparation, however no study has been large enough to report a statistically significant result in terms of complication rate or failure rate. Unreported data from our unit of a randomized double blind placebo controlled trial of danazol and placebo, given for 6 weeks prior to resection at a dose of 200 mg, three time a day, showed a statistically significant greater reduction in measured menstrual blood loss following TCRE in the group who had danazol.

GnRH analogues such as decapeptyl are useful prior to hysteroscopic myomectomy. They reduce fibroid size and vascularity, so facilitating surgery. These agents do add to the cost of the procedure, and their use will vary depending on health funding.

Analogues reduce uterine size and cervical dilatation prior to surgery may be difficult. The use of laminaria may facilitate cervical dilatation, this is especially the case in nulliparous patients.

OPERATIVE TECHNIQUE

The monitor and electrosurgical generator are on the patient's right, positioned so that the surgeon can see the screen (Fig. 14.1). The fluid inflow and outflow systems are on the patient's left. This is necessary as the assembled resectoscope has five cables attached (light, camera, power, inflow and outflow) and without a system, a tangle ensues.

The patient is placed in the lithotomy position, cleaned, draped and a bi-manual examination carried out. The uterus is sounded and then dilated to

Hegar 10, for a standard resectoscope. The hysteroscope should be introduced into the uterus under direct vision. The ostia should be identified, prior to endometrial ablation. An elongated cervix may catch out the unwary surgeon. A number of operative techniques have been described.

The authors' technique for TCRE involves rollerball to the fundus and cornual region, creating a repository at the top of the uterus (Magos et al 1989). A 2 mm diameter rollerball is used, the ball should be kept moving at all times when activated. This repository extends from the fundus to just below the cornua and is a store for resected chips of endometrium. The remainder of the cavity is now systematically resected, starting at the 9 o'clock position and resecting in an anti-clockwise direction. The posterior uterine wall is resected before the anterior wall as the resected chips would otherwise obstruct the view. The loop is extended, buried in the endometrium and the cutting pedal activated. The loop is drawn back into the sheath, the diathermy must be kept active until the loop is within the sheath or the tissue will not be fully resected and pseudopolyps result. The amount of tissue resected is that distance that the loop traverses when extended. It is usually necessary to repeat the procedure at 2 or 3 levels to excise all endometrium. The importance of being systematic cannot be over stressed.

The resection should stop at the level of the internal os. Resecting into the canal runs the immediate risk of haemorrhage due to damage to the cervical branch of the uterine artery, and the long term risk of cervical stenosis with its sequelae. The resected chips are now removed with ovum forceps or a flushing

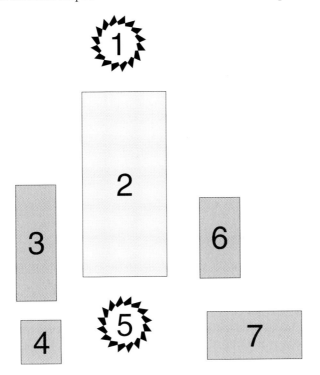

Fig. 14.1 Layout
(1) Anaesthetist; (2) patient; (3) monitor and light source; (4) electrosurgical generator; (5) surgeon; (6) fluid system; and (7) scrub trolley.

curette. Leaving a small rim of endometrium above the internal os is recommended by some authors. The patient is likely to continue to menstruate, albeit lightly, but there is also a higher chance of needing further surgery than when a total resection is performed. Unpublished data from our unit suggest that over-dilatation of the cervix after completion of the procedure helps prevent subsequent development of haematometra.

When resecting fibroids, the chips are brought out as they are cut. This is necessary in all but the smallest fibroids to maintain a clear view, thereby helping with orientation.

ANAESTHESIA

General anaesthesia, regional anaesthesia (spinal or epidural) or a combined local anaesthetic/sedo-analgesia technique can be used. Those suitable for local anaesthesia can usually be selected from the outpatient hysteroscopy clinic. Local anaesthetic is injected into the cervix using a dental syringe, a para-cervical block is given and the endometrium or lesion to be removed is injected with 1 ml aliquots of local anaesthetic. The cornual region is most sensitive. This is supplemented with intravenous medazolam and fentanyl. The patient needs to be closely monitored by an anaesthetist, 1–2% of patients will need conversion to general anaesthesia.

HYSTEROSCOPIC SURGICAL PROCEDURES

Operative hysteroscopy covers a range of procedures. The novice should undertake simple procedures gradually progressing to more advanced surgery.

Certain minor operative procedures can be undertaken at the time of diagnostic hysteroscopy. Small polyps can be removed, lost intra-uterine devices removed, filmy adhesions broken down with the endoscope or scissors and, in the near future, hysteroscopic sterilization will be available. Hysteroscopic myomectomy, endometrial ablation and adhesiolysis require greater skill levels. Repeat ablation, treatment of Asherman's syndrome and larger fibroids are expert procedures.

Equipment and instrumentation

A wide range of endoscopic equipment is now available. A number of systems should be tried before purchasing a set. Gynaecologists have their own preferences and reasons for preferring one system over another. The operating hysteroscope combines a rigid rod lens telescope with a continuous flow sheath. The distal end of the outer sheath of the continuous flow system should have perforations all around for suction. If this is not the case, it will cause problems with removing bubbles from the anterior wall of the uterus when resecting this portion of the cavity. The modified urological resectoscope is a passive system in that the loop is within the sheath at rest. The surgeon pushes the electrode out using the handle mechanism. This adds to the safety of the design. The active resectoscope has an electrode that is outside the sheath at rest, and there is the risk of inadvertent perforation.

The telescope used should have either a 12 or 30 degree lens. The 12 degree telescope has the advantage that when doing an endometrial resection, the fully extended loop can be visualized at all times; whereas with the 30 degree telescope, because of its angulation, the loop when extended is often not visible. The surgeon should appreciate the different properties of a 0 degree, 12 and 30 degree hysteroscope. The design of most rigid angled hysteroscopes is such that, in the neutral position, the light lead inserts into the base of the telescope with the lens pointing upwards. Therefore when the light lead is rotated to the 12 o'clock position the lens is pointing down and, therefore, the posterior wall of the uterus is viewed. Likewise, when the light lead is rotated to the 3 o'clock position, the right side of the uterus is preferentially viewed, i.e. an angled scope inspects that area of the uterus opposite to the direction of the light lead. This presupposes that the camera is always maintained in the neutral position and does not rotate as the telescope is rotated.

Ideally, the camera and light source should be from the same manufacturer. It is possible to mix systems but invariably the picture is not as clear as when a single system is assembled. Using a camera and operating off a colour monitor is more comfortable for the surgeon and facilitates training.

A modern electrosurgical generator with cut, coagulation, blend modes and return electrode monitoring should be chosen. Many systems are available and one that can be used for laparoscopic or open surgery is preferred for economic reasons. Safety is paramount and the system chosen should not operate if a fault is detected in the circuit as created by the patient, electrosurgical generator, return electrode and active electrode.

Fluid monitoring is a vital part of any operation. The inflow and outflow volumes should be calculated and a running balance kept. A gravity feed system or a hysteromat can be used to control the inflow.

The Nd:YAG laser is the most commonly used laser for operative hysteroscopy (Erian 1994) . Unlike the carbon dioxide laser, it passes through clear fluids. The hysteroscope has a working channel through which a quartz laser fibre is guided.

Laser and rollerball ablation may be safer for less experienced endoscopists than resection, but the results are not as good (MISTLETOE 1993).

Complications

The complication profile differs from conventional surgery (Table 14.2). Patients should recover rapidly from hysteroscopic surgery, an undetected complication must be considered if recovery is slow.

Fluid overload

Fluid is infused into the uterine cavity under pressure in order to distend the uterus and maintain a clear operative view. A continuous flow system is used and, therefore, the volume of fluid infused and the volume that has returned from the uterus can be calculated, giving a fluid balance or deficit. The choice between gravity feed and a hysteromat for distention is a matter of individual

Table 14.2 Complications

Intra-operative		Postoperative	
	Early	Intermediate	Late
Perforation	Haemorrhage	Pain	Treatment failure
Fluid overload	Infection	Menorrhagia	Pregnancy
Haemorrhage	'Acute abdomen'	Haematometra	?Adenomyosis
			?Endometrial Ca

preference. In a case where the endometrium is well prepared and the uterus of normal size, both systems are equally good. However, for difficult cases, the inflow rate and inflow pressure can be more easily altered to maintain a clear operative view using a hysteromat. Furthermore, there is evidence that fluid deficit is less when a hysteromat is used.

When gravity feed is used, the infusion bag should be approximately 1 m above the patient, an orthopaedic pressure cuff wrapped around the 3 l bags helps to alter the pressure. The fluid pump chosen should be one with variable flow and pressure.

Fluid balance can easily be monitored by hanging the instillate from a simple spring weight. The weight in grams correlates roughly with the volume (3 kg = 3 l). The deficit can be calculated at any time by measuring the outflow and subtracting this from the inflow (calculated from the initial weight of the bag less the present weight), and allowing for leakage. The fluid balance should be checked every 5 min, giving a running balance. This is preferable to calculating the deficit at the end of the procedure. Some of the newer pumps incorporate a fluid management system which collects leakage and displays the running deficit. Ethanol added to the instillate can be measured in the expired breath and this can be used to measure fluid balance accurately.

Electrolyte free solution is used in electrosurgery. Glycine, sorbitol, dextran 70 and dextrose 5% have all been used. Glycine 1.5%, inherited from the urologists, is most commonly used. It provides an optically clear view, however it is hypo-osmolar and has toxic metabolites. Dextran 70 is viscous and difficult to work with. Unless instruments are cleaned properly after surgery the dextran caramelises and will damage the mechanism (Ruiz et al 1992). Fatal anaphylactic reactions have been reported.

Glycine when absorbed in excess causes intravascular volume expansion, dilutional effects and potential effects from ammonia, the breakdown product of glycine (Istre 1992). This is the so called TURP syndrome.

Volume expansion can lead to pulmonary oedema, this is compounded by the depressant effect of anaesthesia and glycine on the myocardium. This potentially fatal complication can be corrected by diuretics. Equally serious are the sequelae of dilutional hyponatraemia and hypokalaemia. These include cardiac arrythmias, cerebral oedema, coma and death. The management of fluid overload is outlined in Table 14.3.

Normal saline or Hartmann's solution can be used in laser surgery. These solutions are undoubtedly safer than those for electrosurgery, as they are iso-osmolar. Volume overload can still occur.

Fluid overload complicates 1–3% of operative procedures. In theory it is preventable by maintaining a running balance. However, even then, if the

Table 14.3 Management of fluid overload

Deficit (ml)	Management
< 500	Continue surgery
500–1000	Continue surgery
1000–1500	Expedite procedure
	Check urea and electrolytes
	? Give frusemide intravenously
	Catheterise
1500–2000	As above
	Give frusemide 40 mg intravenously
	? Terminate procedure
> 2000	As above
	Terminate procedure

depth of tissue destruction is such that large vessels deep in the myometrium are breached, large volumes can be absorbed rapidly. Irrespective of what operative procedure is being performed, a running balance should be standard practice.

Uterine perforation

Perforation complicates 1–2% of procedures (Hulka et al 1995). Approximately 50% of perforations occur during the operator's first three cases. The corollary though is that the remainder occur when more experience has been gained and care must be exercised at all times. Perforation can occur at dilatation, retrieval of tissue or during surgery. The most serious situation is where perforation occurs with the active electrode. Perforation should be suspected when the view or fluid balance deteriorates, or if there is heavy bleeding. The cornual region is most at risk as the myometrium is only 5 mm thick at this site. Perforation is more common with the loop electrode, but full thickness burns of the myometrium can occur with laser fibres and rollerball electrodes. Perforation with the active electrode requires at least a laparoscopy, and, if the surgeon is not an expert laparoscopist, then a laparotomy is mandatory. Bowel, major vascular and urinary injuries have been reported. The great danger at laparoscopy is of missing a diathermy bowel injury, with the patient presenting some days later with peritonitis.

Perforation at retrieval of tissue at the end of the procedure can often be managed conservatively with observation and antibiotics. If there is heavy bleeding following the perforation, then laparoscopy to define and treat the injury is usually all that is required. Bleeding can be controlled by suturing or diathermy. Perforation at the start of the procedure should be managed conservatively with surgery scheduled for some time in the future.

Uterine perforation at hysteroscopic myomectomy where fertility is preserved or enhanced may increase the risk of uterine rupture during the third trimester. There are a number of case reports in the literature. Such serosal defects should be sutured and the patient observed closely in any subsequent pregnancy.

Patients should recover rapidly following hysteroscopic surgery. Positive findings on abdominal examination should be treated with suspicion, as perforation is not always recognised at the time of surgery.

Air embolism

This is a rare complication (Brooks 1997). When performing hysteroscopic surgery and changing from one electrode to another, the entire resectoscope should be removed, rather than leaving the sheath in situ and just removing the handpiece. Gas cooled sapphire laser tips have been responsible for some fatalities.

Haemorrhage

Endometrial ablation destroys endometrium and superficial myometrium, usually avoiding the deeper vascular layers. The effect of heat destruction is to seal superficial vessels and, therefore, bleeding is not generally a problem. If more than one pass is required to remove all the endometrium, then there is the danger of encountering larger vessels. By and large, if a `bleeder' is noted it can be coagulated immediately, while in view. At the end of the procedure, haemostasis is checked, with a rollerball electrode. The distention pressure can be lowered, permitting visualization of bleeding vessels. If a high pressure is used, then there is a net inflow into these vessels. If bleeding is still a problem then a Foley balloon, inserted into the uterus and distended with 20–30 ml of water will tamponade the vessel. It is rare to have to do an hysterectomy for intractable haemorrhage.

Infection

It is our practice to cover all patients with antibiotics (augmentin, 1.2 g) at the time of surgery. Infection is unusual and certainly the randomized trials comparing endometrial ablation with hysterectomy report less infection in the ablation arm. When infection does occur it should be managed along conventional lines.

Pregnancy and contraception

Endometrial ablation does not guarantee sterility, and pregnancies have been reported following ablation. Those who continue to menstruate are at greatest risk. In our series, approximately 40% of our patients had already been sterilized and another 10% opted for sterilization at the time of surgery. The remainder need to be counselled about the need for barrier contraceptives. Those who are amenorrhoeic following ablation and have not been sterilized may worry about pregnancy and do repeated urinary HCG tests. Patients may rarely develop tubal pain following combined endometrial resection and clip sterilization (Townsend et al 1993).

Those pregnancies that have been reported have had a variable outcome. There is an increased risk of intra-uterine growth retardation and problems with placentation. Many of the reported pregnancies have been terminated.

Combined oestrogen/progesterone preparations should be used. Biopsies from women with amenorrhoea following endometrial ablation show that up to 25% have residual endometrium on biopsy. Indeed, endometrial ablation may be offered to women who have heavy bleeding on HRT which is refractory to medical treatment (Spaulding et al 1994). The endometrium must be sampled prior to such a procedure.

Endometrial cancer has been reported following ablation (Dwyer et al 1993) and one of the early concerns was that such cancers might present later because the cancer might be walled off behind adhesions. Another concern is that of operating on an occult cancer or indeed atypical hyperplastic endometrium. Ideally, all women should have endometrial sampling prior to surgery or, at the very least, a sample sent for routine analysis at the time of surgery. This is one of the advantages of resection over rollerball or laser ablation. DeCherney reported a case of endometrial cancer developing 5 years following a rollerball ablation in a woman with hyperplastic endometrium without atypia. She had a stage 1 moderately differentiated, superficially invasive adenocarcinoma arising from an endometrial polyp. The Bristol study reported one case of endometrial cancer diagnosed on histological examination of the resected chips; she had had a normal pre-operative hysteroscopy and biopsy. At hysterectomy no residual cancer was found in the uterus.

Many thousands of resections have been performed to date, as yet there are only a few cases of endometrial cancer in the literature and their treatment and survival would not appear to have been compromised by the ablation. Although we cannot as yet be definite, it is unlikely that endometrial ablation leads to an increase in endometrial cancer or to a worse outlook for those who develop it.

Cyclical pain and haematometra

Cyclical pain is reported in up to 25% of patients with Asherman's syndrome and intra-uterine adhesions following surgery may be a factor. It is less common following rollerball ablation than endometrial resection. Haematometra should be excluded by ultrasound. This is most commonly seen in the cornua where incompletely treated endometrium buried behind scar tissue bleeds monthly. If small, this may be difficult to visualize. Over dilatation of the cervix, to Hegar 16 at the end of the ablation can help reduce the incidence of this complication. Haematometra can be drained hysteroscopically and the cavity re-ablated. Where no haematometra is found, simple analgesics with non-steroidal anti-inflammatory medication, such as diclofenac 100 mg suppository 16 hourly, may suffice, but many women will request hysterectomy. Some authors have suggested that adenomyosis may develop de novo following endometrial ablation. In our series of 525 consecutive TCREs, 80 patients had a deep myometrial biopsy after resection. Adenomyosis was seen in 10 patients, yet their long term follow up was no different to the rest of the group. Other authors have found that adenomyosis is an important determinant of outcome (McCausland et al 1996). Adenomyosis is seen in 14% of hysterectomy specimens following failed ablation.

Those patients with menstrual pain as a significant feature of their presenting complaint should have a laparoscopy at the same time to exclude endometriosis or pelvic inflammatory disease. The endometriosis can be laser ablated. Those patients with a normal pelvis but significant pain may benefit from a laparoscopic uterine nerve ablation, where the uterosacral ligaments are transected. To date, there is no long term follow-up of these patients and so this cannot recommended as routine clinical practice, but considered on a case-by-case basis.

Treatment failure

The long term results of endometrial ablation show that it is a worthwhile procedure (Derman et al 1991, Baggish et al 1996), the majority of women avoid further gynaecological surgery and there are savings to the health service. A 5 year life table analysis of TRCE revealed that 9% underwent hysterectomy and, overall, 80% avoided further gynaecological surgery, with 98% of repeat surgery occurring in the first three years. Depending on the years of follow-up, 26–40% had amenorrhoea and 79–87% were satisfied with their surgery. Although these results are from a single centre with particular expertise, they are in keeping with the reports from other centres and, indeed, the Medical Research Council funded multi-centred trial of TCRE and hysterectomy had similar follow up at three years (O'Connor et al 1997).

This study included data on psychosocial outcomes and on use of general practitioner services. Re-assuringly, psychosocial variables improved in the TCRE and hysterectomy groups; this improvement was maintained over the three years of follow-up reported and there was no difference between the two procedures. Likewise, there was no significant difference between the two procedures for general practitioner visits, scripts or sick notes for gynaecological and non-gynaecological problems.

CONCLUSION

Hysteroscopy is a safe and effective modality in the management of benign gynaecological pathology. The key to avoiding complications is training leading to a thorough understanding of diagnostic hysteroscopy and the equipment used combined with careful patient selection.

Key points for clinical practice

- Attend a recognised course in basic hysteroscopy early in training.
- Attend a recognised course in advanced hysteroscopy.
- Select easy cases initially and pharmacologically thin the endometrium.
- Rollerball the endometrium initially, until more experienced.
- Monitor fluid balance.
- Never cut away from the sheath, always cut toward the sheath.

References

Baggish M, Eddie H 1996 Endometrial ablation: a series of 568 patients treated over an 11 year period. Am J Obstet Gynecol 174: 908–913

Brooks P 1997 Venous air embolism during operative hysteroscopy. J Am Assoc Gynecol Laparosc 4: 291–292

DeCherney A, Diamond M, Lavy G, Polan M 1987 Endometrial ablation for intractable uterine bleeding: hysteroscopic resection. Obstet Gynecol 70: 668–670

Derman S, Rehnstrom J, Neuwirth R 1991 Long term effectiveness of hysteroscopic treatment of menorrhagia and leiomyomas. Obstet Gynecol 77: 591–594

Dwyer N, Hutton J, Stirrat G 1993 Randomised, controlled trial comparing endometrial resection with abdominal hysterectomy for the surgical treatment of menorrhagia. Br J Obstet Gynaecol 100: 237–243

Erian J 1994 Endometrial ablation in the treatment of menorrhagia. Br J Obstet Gynaecol; 101 (Suppl 11): 19–22

Fraser I, Healy D, Torode H, Song J, Mamers P, Wilde F 1996 Depot goserlin and danazol pre-treatment before rollerball endometrial ablation for menorrhagia. Obstet Gynecol 87: 544–550

Garry R 1995 Good practice with endometrial ablation. Obstet Gynecol 85: 144–151

Gimpelson R, Kaigh J 1992 Mechanical preparation of the endometrium prior to endometrial ablation. J Reprod Med 37: 691–694

Hulka J F, Peterson H A, Phillips J M, Surrey M W 1995 Operative hysteroscopy: American Association of Gynecologic Laparoscopists' 1993 membership survey. J Am Assoc Gynecol Laparosc 2: 131–132

Indman P 1993 Hysteroscopic treatment of menorrhagia associated with uterine leiomyomas. Obstet Gynecol 81: 716–720

Istre O 1992 Changes in serum electrolytes after transcervical resection of the endometrium and submucous fibroids with use of glycine 1.5% for uterine irrigation. Obstet Gynecol 80: 218–222

Lefler H, Sullivan G, Hulka J 1991 Modified endometrial ablation: electrocoagulation with vasopressin and suction curettage preparation. Obstet Gynecol 77: 949–953

McCausland A, McCausland V 1996 Depth of endometrial penetration in adenomyosis helps determine outcome of rollerball ablation. Am J Obstet Gynecol 174: 1786–1794

Magos A, Baumann R, Turnbull A 1989 Transcervical resection of endometrium in women with menorrhagia. BMJ 298: 1209–1212

Magos A, Baumann R, Lockwood G, Turnbull A 1991 Experience with the first 250 endometrial resections for menorrhagia. Lancet 337: 1074–1078

MISTLETOE 1993 Update October 1993 (Newsletter). Manchester: RCOG Audit Unit

O'Connor H, Magos A 1996 Endometrial resection for the treatment of menorrhagia. N Engl J Med 335: 151–156

O'Connor H, Broadbent J, Magos A, McPherson K 1997 Medical Research Council randomized trial of endometrial resection versus hysterectomy in the management of menorrhagia. Lancet 349: 897–901

Pinion S, Parkin D, Abramovich D 1994 Randomized trial of hysterectomy, endometrial laser ablation, and transcervical endometrial resection for dysfunctional uterine bleeding. BMJ 309: 979–983

Raiga J, Mage M, Glowaczower E et al 1995 Factors affecting risk of failure after endometrial resection. J Gynecol Surg 11: 1–6

RCOG 1994 Report of the RCOG working party on training in gynaecological endoscopic surgery. Manchester: RCOG Press

Ruiz J, Neuwirth R 1992 The incidence of complications associated with the use of hyskon during hysteroscopy: experience in 1793 consecutive patients. J Gynecol Surg 8: 219–224

Spaulding L 1994 Endometrial ablation for refractory post menopausal bleeding with continuous hormone replacement therapy. Fertil Steril 62: 1181–1185

Townsend D, McCausland V, McCausland A, Fields G, Kauffman K 1993 Post ablation tubal sterilisation syndrome. Obstet Gynecol 82: 422–424

Wallwiener D, Rimbach S, Bastert G 1994 The hysterotrainer, a simulator for diagnostic and operative hysteroscopy. J Am Assoc Gynecol Laparosc 1: 61–63

Wamsteker K, Emanuel M, de Kruif J 1993 Transcervical hysteroscopic resection of submucous fibroids for abnormal uterine bleeding: results regarding the degree of intramural extension. Obstet Gynecol 82: 736–740

Index

A

Abortion, folate status, 16
Absent end-diastolic flow velocity, 70
Acardiac twin gestation, 72–3
Activated protein C *see* APC
Acute chest syndrome, in sickle cell disease pregnancy, 31
Adenomyosis, 211
Adhesiolysis, 203
Air embolism, 210
Alcohol abuse, folate status, 17
Allopurinol, 162
Alpha interferon, 175
Amenorrhoea, 23
Amniocentesis, twin, 67
Amnionitis, 99
Ampicillin, 102
Anaesthesia
    see also Epidural anaesthesia
    hysteroscopic surgery, 206
    pre–eclampsia caesarian section, 121
Analgesia
    delivery in coagulation disorders, 44
    delivery in thrombophilic defects, 59
    in labour with sickle cell disease, 31–2
Anaphylaxis, 147
Anencephaly, 9
    detection, 67
Aneuploidy, 67
Antenatal corticosteroids, 81–95
    economic effects, 89
    effect of gender, 85–6
    evidence of efficacy, 83–92
    extrapulmonary effects, 82–3
    intraventricular haemorrhage, 86–7
    maternal risks, 92
    mode of action, 82–3
    neonatal mortality, 83, 84–5
    postnatal surfactant, 86
    pulmonary effects, 82

    respiratory distress syndrome, 83–5, 86–7
    single versus multiple doses, 91–2
    systematic review of therapy, 83–7
Antenatal Day Assessment Unit, 113
Antibiotic therapy
    peritoneal irrigation, 147
    in preterm labour, 102
        high risk, 102
    in preterm prelabour rupture of membranes, 102–3
Anticoagulant prophylaxis, fetal complication risk, 56
Anticonvulsant drugs
    folic acid supplements, 17
    use, 115–16
Antiphospholipid antibodies and thrombosis, 53
Antithrombin, 37
    activity screening, 55
    deficiency, 48, 49–50
        prevalence, 49
APC resistance
    and factor V Leiden, 51
    and pregnancy related thrombosis, 54
    screening, 51
APC resistance test, 37, 55
Asherman's syndrome, hysteroscopic surgery, 203, 206, 211
Asphyxial damage to brain, 154
Aspiration syndrome, in pregnancy, 112
Atosiban, 104
Augmentin, 103, 210
Azoospermia, 23

B

B–Lynch Brace Suturing Technique, 145
Bacterial endotoxins, 99–100
Bacterial vaginosis, 100, 102, 146
Bacteroides spp., 100
Beta thalassaemia, carrier state, 21

Beta thalassaemia major
  endocrine complications, 23
  labour management, 27
  management, 22–3
  in pregnancy, 26–7
  pre–pregnancy assessment and care, 24–5
Betamethasone, preterm birth trial, 81
Birth
  asphyxia and cerebral palsy, 162–3
  place role, 106
Bladder, caesarian section damage, 149
Bleomycin, 175
Blood group antibodies
  in β-thalassaemia major, 25
  in sickle cell disease, 30
Blood transfusion
  in β-thalassaemia pregnancy, 26–7
  in caesarian section, 143
  in sickle cell disease pregnancy, 31
  in thalassaemia, 22
Body mass index, preterm birth, 98
Bone pain, in sickle cell disease pregnancy, 31
Booking visit
  in β–thalassaemia pregnancy, 26
  in sickle cell disease pregnancy, 30–1
  ultrasound examination, 65
Bowel
  caesarian section damage, 149
  diathermy injury, 209
Bowenoid papulosis, 171
Brain
  early development, 153–4
  injury timing, 154
  neuropathological study, 154–5
  non–invasive study methods, 155–6
  ultrasonography, 155
Breast feeding
  in β-thalassaemia, 28
  in sickle cell disease, 32

C

Caesarian section
  in β-thalassaemia, 27
  blood loss reduction, 144
  complication reduction, 141–53
  elective, 126
  factor replacement in coagulation disorders, 45
  fetus delivery, 149
  haemophilia carrier, 44
  infection, 145–6
    prophylaxis, 146–7
  maternal mortality, 142
  postoperative measures, 150–1
  in pre–eclampsia, 121
  preterm delivery, 106–7
  risk factors, 141
  skin incision and entry, 148
  surgical techniques, 148–51
  twin gestation, 72, 73–4
    technique, 74–5
  urinary tract and bowel injury, 149
  uterine incision, 148–9

Calcium in flour, 13
Carboplatin, 179
Cardiac function
  in β-thalassaemia major, 24
  in β-thalassaemia pregnancy, 26
Cardiotocography, 119–20
Cefotaxime, 147
Cefoxitin, 147
Cephalhaematoma, 128, 129
Cerebral palsy
  birthweight, 159
  known causes, 157
  pregnancy and delivery relationship, 153–64
  and preterm birth, 159–60
  in preterm infants, 107
  rate/1000 survivors, 158
  risk factors, 157–64
Cerebral vascular accident in pregnancy, 112
Cervical cerclage, preterm birth prevention, 104–5
Cervical incompetence and preterm birth, 98
Cervical intra–epithelial neoplasia (CIN), 168–9
Cervix
  assessment in preterm birth risk, 101
  incompetence, twin pregnancy, 68–9
  neoplasia, in VIN, 172
  transvaginal ultrasound assessment, 69
Children, long–term effects of antenatal corticosteroids, 87–8
Chorioamnionitis, 161
Chorionic villus sampling
  for aneuploidy, 67
  clotting factor deficiency, 42
Chorionicity, diagnosis and determination, 65–7
CHUMS trial, 101–2
Cigarette smoking, in VIN, 169
Cisplatin, 179
Cisplatin/cyclophosphamide, 180
Clindamycin, 102
Clinical practice key points
  antenatal corticosteroid therapy, 92
  caesarian section, 151
  cerebral palsy, 163
  folate status in pregnancy, 18
  hysteroscopic surgery complication avoidance, 201–14
  laparoscopy complication avoidance, 200
  ovarian cancer with paclitaxel treatment, 186
  pregnancy in major haemoglobino pathies, 33
  pregnancy management with coagulation disorders, 61–2
  preterm labour, 108
  severe pre-eclampsia and antihyper tensive therapy, 122
  twin pregnancy fetal assessment and labour management, 77
  vacuum extraction, 136

vulval intra-epithelial neoplasia, 176
Clitoris, intra–epithelial neoplasia, 174
Coagulation factors
    also under individual factors
    in pregnancy, 35, 36–37, 38
Coagulation screening, 55
Cocaine, and preterm birth, 98
Comprehensive Care Haemophilia Centre, 41
Computerized tomography, neonatal brain, 155
Confidential Enquiry into Maternal Deaths in the UK (1991–1993), 142
Congenital anomalies and cerebral palsy, 157–8
Congenital coagulation diseases, 38–47
    management
            of delivery, 43–4
            during pregnancy, 43
            post partum, 46–7
    and thromboembolism, 142
Congenital thrombophilic defects, 47–8
Contraception
    after hysteroscopic surgery, 210
    in β-thalassaemia, 28
    for inherited coagulation diseases, 41–2
    in sickle cell disease, 32
Convulsions
    postnatal, 122
    in pregnancy, 112
Cooley's anaemia, 22
Corticosteroids
    antenatal, 81–95
    effects, 88
    lung maturity enhancement, 105–6
    in preterm labour, 102
Coumarin, fetal complication risk, 56
Counselling
    see also Genetic counselling
    hysteroscopic surgery, 202
    inherited coagulation diseases, 41–2
Cyclical pain after hysteroscopic surgery, 211

D

Dalteparin, 58
Decapeptyl, 204
Delivery
    see also Preterm delivery
    assisted, avoidance, 126
    in inherited coagulation diseases, 43–4
    instrumental vaginal, long-term effects, 130
    intervention rates, 125–6
    maternal morbidity, 127–8
    neurological injuries, 129–30
    in pre-eclampsia, 121
    in severe pre-eclampsia, 117
    in sickle cell disease, 32
Desamino-8-D-arginine vasopressin (DDAVP), 38–40
    infusion, 46
Desferrioxamine, 22, 23, 25
    in puerperium, 28
    risk in β-thalassaemia pregnancy, 26
Dexamethasone, 117

Dextran, 70, 208
Diazepam, 115
Diclofenac, 211
Diet and NTDs, 12–13
DNA
    haemophilia carrier diagnosis, 42
    neonatal analysis for heritable thrombophilic defects, 60
DNA cycle
    folate cofactors role, 4
    in folate deficiency, 5
Docetaxel, 186
Doppler cerebral blood flow in fetus and newborn, 156
Doppler scans in fetal twin growth, 70
Double-puncture amniocentesis, 67
Down's syndrome, nuchal translucency screening, 67
Dysfibrinogenaemia, 48

E

Echocardiography 24
Effects of Corticosteroids for Fetal Maturation on Perinatal Outcomes (NIH 1995), 81–2
Endometrial ablation, hysteroscopic surgery, 202, 203
Endometrial carcinoma, 211
Endometriosis, 212
Endometritis, 145–6
Enoxaparin, 58
Enterococcus faecalis, 146
EPICURE study, 107
Epidural anaesthesia
    antenatal heparin, 59
    twin delivery, 74, 75
Erythromycin, 102–3
Escherichia coli , 100, 146
Ethanol , 208
Ethnic origin, and preterm birth, 98
Exomphalos diagnosis, 67

F

Facial nerve palsy after forceps delivery, 128
Factor 20210A, 48, 51–2
    prevalence, 49
    variant screening, 55
Factor IXC, in pregnancy, 45
Factor V Leiden, 48
    APC resistance, 51
    prevalence, 49
    screening, 55
Factor VIIC, 37
Factor VIII, thrombotic risk factor, 48
Factor VIII complex, 37
Factor VIIIC
    activity, 52
    in pregnancy, 44–5
Factor XI
    at delivery, 45
    deficiency, 41
Ferritin, 25
    in β-thalassaemia pregnancy, 27

in sickle cell disease, 30
Fertility
  in β-thalassaemia, 23
  in sickle cell disease, 29
  treatment in β-thalassaemia major, 25
Fetal alcohol syndrome, 17
Fetus
  assessment
      after 20 weeks, 68–9
      in pre–eclampsia, 119–21
  brain neuro–imaging, 155
  cerebral haemodynamics and function
  study, 155–6
  delivery by caesarian section, 149
  dichorionic gestation, 70
  growth, 70–1
  monochorionic gestation, 70–1
  recurrent loss, prophylactic
  anticoagulation, 60
  scalp sampling, 126
  structural abnormalities, 67–8
  surveillance in β-thalassaemia
  pregnancy, 27
  ultrasound assessment, 120
Fibrinogen, thrombotic risk factor, 48
Fibrinolytic system, changes in pregnancy, 38
Fibroids
  classification, 204
  hysteroscopic surgery, 202, 203, 206
Fibronectin, and preterm birth, 99–100
Flour additives, 13–14
Fluid overload
  in hysteroscopic surgery, 207–9
  management, 209
Fluorescent in situ hybridisation (FISH), 67
Folate
  cellular turnover, 6
  deficiency, 5–6
  functions, 3, 4–5
  NTD prevention recommendations, 11
  and pregnancy, 6, 8–9
  role in pregnancy, 1–19
  structure, 2, 3
Folate status, reduced, effects on
  pregnancy, 18
Folic acid
  in β-thalassaemia pregnancy, 26
  fortification option, 13–15
  neuropathy development, 15
  NTD prevention recommendations, 11
  in pernicious anaemia, 15
  role in pregnancy, 1–19
  structure, 2–3
  supplement option, 13
  supplement use indications, 7, 9
Forceps
  effects on fetus/neonate, 128–30
  maternal morbidity, 127–8
  rare adverse neonatal events, 130
Frusemide, 122

G

Gardnerella vaginalis, 100
Genetic counselling

in β-thalassaemia major, 25
inherited coagulation diseases, 42–3
in sickle cell disease, 30
Genetic factors in cerebral palsy, 157
Glyceryl trinitrate transdermal patches 104
Glycine, 208
Gynaecology, laparoscopic techniques and
  complications, 190

H

Haemabate, 145
Haematoma, subaponeurotic, 128–9
Haematometra, 211
Haemoglobin, globin changes in
  thalassaemias, 22
Haemoglobinopathies
  carrier identification, 21
  classification, 21
  effects on pregnancy, 21–34
  populations distribution, 21
Haemolysis elevated liver enzymes and
  low platelets see HELLP syndrome
Haemophilia
  blood factors in pregnancy, 44–5
  counselling, 41–2
  prenatal diagnosis, 42
  types, 38–9
Haemophilia Centre, 41–2
  Royal Free Hospital, London, 44
Haemorrhage
  at caesarian section, 143
    control strategies, 144–5
  in hysteroscopic surgery, 210
  intracranial, 129
  intraventricular, corticosteroid therapy,
  86–7
  post–partum, 112
    twin delivery, 77
  retinal, after vacuum extraction, 128
Haemostasis, normal pregnancy, 35, 37–8
Hasson's approach, 193
Headache, in pregnancy, 112–13
HELLP syndrome, 112, 119
Heparin, 142–3
  in pregnancy, risk, 56–7
  pregnancy management, 57–8
Hepatitis B
  immunisation, 25
  immunisation in pregnancy, 43
Heroin and preterm birth, 98
Herpes simplex virus in VIN, 169
HIV
  immunisation, 25
  infection, 169
Homocysteine, 18
Homozygous β-thalassaemia, 22
Hormonal replacement therapy, 211
  in β-thalassaemia, 28
Hydrallazine, 113–14
Hyperhomocysteinemia, 52–3
  thrombotic risk factor, 48
Hyperreflexia, 115
Hypertension, in pregnancy
  assessment, 117–19

control agents, 113–15
follow–up, 123
management, 118
maternal sequelae, 112
regime, 114
screening, 112–13
stepwise management, 114
Hypogonadotrophic hypogonadism, 23
Hypokalaemia sequelae, 208
Hyponatraemia sequelae, 208
Hypothyroidism in β-thalassaemia major, 24
Hypothyroxinaemia, 158
Hypovolemic shock, 129
Hypoxic–ischaemic damage, brain, 154
Hysteromat, 208
Hysteroscopic myomectomy, uterine
  perforation, 209
Hysteroscopic surgery
  complication avoidance, 201–14
  complications, 207, 208–12
  counselling/consent, 202
  endometrial preparation, 204
  equipment and instrumentation, 206–7
  and fertility, 203
  fluid monitoring, 207
  operative technique, 204–6
    layout, 205
  patient selection, 203
  surgical procedures, 206–12
  training, 201–2
  treatment failure, 212

I

IgG assay, 55
IgM anticardiolipin assay, 55
Immunisation
  in pregnancy, 43
  for viral infections, 25
Immunodeficiency, in HPV infection and
  anogenital tumours, 169
Immunosuppression, in intra–epithelial
  neoplasia of genital tract, 169–70
Immunotherapy, VIN 175
Impaired glucose tolerance, 24
Indomethacin, 98
  maternal side effects, 103–4
Infection
  caesarian section, 145–7
  in hysteroscopic surgery, 210
  intra-uterine, and brain injury, 158
  and preterm birth, 99–100
  in sickle cell disease puerperium, 32
Insulin growth factors, 162
Interleukin-6, 99
International Normalised Ratio, 59
International Society of Gynaecological
  Pathologists, 167
International Society for the Study of
  Vulvar Disease, 167
Intracranial haemorrhage, 129
  haemophilic newborn, 44
Intrauterine development, folic acid
  supplements, 16
Intrauterine growth restriction, 70

and cerebral palsy, 161
Iodophor, 147
Iron
  in flour, 13
  overload, 22–3

J

Jaundice after vacuum extraction, 128

L

Labetalol, 113–14
  intravenous, 115
Labour
  in β-thalassaemia pregnancy, 27
  dysfunctional, 126
  preterm, 97–110
  in sickle cell disease, 31–2
Lactation, folic acid supplements, 17
Laparoscopy
  abdomen access failure, 190
  abdominal wall
    elevation, 194
    incision repair, 199
  vessel damage, 190
  alternative primary entry sites, 198
  bowel damage, 191
  classic technique, 191
  CO_2 insufflation, 195–6
  complication avoidance, 189–200
  complication incidence, 189–91
  direct insertion, 191–2
  direct vision insertion, 193–8
  gasless, 193
  gastro–intestinal tract damage, 190
  initial skin incision, 194
  intra-abdominal blood vessel damage, 191
  open technique, 192
  post–laparoscopic bowel herniation
    through scars, 190
  primary trocar insertion, 196–8
  secondary trocar insertions, 198–9
  trocar insertion danger, 191
  Veress needle
    insertion, 194–5
    position check, 195
Laser treatment for VIN, 174
Leucovorin, 5
Lissencephaly, 154
Liver
  failure in pregnancy, 112
  function tests in pre-eclampsia, 119
Lung surfactant, 105
Lupus anticoagulant screening, 55

M

Magnesium, 162
  toxicity, 115
Magnesium sulphate, 104, 115–16
Magnetic resonance imaging, neonatal
  brain, 155
Magnetic resonance spectroscopy, phosphorus metabolites in brain tissue, 156

Mannitol, 122
Marmite, 1
Maternal age and cerebral palsy, 158
Maternal death, causes, 113
Maternal diabetes
    in β-thalassaemia major, 24
    respiratory distress syndrome
        prevention, 90
Maternal hypertensive disease, respiratory
    distress syndrome, prevention, 90–1
Maternal infection
    and cerebral palsy, 161–2
    and corticosteroid use, 88
Maternal mortality
    caesarian section, 142
    thromboembolism, 142–3
Maternal pulmonary oedema and
    corticosteroid use, 88–9
Maternal thyroid dysfunction and CP risk,
    158
Maylard incision, 148
Mediterranean anaemia, 22
Megaloblastic anaemia of pregnancy, 6, 8
    prevention, 8–9
    in twins, 17
Menorrhagia, hysteroscopic surgery, 203
Methionine synthase, 4, 14, 15
Methyl folate trap hypothesis, 14
Methylation cycle
    folate cofactors role, 4
    in folate deficiency, 5–6
    neuropathy, 15
Methyldopa, 113
Metronidazole, 102–3
Micro–laparoscopic equipment, 193
Monoamniotic twin gestation, 72
MRC Vitamin Study Research Group, 10,
    12
MUGA scan, 24
Multiple pregnancy
    and cerebral palsy, 160
    folate status, 17–18
    respiratory distress syndrome prevention,
        91

N

Nd:YAG laser, 207
Near infrared spectroscopy, cerebral blood
    flow, 156
Necrotising enterocolitis, corticosteroid
    use, 87
Neonatal brain neuro-imaging, 155
Neonatal heritable thrombophilic defects,
    management, 60
Neonatal lateral rectus paralysis, 129
Neonatal mortality, antenatal
    corticosteroids therapy, 83, 84–5
Neonatal post–partum care in inherited
    coagulation disorders, 47
Neonatal scalp after vacuum delivery, 128
Neural tube defects (NTDs), 9–15
    folate prevention, 1
    genetic predisposition, 9
    prevention, 10, 11–12

recurrence risk, 9–12
Neuro-imaging
    fetal and neonatal, 155–7
    later childhood, 156
Neuronal migration disorder, 154
NHANES II, 9
Niacin in flour, 13
Nifedipine, 104, 113–14
Nifedipine/magnesium sulphate, 114

O

Occipital lobe blindness, in pregnancy, 112
Oedema, in pregnancy, 112
Oliguria, pre–eclampsia post–delivery,
    121–2
ORACLE trial, 103, 162
Oral contraceptives, folate status, 17
Oral glucose tolerance test, 24
Orofacial clefts, 16
Osteopenia, heparin in pregnancy risk,
    56–7
Ovarian cancer
    incidence, 179
    paclitaxel treatment, 179–88
Oxytocin, 76–7
Oxytocin receptor blockers, 104

P

Paclitaxel
    anti–tumour activity, 181
    dose and scheduling, 182
    early clinical trials, 180–1
    high dose chemotherapy, 185–6
    identification, 180
    mode of action, 180
    toxicity, 181
Paclitaxel/carboplatin, 184
Paclitaxel/cisplatin
    versus paclitaxel/carboplatin, 185
    versus single agent paclitaxel, 183
    versus standard treatment, 182–3
Paclitaxel/platinum, randomised studies,
    185
Paget's disease of the vulva, 167, 175–6
Palmar creases, abnormal, 157
Perianal skin, intra–epithelial neoplasia, 174
Peritoneal antibiotic irrigation, 147
Periventricular leucomalacia, 154
Pernicious anaemia
    and folic acid, 15
    malabsorption, 14
Pfannenstiel incision, 148
Phenytoin, 115–16
Phospholipase A2, 100
Placenta
    blood flow in pre-eclampsia, 120
    expulsion at caesarian section, 144
Plasminogen activator inhibitors, 38
Platelet count in pre-eclampsia, 118–19
Polyhydramnios, 70–1, 98
Polymicrogyria, 154
Post partum haemorrhage, 112

Pre-eclampsia
  care after delivery, 121–3
  and cerebral palsy, 160–1
  delivery plan, 121
  fetal assessment, 119–21
  maternal mortality, 112
  monitoring protocol, 120
  severe
    management, 111–24
    management plan, 117
  in sickle cell disease pregnancy 31
Pregnancy
  after hysteroscopic surgery, 210
  in β-thalassaemia, 23–4
    management, 26–7
  coagulation factors, 35, 36–7, 38
  complications in inherited coagulation
  disorders, 47
  continuation in pre-eclampsia, 116–17
  folic acid/folate role, 1–19
  haemoglobinopathies effects, 21–34
  haemostasis, 35, 37–8
  hepatitis B immunisation, 43
  management in [beta]–thalassaemia,
  26–7
  multifetal reduction, 71
  in sickle cell disease, 29–30
    management, 30–1
  thrombotic risk in heritable
  thrombophilias, 53–4
  and venous thrombosis, 48
  in von Willebrand's disease, 40
Pregnavite Forte F, 10
Premature infants, folic acid supplements,
  16
Prenatal diagnosis, inherited coagulation
  diseases, 42
Preterm birth
  aetiology and prediction, 97–100
  and cerebral palsy, 159–60
  cervical cerclage prevention, 104–5
  prevention, 100–3
  sociodemographic variables 97–8
Preterm delivery
  optimum mode, 106–7
  prevention by tocolytic therapy, 103–4
Preterm labour, 97–110
  bacterial pathogens, 100
  monitoring, 107
Preterm prelabour rupture of membranes
  antibiotic use, 102–3
  respiratory distress prevention, 89–90
Protein C 37
  activity screening, 55
Protein C deficiency, 48, 50
  prevalence, 49
Protein S, 37
  antigen screening, 55
Protein S deficiency, 48, 50–1
  prevalence, 49
Proteinuria in pregnancy, 112–13, 118
Proteus mirabilis, 146
Prothrombin, 37
Prothrombin gene mutation see Factor
  20210A

Pruritus, in VIN, 171
Puerperium
  in β-thalassaemia, 28
  in sickle cell disease, 32
Pulmonary embolism in pregnancy, 48
Pulmonary oedema
  and hysteroscopic surgery, 208
  pre–eclampsia post–delivery, 121–2
  in pregnancy, 112
Pulse–oximeter, 122
Pump twin, 72

R

Red cell folate level, 9
Renal failure, in pregnancy, 112
Resectoscope, 203, 205
Respiratory distress, preterm birth and
  corticosteroid trial, 81
Respiratory distress syndrome, 81, 82, 83–5
  antenatal steroids reduction, 105
  prevention in clinical situations, 89–91
Retinal haemorrhage, after vacuum
  extraction, 128
Richter's herniation, 199
Ristocetin cofactor, 37, 39
Ritodrine, 104

S

Sickle cell β-thalassaemia, 28
Sickle cell disease
  haemoglobin variants, 28
  labour in, 31–2
  management, 29
    pregnancy, 30–1
  pre–pregnancy assessment and care, 30
  puerperium, 32
Sickle cell haemoglobin, carrier state, 21
Sickle cell haemoglobin C disease, 28
Sickle cell syndromes, world distribution,
  28–9
Spina bifida, 9
Splenectomy, 22
  in β-thalassaemia pregnancy, 27
Staphyloccus aureus, 146
Staphylococcus aureus, methicillin–resistant,
  147
Staphylococcus epidermis, 146
Streptococcus Group B, 100, 146
Stress and preterm birth, 98
'Stuck–twin' delivery, 74
Subacute combined degeneration, 6, 14
Subgaleal haematomata, 128–9
Sulindac, 104
Surfactant
  effects, 88
  lung, 105
  therapy trials, 81
Surgical techniques, for caesarian section,
  148–51
Survanta prevention and rescue trials, 86, 88
Syntocinon, 121, 126

T

Taxanes, 180–6
Termination, selective, 67–8, 71
Thalassaemia
  homozygous, 22
  world distribtuion, 22
Thiamin in flour, 13
Thromboembolism
  maternal mortality, 142–3
  risk factors, 143
  venous, 47–8
Thrombophilia
  childhood screening, 60
  complex defects, 52–3
  heritable, screening, 55
  heritable defects
    and antiphospholipid antibodies, 53
    multigene, 52
    pregnancy and thrombotic risk, 53–4
Thrombophilia Clinic, 56, 57
Thrombophilias, heritable, 48–53
  management
    of delivery, 58–9
    in pregnancy, 57–8
  post partum follow–up, 59–60
  prenatal diagnosis, 57
  prevalences, 49
Thrombosis
  pregnancy related in heritable
    thrombophilias, 53–4
  risk assessment, 54–5
  venous, and pregnancy, 48
Thyroid dysfunction, maternal, 158–9
Thyroid stimulating hormone, antenatal,
  105–6
Thyrotrophic releasing hormone, preterm
  labour risk, 159
Thyrotropin releasing hormone, 91
Thyroxine and cerebral palsy, 158
Tocodynamometry, ambulating, 101
Tocolytics
  side effects, 103
  therapy in preterm delivery prevention,
    103–4
Tooth enamel defects with cerebral palsy,
  157
Toxins, intra–uterine exposure, and
  cerebral palsy, 158
Tumour necrosis factor, 99–100, 161
TURP syndrome, 208
Twin, acardiac, 68
Twin pregnancy
  abnormality and selective termination,
    67–8
  acardiac, 72–3
  co-twin death, 71
  extreme preterm delivery of one twin, 73
  fetal assessment, 65–71
  induction of labour, 73
  labour management, 73–7
  labour management at University
    College London, 75–6
  monoamniotic, 72
  post-partum haemorrhage, 77
  prenatal diagnosis issues, 65–8
  timing and mode of delivery, 73–7
Twin reversed arterial perfusion, 72
'Twin-peak' sign, 66–7
Twin-to-twin transfusion syndrome
  co-twin death, 71
  diagnosis, 67
  ultrasound monitoring, 70

U

UK Ten Centre trial, 81
Ultrasound
  at booking visit, 65
  in β–thalassaemia pregnancy, 27
  fetal assessment, 120
  fetal brain, 155
  infant intracranial, 129
  newborn brain, 155
  in prediction of chorionicity, 66
  in sickle cell disease pregnancy, 31
  transvaginal cervical, 69
Umbilical Doppler artery assessment, 120
Ureter, caesarian section damage, 149
Urethral meatus, intra-epithelial neoplasia,
  174
Uric acid measurement in pre-eclampsia,
  118
Urinalysis, in sickle cell disease pregnancy,
  31
Urogenital infection, 100
  eradication, 102
US Exosurf trial, 81
Uterus
  activity monitoring, 101
  caesarian section incision, 148–9
  excessive activity and preterm birth, 99
  haemorrhage at caesarian section, 144
  perforation by hysteroscopic surgery,
    209–10
  surgical closure, 149–50

V

Vacuum extraction
  advantages, 127–8
  effects on fetus/neonate, 128–30
Vacuum extractor
  application, 131–2
  delivery, 125–39
  and forceps delivery, trials, 127
  indications and contra–indications,
    130–1
  medico–legal risks, 134–5
  metal cup, 129, 131–2
  pumps, 131
  rare adverse neonatal events, 130
  silicone rubber cup, 129, 131–2
  special indications, 133–4
  technique, 134
  training in use, 136
  use by midwife, 136–7
Vaginal flora and endometritis, 146
Vaginosis, bacterial, 100, 102, 146
Varicella–zoster virus screening, 25

Venous thromboembolism, 47–8
  familial, 48
  risk assessment, 56
Venous thrombosis
  and pregnancy, 48
  in pregnancy, 112
  risk in APC resistance, 51
Ventouse extraction, risks in inherited
  coagulation diseases, 44
Viral infections, in sickle cell disease, 30
Viral screen, in β-thalassaemia major, 25
Vitamin B12, deficiency, 14
Vitamin B12–associated neuropathy, 14–15
Vitamin C, risk in β-thalassaemia
  pregnancy, 26
Vitamin K dependent clotting factors, 37,
  40–1
Von Willebrand factor, 37
Von Willebrand's disease, 39–41
  blood factors in pregnancy, 44–5
  classification, 39
  counselling, 41–2
  delivery management, 44
  post–partum haemorrhage risk, 46
  pregnancy complications, 47
Vulva
  early invasive carcinoma, 176
  intraepithelial melanoma, 167, 176
  melanoma *in situ see* intraepithelial
    melanoma
Vulval intra-epithelial neoplasia
  angiogenic phenotype switch, 171
  classification, 167–8
  clinical features, 171–2
  diagnosis and management, 167–78
  eponyms, 167
  follow–up, 175
  increasing incidence, 170
  local excision, 173
  medical therapy, 174–5
  natural history, 170–1
  pathology and pathogenesis, 168–70
  treatment, 172–5
Vulvectomy, 173–4

W

Warfarin prophylaxis, and pregnancy, 57
Watershed zones, 154

X

X–linked recessive disorders, 38–9